# Phytomedicine and Phytotherapy

# Phytomedicine and Phytotherapy

Edited by Dominic Patterson

hayle
medical

New York

Hayle Medical,
750 Third Avenue, 9th Floor,
New York, NY 10017, USA

Visit us on the World Wide Web at:
www.haylemedical.com

ISBN: 978-1-63241-784-8

**Cataloging-in-Publication Data**

Phytomedicine and phytotherapy / edited by Dominic Patterson.
    p. cm.
Includes bibliographical references and index.
ISBN 978-1-63241-784-8
1. Herbs--Therapeutic use. 2. Materia medica, Vegetable. 3. Medicinal plants.
4. Botany, Medical. I. Patterson, Dominic.
RM666.H33 P49 2019
615.321--dc23

# Table of Contents

# Preface

Phytomedicine refers to the study of botany that is concerned with the use of plants intended for medicinal and therapeutic purposes. Panax ginseng and Panax quinquefolium are common types of plants used for their therapeutic properties. The alternative practice of using unrefined plant or animal extracts for medicinal purposes is called phytotherapy. Such plant-derived or animal-derived medicines require very less processing. They are believed to be safer and more effective than other pharmaceutical drugs. Herbal dietary supplements are one of the most common examples of such plant-derived medicines. This book is a valuable compilation of topics, ranging from the basic to the most complex advancements in the field of phytotherapy and phytomedicine. The various studies that are constantly contributing towards advancing technologies and evolution of these fields are examined in detail. This book includes contributions of experts and researchers, which will provide innovative insights into this field.

The information shared in this book is based on empirical researches made by veterans in this field of study. The elaborative information provided in this book will help the readers further their scope of knowledge leading to advancements in this field.

Finally, I would like to thank my fellow researchers who gave constructive feedback and my family members who supported me at every step of my research.

**Editor**

# Canephron® N in the treatment of recurrent cystitis in women of child-bearing Age

Maksim Sabadash[1*] and Alexander Shulyak[2]

## Abstract

**Background:** The aim of this study was to investigate the effect of the herbal medicine Canephron®N, particularly regarding its ability to prevent recurrences of cystitis, associated with E.Coli in women of child-bearing age.

**Methods:** Ninety patients were randomised into two treatment groups. Both, the test group ($n = 45$) and the control group ($n = 45$), received an antibacterial therapy (fluoroquinolones) for 7 days determined by urine culture. Furthermore, in both groups general recommendations on preventing cystitis were made (sufficient liquid consumption, avoidance of hypothermia etc.). The test group received an additional Canephron®N therapy for 3 months (2 tablets, three times a day).
Control examinations were conducted on day 7 and after 3, 6 and 12 months; or immediately in the case of a recurrent episode. The following cystitis symptoms were recorded at each time point: pain in the bladder, burning and stinging during urination, urinary urgency and frequent urination in small amounts. The criteria for defining a recurrent episode of cystitis were rebound lower urinary tract infection symptoms with pyuria and positive bacteriological urine culture.

**Results:** Canephron®N in addition to fluoroquinolones helps to reduce cystitis symptoms after 7 days better compared to treatment with fluoroquinolones only, as well as pyuria after 3, 6 and 12 months and urine levels of *E. coli* at 3 and 12 months.
The frequency rate of recurrent episodes of cystitis was in the test group always lower than in the control group with a statistically significant difference at 6 months (8.9% vs. 17.8%) and at 12 months (15.5% vs. 35.5%). At 12 months, the mean score of the LUTI Symptom Severity Index was 6 ($p \leq 0.05$) in the control patients and 3 ($p \leq 0.05$) in the test patients. This may indicate that the relapses were less severe in the test group.

**Conclusion:** Treatment with the herbal medicine Canephron®N is a novel treatment method of alleviating the symptoms of cystitis and especially for reducing the rate of recurrent cystitis episodes.

**Keywords:** Herbal medicine, Cystitis, Pyuria, Canephron®N

## Background

Cystitis is an infectious and inflammatory process in the bladder wall, primarily localised in the mucosa. This is usually associated with lower urinary tract infection (LUTI) [1]. Cystitis is an unpleasant condition, but never causes death or irreversible bladder changes [2]. Typical signs of cystitis are inconvenient and frequent urges to urinate. The patients may also experience pain in the lower abdomen, haematuria and urinary urgency. Furthermore, the urine may be turbid and have an unpleasant odour.

*Escherichia coli* is the main pathogen causing cystitis in 85% of community-acquired LUTIs and 50% of hospital LUTIs. Bladder infections are normally treated by antibiotic therapy [1, 3]. If the symptoms are mild, antibacterials may be prescribed upon completion of a bacterial urine culture.

In men with normal urinary tract anatomy LUTIs are rare [4], but one third of women under 24 years have had

* Correspondence: Sobodash@ukr.net; maxsabadash@i.ua
[1]Institute of Urology of NAMS of Ukraine, 04053Str. V. Vinnichenko, 9-a, Kiev, Ukraine
Full list of author information is available at the end of the article

at least one LUTI episode requiring antibiotic treatment in their life. About half of all women suffer from cystitis at least once during their lifetime, and more than half of them develop one or two recurrences. In most cases, recurrent episodes occur because of sexual intercourse, and may also be associated with the use of spermicides, but in certain cases the underlying causes are unclear. Recurrent episodes may be prevented with prophylactic antibiotics, although there is a risk that resistances may be developed [5, 6].

Herbal medicines may be used to circumvent the development of antibiotic resistance, particularly in long-term prevention of episodes of recurrent cystitis. One of the herbal medicines for the prevention of recurrent episodes of UTI is Canephron®N (Bionorica, SE, Germany). This is a fixed combination of herbal medicine components – century grass, lovage root and rosemary leaves – and acts against infection and inflammation in the urinary tract. It exhibits in-vitro both bactericidal and bacteriostatic effects on a wide range of uropathogens and inhibits bacterial adhesion to the urothelium, improves urodynamics and inhibits inflammatory reactions [7, 8]. The improvements in urodynamics are linked to mild diuresis [9] and spasmolysis [10].

Canephron®N has been shown to exhibit high efficacy in the prevention of chronic/recurrent infectious and inflammatory pathology of the urinary tract [reviewed in [10]]. We now present the first randomised long-term study of Canephron®N in the prevention of recurrent episodes of cystitis in women of child-bearing age.

## Methods

The aim of this study was to investigate the effect of the herbal medicine Canephron®N on the clinical course of acute recurrent cystitis in women of child-bearing age, associated with E.Coli. The study was designed as open labeled, randomised controlled study, in which the standard treatment with fluoroquinolones (ofloxacin) – the control group – was compared with standard treatment plus Canephron®N.

The study enrolled 90 women aged from 18 to 45 years. All of them had been diagnosed with acute recurrent cystitis caused by *E. coli* (with episode rates of up to twice every 6 months or 3 times a year). The patients were examined and treated at the SE "Institute of Urology of the NAMS of Ukraine".

The study was conducted in accordance with the principles laid down in the Declaration of Helsinki and approved by local Ethics committee.

The following methods of examination were used on admission:

- blood chemistry and urine analysis;
- standard bacterial urine culture and antibacterial susceptibility test;

- ultrasound examination of bladder and kidneys;
- LUTI Symptom Severity Index (see Table 1).

Patients were excluded from study participation if they exhibited:

- malformation of the urinary system;
- intracellular sexually-transmitted pathogens, and pathogens other than *E. coli*;
- individual intolerance of Canephron® N components;
- calculi impairing urodynamics, dendritic urolithiasis;
- type 1 or type 2 diabetes mellitus;
- hematuria, chronic renal impairment and other pathologies of the urinary system that might enhance the risk of relapse;
- ≤3 or ≥ 9 points in total on the main 3 LUTI Symptom Severity Index (see Table 1).
- Association of cystitis with sexual activity (postcoital cystitis)

The patients were randomly assigned to test ($n = 45$) and control ($n = 45$) groups.

Both, the test group and the control group received an antibacterial therapy (ofloxacin 200 mg/2 times daily) for 7 days determined by urine culture. Furthermore, in both groups general recommendations on preventing cystitis were made (sufficient liquid consumption, avoidance of hypothermia etc.).

Additional to these standard treatments, the patients in the test group received a Canephron®N therapy for 3 months (2 tablets TID for 3 months),

After the initial examination, all patients returned for a control examination on day 7 and for further examinations at 3, 6 and 12 months; or immediately in case of a recurrent episode. The following cystitis symptoms were recorded at each time point: pain in the bladder, burning and stinging during urination, urinal urgency and frequent urination in small amounts.

Pyuria was measured up to 12 months. A bacterial count for E.coli was conducted on culture at each examination and the relapses of cystitis were recorded for a follow-up period of up to 12 months.

**Table 1** LUTI Symptom Severity Index

| Points | Assessment of background symptoms [a] |
|--------|----------------------------------------|
| 0 | None |
| 1 | Mild (causing no effect upon daily activities or sleep) |
| 2 | Moderate (minor effect upon daily activities or sleep) |
| 3 | Severe (major effect upon daily activities or sleep) |
| 4 | Very severe (daily activities or sleep is impossible) |

[a] *Background symptoms: dysuria, pollakiuria (frequency), urgency*

**Table 2** Cystitis symptoms in the two treatment groups, on admission and after 7-day treatment

| Groups | Test group n = 45 | | Control group n = 45 | |
|---|---|---|---|---|
| Examination time Symptoms | On admission | After 7-day treatment course | On admission | After 7-day treatment course |
| Pain in the bladder | 26 (57.7%) | 3 (6.7%) | 23 (51.1%) | 5 (11.1%) |
| Burning and stinging during urination | 45 (100%) | 6 (13.3%) | 45 (100%) | 9 (20%) |
| Urinal urgency | 38 (84.4%) | 2 (4.4%) | 39 (86.6%) | 5 (11.1%) |
| Frequent urination in small amounts | 45 (100%) | 6 (13.3%) | 45 (100%) | 9 (20%) |

The criteria for recurrent episodes of acute cystitis were rebound LUTI symptoms with a positive bacteriological urine culture.

To prevent distortion of the results due to errors with urine sampling technique, urine samples for bacterial culture in acute cystitis were taken using Nelaton Fr 6 catheter. At month 3, 6 and 12 - midstream urine was taken without catheter.

All results were expressed as quantities and percentages, if appropriate. Statistical comparisons were conducted using the Student's $t$ test, with a two-sided 95% confidence interval (95% CI), $p \leq 0.05$.

## Results

The incidence of the main symptoms of cystitis (pain in the bladder, burning and stinging during urination; urinal urgency; frequent urination in small amounts) were essentially the same in the test and control groups (Table 2), which confirmed the comparability of the groups. All four symptoms improved in both groups after 7 days of treatment, although there was a tendency for a greater improvement in the test group than in the control group. The only statistically significant difference between the two groups was in the symptom of urinal ssurgency.

Pyuria (6 or more leucocytes in the field of view of the microscope) was initially present in all patients in both groups. During the follow-up period, pyuria was always more frequent in the control group than in the test group (see Fig. 1). This difference was statistically significant at 3 months (31.1% vs. 6.7%, $p \leq 0.05$), 6 months (31.1% vs. 6.6%, $p \leq 0.05$) and 12 months (31.1% vs. 4.4%, $p \leq 0.05$). The differences between the groups remained constant after 3 months.

The culture data for *Escherichia coli* were analysed separately for bacteriuria (E. Coli titer $\geq 10^3$ CFU/ml) and for no bacteriuria.

Initially, all patients in both groups (100%) showed bacteriuria. During the follow-up were constantly fewer patients with bacteriuria in the test group than in the control group. This difference was statistically significant at 3 months and at 12 months (Table 3).

The rate of recurrent episodes of acute uncomplicated cystitis was always lower in the test group than in the

control group (see Fig. 2). This difference was statistically significant at 6 months (8.9% vs. 17.8%) and at 12 months (15.5% vs. 35.5%).

During the 12-month period, the mean score of the LUTI Symptom Severity Index of the recurrent cystitis episodes was 6 in the control patients and 3 in the test patients.

## Discussion

This randomised controlled study was performed in women of child-bearing age who were suffering from an acute episode of recurrent cystitis. Patients in the test group received an identical treatment as patients in the control group, but were additionally treated with the herbal medicine Canephron®N (2 tablets TID for 3 months).

During the first 7 days of treatment, the symptoms of cystitis improved in both groups. There was a tendency for better results for the test group than for the control group but the difference was only statistically significant in symptom of urgency (4.44% vs. 11.1%).

Pyuria was significantly lower in the test group 3, 6 and 12 months after the end of antibiotic treatment (Fig. 1). Presence of bacteriuria was also lower during this period (Table 3). Finally, the rate of recurrent episodes of acute cystitis was also lower in the test group after 6 and 12 months (Fig. 2).

During the 12-month period, the mean score of the LUTI Symptom Severity Index of the recurrent cystitis

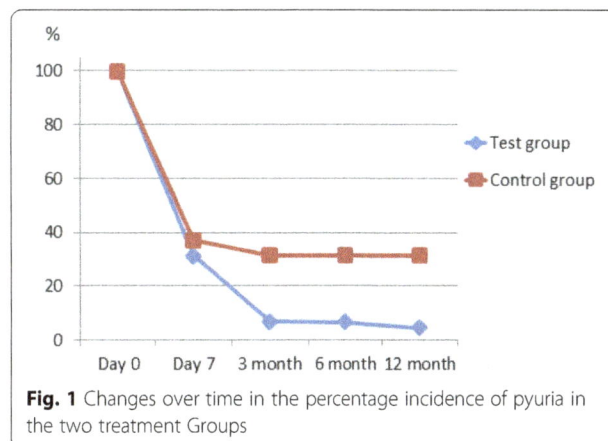

**Fig. 1** Changes over time in the percentage incidence of pyuria in the two treatment Groups

**Table 3** Prevalence of bacteriuria and no bacteriuria (*E. coli* titer $> 10^3$ CFU/ml) in the two treatment groups

| Groups | Test group $n = 45$ | | | | Control group $n = 45$ | | | |
|---|---|---|---|---|---|---|---|---|
| Examination time Day | Day 7 | Month 3 | Month 6 | Month 12 | Day 7 | Month 3 | Month 6 | Month 12 |
| Prevalence of bacteriuria | 33.3 | 13.3 | 13.4 | 13.4 | 42.2 | 28.9 | 33.3 | 47.2 |
| No bacteriuria (*E. coli*) | 66.7 | 86.7 | 86.6 | 86.6 | 57.8 | 71.1 | 66.7 | 52.8 |

episodes was 6 in the control patients and 3 in the test patients. This may indicate that the recurrences were less severe in the test group than in the control group.

These effects may be related to the pharmacological activity possessed by Canephron®N, including diuretic, spasmolytic, anti-inflammatory, antibacterial and nephroprotective effects [10]. Taking into account the variability of chemotypes of medicinal plants and methods of production of herbal remedies it is important to note, that Canephron® N is a fixed combination of standardised herbal medicine components – centuary grass, lovage root and rosemary leaves in which special attention is paid to question about standardization and reproducibility of ingredients. It is more difficult to explain the differences between the groups at 6 and 12 months after treatment, when the patients were no longer receiving Canephron®N. It might be postulated that the physiological effects caused by Canephron®N (e.g. less inflammation) last for longer than the immediate presence of the components of the herbal medicine. Anyway reducing the frequency of recurrent episodes of cystitis can be explained by sustained positive changes in the urinary tract and possibly a change in the nature of the relationship microorganism/macro-organism. This issue could be investigated by further pharmacokinetic studies.

The limitations of this study include the lack of blinding to the patients and the physician at any time, the lack of characterisation of the individual components of the herbal medicine and the lack of more detailed studies of urological function.

## Conclusion

In women of child bearing age suffering from acute recurrent cystitis, the herbal medicine Canephron®N can reduce the rate of episodes of recurrence, as well as bacteriuria and pyuria. To generalize the results, additional studies are needed, including longer-term studies and studies in older women.

The present data indicate that Canephron®N is a novel and effective treatment of recurrent cystitis. Because of the complex composition of Canephron®N, there may be less risk that bacterial resistance will develop than during antibiotic treatment of the same condition. This possibility should be also examined.

## Abbreviation
LUTI: Lower urinary tract infection

## Authors' contributions
MS performed the selection of patients, conducted treatment and observation during the period of the study, collected of the study results data, participated in writing of the manuscript. AS developed the study design, performed statistical analysis, monitoring of the study. Conducted analysis and review of study-results, participated in writing of the manuscript. All authors read and approved the final manuscript.

## Competing interests
The authors declare that they have no competing interests.

## Author details
[1]Institute of Urology of NAMS of Ukraine, 04053Str. V. Vinnichenko, 9-a, Kiev, Ukraine. [2]Institute of Urology Cystitis in Women, 04053Str. V. Vinnichenko, 9-a, Kiev, Ukraine.

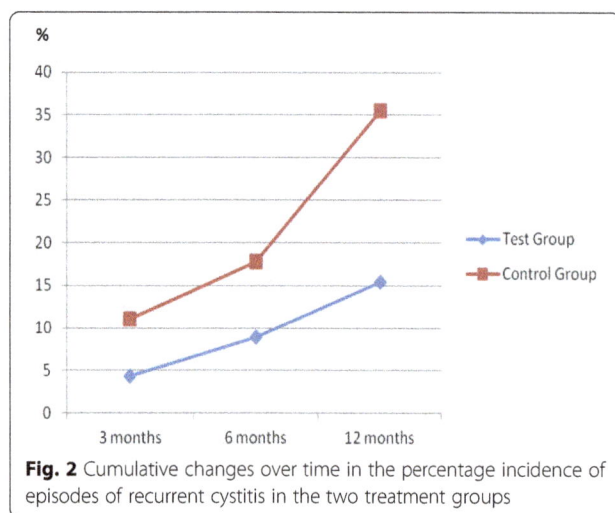

**Fig. 2** Cumulative changes over time in the percentage incidence of episodes of recurrent cystitis in the two treatment groups

## References
1. Nickel JC, Shoskes DA, Irvine-Bird K. Prevalence and impact of bacteriuria and/or urinary tract infection in interstitial cystitis/painful bladder syndrome. Urology. 2010;76:799–803.
2. Gupta K, Hooton TM, Naber KG et al. International clinical practice guidelines for the treatment of acute uncomplicated cystitis and pyelonephritis in women: a 2010 update by the Infectious Diseases Society of America and the European Society for Microbiology and Infectious Diseases. Clin Infect Dis. 2011;52(5):e103–20. https://academic.oup.com/cid/article-lookup/doi/10.1093/cid/ciq257.
3. Johansen TEB, Naber KG. Urinary tract infections. Antibiotics (Basel). 2014;3:375–7.

4.   Grabe M, Bartoletti R, Bjerklund Johansen TE, Cai T, Çek M, Köves B, Naber KG, Pickard RS, Tenke P, Wagenlehner F, Wullt B. EAU guidelines on urological infections. European Association of Urology 2015: Arnhem; 2015. p. 1–78.

5.   Stanford E, McMurphy C. There is a low incidence of recurrent bacteriuria in painful bladder syndrome/interstitial cystitis patients followed longitudinally. Int Urogynecol J Pelvic Floor Dysfunct. 2007;18:551–4.

6.   Abdul-Ghani AS, El-Lati SG, Sacaan A, et al. Anticonvulsant effects of some Arab medicinal plants. Int J Crude Drug Res. 1987;25:39–43.

7.   Gracza L, Koch H, Löffler E. Isolierung von rosmarinsäure aus symphytum officinale und ihre antiinflammatorische wirksamkeit in einem in-vitro model. Arch Pharm. 1985;318:1090–5.

8.   Haloui M, Louedec L, Michel B, Lyoussi B. Experimental diuretic effects of Rosmarinus officinalis und Centaurium erythrea. J Ethnopharmacol. 2000;71:465–72.

9.   Kumarasamy Y, Nahar L, Sarker SD. Bioactivity of gentiopicroside from the aerial parts of Centaurium erythrae. Fitoterapia. 2003;74:151–4.

10.  Naber G. Efficacy and safety of the phytotherapeutic drug canephron® N in prevention and treatment of urogenital and gestational disease: review of clinical experience in eastern Europe and central Asia. Res Rep Urol. 2013;5:39–46.

# 2

# Evaluation of central nervous system (CNS) depressant activity of methanolic extract of *Commelina diffusa* Burm. in mice

Tania Sultana, Md. Abdul Mannan[*] and Tajnin Ahmed

## Abstract

**Background:** *Commelina diffusa* Burm. (Family: Commelinaceae) is usually known as "climbing dayflower or spreading dayflower" in Bangladesh. The plant is used in fever, malaria, insect, bug bites, rheumatoid arthritis, gonorrhea, influenza, and bladder infection etc. The present investigation was undertaken which deals with the evaluation of central nervous system (CNS) depressant activity of methanolic extract of *C. diffusa* in mice models.

**Methods:** The central nervous system (CNS) depressant activity of *C. diffusa* was evaluated by the classical models of depression as open field, hole cross, forced swimming, tail suspension, and thiopental sodium induced sleeping time tests in mice. The animals were divided into control, positive control, and three test groups containing five mice each. The test groups received extract at the doses of 50, 100, and 200 mg/kg body weight orally where as the control group received distilled water (0.1 mL/mouse, p.o.). Diazepam (1 mg/kg, i.p.) was used as standard drug.

**Results:** It is clear that the plant extract significantly decreased the locomotor activity of mice in open field and hole cross tests when compared to the control ($p < 0.05$). It is observed that the extract showed significantly ($p < 0.05$) increased in immobility time in forced swimming and tail suspension tests in mice. In addition, the extract produced prolongs the sleeping time with onset of action in contrast to the control group.

**Conclusions:** The present work depicts the evaluation of possible CNS depressant activity of *C. diffusa* in mice models. The obtained results provide support for the use of this species in traditional medicine and warrants further pharmacological investigations that could lead to novel leads in future.

**Keywords:** *Commelina diffusa*, CNS depressant, Extract, Diazepam

## Background

Depression is a widespread psychiatric ailment [1]. It is already expected to constitute the second largest source of global burden of disease after heart disease in 2020 [2]. The monoaminergic hypothesis of depression does not provide a full understanding of the progression, causes, and pharmacotherapy of depression [3]. Most accepted hypothesis of depression is postulated, and oxidative stress is suggested to be involved in the pathophysiology of depression [4]. According to WHO estimated, 121 million people suffer from clinical depression [5]. It occurs usually in the early adult life of patients with decrease in monoamine neurotransmitters [6]. Medicinal plants therapies may be effective alternatives in the treatment of depression. It possesses least side effects compared to synthetic medicines [7]. It has contributed significantly towards the development of modern medicine. Recently, traditional medicine is being re-evaluated by extensive research on different plant species and their active therapeutic principles in worldwide. The rich wealth of plant kingdom can represent a novel source of newer compounds with significant therapeutic activities. The most important merits of herbal medicine seem to be their perceived efficacy, low adverse effects, and low cost [8].

*Commelina diffusa* Burm. (Family: Commelinaceae) is a pan tropical herbaceous plant, which is known as "climbing dayflower or spreading dayflower" in Bangladesh. [9, 10]. This herb is widely distributed

* Correspondence: manna.034@gmail.com
Department of Pharmacy, Stamford University Bangladesh, 51, Siddeswari Road, Dhaka -1217, Bangladesh

throughout in Bangladesh and other South Asian countries. It is widely used in urinary tract infections, swellings, inflammation, diarrhoea, hemorrhoids, enteritis, eye irritation, conjunctivitis and ophthalmia. The juice of stem is used in laryngitis, sore throats, acute tonsillitis, pharyngitis, otitis media, and nose bleeding. Topically or internally, the plant is used in abscess, boils, fever, malaria, insect, snake, bug bites, rheumatoid arthritis, mumps, gonorrhea, common cold, cough, coughing up blood, influenza, bladder infection, and edema. Throughout Latin America, the plant parts are used in dermatitis and burns [11]. In Nepal, it is used to treat hemorrhoids, inflamed uterus, laryngitis, leprosy, malaria, mumps, otitis media, painful menses, pharyngitis, rheumatoid arthritis, sore throats, snake bites, tonsillitis and tumors. In Egypt, the weed is used as a refrigerant, tonic for treating stomach and groin problems [12]. In Caribbean Indians, the plant is used as a tea to ward off influenza and medicinal baths. In Mexico, it is used for the treatment of conjunctivitis, dermatitis, dysmenorrheal. In Paraguay, it is used for enteritis, gonorrhea, and infertility treatments. In the Dominican Republic, Haiti, and South America, it is used for kidney ailments, leucorrhea, malaria, nervous conditions, post partum discomfort, tuberculosis, tumors, and venereal diseases. The tiny blue flowers are boiled in Ecuador and Peru to make a tea for the relief of headaches [13]. In Trinidad, it is used as a depurative, bladder infection and cooling medicinal infusions. In the Windward Islands and Cuba, it is used for the treatment of jaundice in young children [14]. According to previous studies; *C. diffusa* exhibited good antimicrobial activity against a range of Gram-positive and Gram-negative bacteria as well as fungi [15]. The anti-inflammatory activity of the extract tested using the chick carrageenan-induced foot oedema model. [16]. It also demonstrated protection of MRC-5 cells against oxidation by reactive oxygen species [17]. Another study mentioned that the extract is used for the treatment of cancer [18], antidiabetes [19], leprosy, and nervous system related disorders [20].

However, there is lack of scientific report to support these supposed central nervous system (CNS) depressant activity in mice. The present investigation was undertaken which deals with the evaluation of central nervous system (CNS) depressant activity of methanolic extract of *C. diffusa* Burm. in mice models.

## Methods
### Chemicals
The following drugs and chemicals were used in this study: Diazepam (Square Pharmaceutical Ltd., Bangladesh), Thiopental sodium (Gonoshastha Pharmaceuticals Ltd., Bangladesh), Methanol (Sigma Chemicals Co., USA). Diazepam (1 mg/kg i.p.) was used in open field, hole

cross, forced swimming, tail suspension and thiopental sodium-induced sleeping time tests. The drugs were intraperitoneally (i.p.) administered 15 min before the experiment. The extract was orally administered 30 min before the experiment (Except open field, and hole cross tests) at the doses of 50, 100, and 200 mg/kg, where as the animal of control group received distilled water (0.1 mL/mouse, p.o.).

### Collection of plant materials
The plant was accumulated from the village of Roypur of Chuadanga district in January 2016 when weed beds were in their maximum densities. The whole plant with leaves, stems and roots was collected and analyzed by the proficient of Bangladesh National Herbarium, Mirpur, Dhaka, Bangladesh, where a voucher specimen (Accession No: 42,861) has been deposited for future reference.

### Preparation of extraction
The whole plant was intensively washed with water. The adulterants were removed to obtain fresh sample. The collected samples were cut and sliced, if necessary. The samples were dried for 7 days in hot air oven at laboratory conditions. After drying, the dried samples were grounded to coarse powder with an electrical grinder. The powder sample was soaked in adequate amount of methanol for three days at room temperature with infrequent stirring and shaking. The solvent was filtered 3 times through a Whatman No. 1 filter paper and sterilized cotton bed. Then, the solvent was fully removed and obtained crude extract, which was used for the investigation of phytochemical screening and evaluation of central nervous system (CNS) depressant activity in mice models.

### Test animals
Swiss albino mice, 3–4 weeks of age, weighing between 20 and 25 g, were used in this study. These mice were collected from Pharmacology Laboratory, Jahangirnagar University, Savar, Dhaka, Bangladesh. Animals were kept in polyvinyl cages with soft wood bedding materials. Animals were well maintained under standard environmental conditions (temperature: $25 \pm 2$ °C, relative humidity: 55–65% and 12 h light/dark cycle). The animals were habituated to the laboratory environment for a period of 14 days prior to performing the experiments. All the experimental mice were treated following the Ethical Principles and Guidelines for Scientific Experiments on Animals (1995) formulated by The Swiss Academy of Medical Sciences and the Swiss Academy of Sciences. The Institutional Animal Ethical Committee (SUB/ IAEC/17.02) of Stamford University Bangladesh approved all experimental rules.

## Acute toxicity test

Mice were divided into a control and three test groups ($n = 5$). The test groups received extract orally at the doses of 500, 1000, and 2000 mg/kg body weight. After administration, the animals were kept in separate cages and were allowed to food and water ad libitum. The animals were then observed for possible behavioral changes, allergic reaction (skin rash, itching) and mortality for the next 72 h [21].

## Phytochemical screening

Methanolic extract of *C. diffusa* was qualitatively tested for the detection of alkaloids, flavonoids, saponins, tannins, cardiac glycosides, carbohydrates, reducing sugars, proteins, glucosides, terpenoids, and steroids [22].

## Pharmacological tests

### Open field test

The open field test is used to measure the locomotion in mice by the number of square cross. The animals were divided into control, positive control and three test groups containing five mice each. The test groups received extract at the doses of 50, 100, and 200 mg/kg body weight orally where as the control group received distilled water (0.1 mL/mouse, p.o.). Diazepam (1 mg/kg, i.p.) used as positive control group. The open field was divided into a series of squares. Each square is separately colored black and white. The apparatus had a wall of 40 cm height. The animals were visited the squares and the number of visited squares were counted for 3 min at 0, 30, 60, 90 and 120 min intervals [23].

### Hole cross test

A case having a size of ($30 \times 20 \times 14$ cm) with a wood partition fixed in the middle was used. The cage had a hole of 3 cm diameter at a height of 7.5 cm in the center. The animals were divided into control, positive control, and three test groups containing five animals in each. The test groups received extract at the doses of 50, 100, and 200 mg/kg body weight orally and the control group received distilled water (0.1 mL/mouse, p.o.). The standard drug diazepam (1 mg/kg, i.p.) was used as positive control group. The mice were passed through the hole from one chamber to another and the number of passage was counted for 3 min at 0, 30, 60, 90, and 120 min intervals respectively [24].

### Forced swimming test

The forced swimming test is commonly used assays of antidepressant-like activity in rodents. Animals were randomly divided into five groups. Thirty minutes later, the treatment with the extract (50, 100, and 200 mg/kg, p.o.) or diazepam (1 mg/kg, i.p.), a standard drug, or distilled water (0.1 mL/mouse, p.o.), mice were individually placed in an open cylindrical container (45 cm height × 20 cm diameter) containing 17 cm of water at 25 °C for 5 min. Mice were recorded as immobile when floating motionless or making only those movements necessary to keep the head above water [25].

### Tail suspension test

This behavior displayed in rodents subjected to unavoidable and inescapable stresses during tail suspension test reflects behavioral despair, which reflects depression in humans. Mice were divided into five groups. Thirty minutes later, the extract (50, 100, and 200 mg/kg, p.o.) was used as test groups. The diazepam (1 mg/kg, i.p.) was used as standard drug when the control group received distilled water (0.1 mL/mouse, p.o.). Mice were suspended 50 cm above the floor using adhesive tape placed approximately 1 cm from the tip of their tails. The duration of immobility time was recorded for 6 min. The mice were considered immobile when they passively hung or stayed motionless [26].

### Thiopental sodium-induced sleeping time test

In this test, the animals were assigned for five groups comprising of five mice in each group. The test groups expected the extract at the doses of 50, 100, and 200 mg/kg when the control group received distilled water (0.1 ml/mouse, p.o.). The standard drug diazepam (1 mg/kg, i.p.) was used as positive control group. After passing thirty minutes, each mouse was treated with thiopental sodium (40 mg/kg, i.p.) to induce sleep. The rodents were monitored by placing them on different chambers for the latent period (time between thiopental sodium administrations to loss righting reflex) and duration of sleeping time (time between the loss and recovery of righting reflex) [27].

## Statistical analysis

The results were presented as mean ± SEM. The statistical analysis was performed using one way analysis of variance (ANOVA) followed by Dunnett's post hoc test as using SPSS 18.00 software. Differences between groups were considered significant at a level of $*p < 0.05$.

## Results

### Phytochemical screening

Phytochemical screening of the methanolic extract of *C. diffusa* revealed the presence of alkaloids, flavonoids, saponins, tannins, cardiac glycosides, terpenoids, and steroids (Table 1).

### Acute toxicity

There was no mortality up to 2000 mg/kg dose. It was observed that there was significant reduction in the activity of animals from ½ h up to 4 h and subsequently

**Table 1** Preliminary qualitative phytochemical screening of methanolic extract of *C. diffusa* (MECD)

| Plant constituents | Inference |
|---|---|
| Alkaloids | + |
| Flavonoids | + |
| Saponins | + |
| Tannins | + |
| Cardiac glycosides | + |
| Carbohydrates | – |
| Reducing sugars | – |
| Proteins | – |
| Glucosides | – |
| Terpenoids | + |
| Steroids | + |

+: Presence; –: Absence

they were normal. Therefore, it can be assumed that MECD possesses a low toxicity profile and the $LD_{50}$ is more than 2000 mg/kg.

### Open field test

The extract significantly decreased the locomotor activity in mice at the doses of 50, 100, and 200 mg/kg body weight ($p < 0.05$) and this effect was evident from the initial observation (0 min) period and continued up to 5th observation period (120 min) (Table 2). Diazepam (1 mg/kg, i.p.) showed a noticeable decrease in locomotion in mice from the 2$^{nd}$ observation period to 5th observation period as expected.

### Hole cross test

Methanolic extract of *C. diffusa* showed significant decrease of movement at the doses of 50, 100, and 200 mg/kg body weight from its initial value at 0 min to 120 min ($p < 0.05$). The number of hole crossed from one chamber to another by mice of the standard drug diazepam (1 mg/kg, i.p.) is decreased from 0 min to 120 min (Table 3). The extract showed dose dependent activity and maximum depressive effect was observed at 5th observation period.

### Forced swimming test

After oral administration, the extract at the doses of 50, 100, and 200 mg/kg significantly increased the immobility times when compared with the control group ($p < 0.05$) (Table 4). Similarly, the standard drug diazepam (1 mg/kg, i.p.), as expected, showed a significant increase in the immobility times ($p < 0.05$).

### Tail suspension test

The extract at the doses of 50, 100, and 200 mg/kg produced a significant increase in the immobility times when compared to control group ($p < 0.05$). The effect of the extract on behavior in this test is shown in Table 5. Diazepam (1 mg/kg, i.p.), the duration of immobility time was compared with control group which showed significant increase in immobility times ($p < 0.05$).

### Thiopental sodium-induced sleeping time test

The plant extract decreased the onset of action time and increased the length of the sleeping time, which was comparable to the control group (Table 6). The extract produced a significant effect on the duration of sleeping times. The standard drug diazepam (1 mg/kg, i.p.), was also showed a statistically significant effect on the onset of sleep and the duration of sleeping times ($p < 0.05$).

### Discussion

The present study was conducted to explicate central nervous system (CNS) depressant activities of the methanolic extract of *C. diffusa* in mice. The CNS depressant effect of *C. diffusa* was studied using five neuropharmacological models namely open field, hole cross, forced swimming, tail suspension, and thiopental sodium induced sleeping time tests. These paradigms are widely used classical models for screening neuropharmacological activity.

The methanolic extract of *C. diffusa* decreased the frequency and amplitude of movements in the open field and hole cross tests in mice. The results of these study provided evidence that the extract reduced locomotor activity confirming its CNS depressant effects. Locomotor activity is considered as an index of alertness and

**Table 2** Effects of *C. diffusa* extract and diazepam on the open field test

| Treatment | Dose (mg/kg) | Number of square crossed | | | | |
|---|---|---|---|---|---|---|
| | | 0 min | 30 min | 60 min | 90 min | 120 min |
| Control | 0.1 mL/mouse | 76.00 ± 1.64 | 72.20 ± 3.48 | 61.00 ± 2.66 | 41.40 ± 1.07 | 32.60 ± 1.36 |
| Diazepam | 1 | 71.80 ± 3.26 | 55.80 ± 2.69* | 30.40 ± 2.04* | 15.00 ± 0.70* | 6.80 ± 0.58* |
| MECD | 50 | 59.80 ± 1.96 | 49.00 ± 4.19* | 44.00 ± 1.22* | 27.60 ± 1.12* | 15.40 ± 0.74* |
| MECD | 100 | 56.40 ± 2.42 | 43.20 ± 1.28* | 40.40 ± 2.06* | 19.60 ± 0.92* | 9.80 ± 0.66* |
| MECD | 200 | 63.60 ± 1.93 | 51.00 ± 1.76* | 33.60 ± 1.83* | 17.40 ± 0.92* | 8.20 ± 0.58* |

Values are presented as mean ± SEM ($n = 5$). MECD = Methanolic extract of *C. diffusa*
* $p < 0.05$, vs. control (Dunnett's test)

**Table 3** Effects of C. diffusa extract and diazepam on hole cross test

| Treatment | Dose (mg/kg) | Number of hole crossed | | | | |
|---|---|---|---|---|---|---|
| | | 0 min | 30 min | 60 min | 90 min | 120 min |
| Control | 0.1 mL/mouse | 16.40 ± 0.92 | 12.40 ± 1.12 | 9.40 ± 0.51 | 6.60 ± 0.81 | 4.00 ± 0.70 |
| Diazepam | 1 | 14.00 ± 1.41 | 5.40 ± 0.51* | 3.40 ± 0.24* | 1.20 ± 0.37* | 0.60 ± 0.24* |
| MECD | 50 | 14.40 ± 1.69 | 7.60 ± 0.40* | 6.20 ± 1.02* | 3.00 ± 0.54* | 2.40 ± 0.51 |
| MECD | 100 | 13.40 ± 0.92 | 6.60 ± 0.74* | 5.00 ± 0.89* | 2.40 ± 0.67* | 1.60 ± 0.51* |
| MECD | 200 | 15.00 ± 0.83 | 6.40 ± 0.51* | 4.20 ± 0.37* | 1.80 ± 0.37* | 1.00 ± 0.31* |

Values are presented as mean ± SEM ($n = 5$). MECD = Methanolic extract of C. diffusa
* $p < 0.05$, vs. control (Dunnett's test)

a reduction of it is an indicative of CNS depressant activity [28]. It is a measurement of the level of excitability of the CNS [29], this decrease in spontaneous motor activity could be attributed to the CNS depressant effect of the plant extract [30]. Both tests significantly decreased locomotion in mice. Gamma amino butyric acid is the major inhibitory neurotransmitter in the central nervous system [31], which is involved in the physiological functions related to the psychological and neurological disorders as epilepsy, depression, parkinson syndrome, and alzheimer's disease [32]. Diverse drugs might modify the GABA system, at the level of the synthesis of it by potentiating the GABA-mediated postsynaptic inhibition through an allosteric modification of GABA receptors. It directly increases in chloride conductance or indirectly by potentiating GABA-induced chloride conductance with simultaneous depression of voltage activated $Ca^{2+}$ channel like barbiturates [33]. Therefore, it is predictable that the extract may act by potentiating GABAergic inhibition in the CNS via membrane hyper polarization leading to a reduction in the firing rate of critical neurons in the brain or it may be due to direct activation of GABA receptors [31]. It may also be due to enhanced affinity for GABA or an increase in the duration of the GABA-gated channel opening [34].

The forced swimming test is widely used for the assessment of antidepressant-like activity in animal models. The shortening of immobility duration indicates antidepressant activity in this model, while prolonged immobility time reflects a CNS depression-like effect

[35]. However, CNS depressant effect was observed in the forced swimming test. Additionally, the experiment was extended to observe the tail suspension test allow as a fast and reliable screening of the psychotropic properties of drugs. Basically, the measuring principle is based on the energy developed by mice trying to escape from their suspension. During this test, the movements of the mice were analyzed in terms of energy and power developed over time. The extract was significantly increased in immobility time which indicated as CNS depressant effects in mice. The standard drug diazepam also indicated CNS depressant effects in mice model. It has been argued that tail suspension test is less stressful than force swimming test and has greater pharmacological sensitivity. The results obtained from tail suspension test is in concordance with the validated forced swimming test by Porsolt et al. Environmental factors and hereditary factors play a major role in producing deficient monoaminergic transmission in the CNS there by producing symptoms of depression [36].

Previous phytochemical investigation suggests that flavonoids and neuroactive steroids are ligands for $GABA_A$ receptors in the CNS which indicates that they can act as benzodiazepine-like agents [37]. It has also been reported that some flavanoids exhibit high affinity binding to the benzodiazepine site of $GABA_A$ receptors. Therefore, the CNS depressant activity may be due to the phytoconstituents present in the extract of C. diffusa. Triterpenoids, and saponins are reported to have agonistic activities at $GABA_A$ receptor complex [33, 38, 39].

**Table 4** Effects of C. diffusa extract and diazepam on forced swimming test

| Treatment | Dose (mg/kg) | Immobility time (s) |
|---|---|---|
| Control | 0.1 mL/mouse | 62.00 ± 2.92 |
| Diazepam | 1 | 177.00 ± 2.55* |
| MECD | 50 | 73.20 ± 1.99 |
| MECD | 100 | 87.20 ± 3.61* |
| MECD | 200 | 141.40 ± 4.25* |

Values are presented as mean ± SEM ($n = 5$). MECD = Methanolic extract of C. diffusa
* $p < 0.05$, vs. control (Dunnett's test)

**Table 5** Effects of C. diffusa extract and diazepam on tail suspension test

| Treatment | Dose (mg/kg) | Immobility time(s) |
|---|---|---|
| Control | 0.1 mL/mouse | 84.80 ± 2.41 |
| Diazepam | 1 | 219.80 ± 3.98* |
| MECD | 50 | 106.00 ± 2.12* |
| MECD | 100 | 130.80 ± 2.22* |
| MECD | 200 | 191.20 ± 2.35* |

Values are presented as mean ± SEM ($n = 5$). MECD = Methanolic extract of C. diffusa
* $p < 0.05$, vs. control (Dunnett's test)

**Table 6** Effects of *C. diffusa* extract and diazepam on thiopental sodium-induced sleeping time test

| Treatment | Dose (mg/kg) | Onset of action (min) | Duration of sleeping time (min) |
|---|---|---|---|
| Control | 0.1 mL/mouse | 4.95 ± 0.41 | 27.00 ± 1.92 |
| Diazepam | 1 | 3.01 ± 0.13* | 91.20 ± 1.93* |
| MECD | 50 | 4.78 ± 0.22 | 38.80 ± 1.36* |
| MECD | 100 | 4.56 ± 0.22 | 46.80 ± 1.28* |
| MECD | 200 | 3.74 ± 0.24* | 76.20 ± 2.15* |

Values are presented as mean ± SEM ($n = 5$). MECD = Methanolic extract of *C. diffusa*
* $p < 0.05$, vs. control (Dunnett's test)

These phytoconstituents may be contributed to the CNS depressant effects in mice. There is no strict evidence which substances are exactly responsible for the CNS depressant effects.

Thiopental sodium belongs to the barbiturate and induces sleep in both humans and rodents. The thiopental sodium induced sleeping time test in mice was used to investigate the sedative–hypnotic drugs [40]. It binds with GABA receptor complex and shows GABA mediated hyper polarization of postsynaptic neurons [40]. It potentiates GABA activity, entering chloride into the neuron by prolonging the duration of chloride channel opening. On the other hand, thiopental can block excitatory glutamate receptors. All of these molecular action lead to decrease of neuronal activity that support the following reference substances which possess CNS depressant action. Our results demonstrate a relationship between the CNS depressant effect of *C. diffusa* and diazepam which could be suggested in this test.

## Conclusions

The present work depicts the evaluation of possible CNS depressant activity of *C. diffusa* in mice models. The obtained results provide support for the use of this species in traditional medicine and warrants further pharmacological investigations that could lead to novel leads in future.

## Acknowledgements
The authors are grateful to Professor Dr. Bidyut Kanti Datta, Chairman, Department of Pharmacy, Stamford University Bangladesh for his permission to use the facilities of the Pharmacology and Phytochemistry Laboratory.

## Authors' contributions
MAM designed and coordinated all laboratory experiments, analyzed and interpreted results. MAM and TS conducted all experiments. MAM did statistical analysis and drafted the manuscript. All authors read and approved the manuscript.

## Competing interests
The authors report no conflicts of interest. The authors alone are responsible for the content and writing of the paper.

## References
1. Ferrari AJ, Charlson FJ, Norman RN, Patten SB, Freedman G, CGL M, Vos T, Whiteford HA. Burden of depressive disorders by country, sex, age, and year: findings from the global burden of disease study 2010. PLoS Med. 2013; 10(11):1–12.
2. Smith AJ, Sketris I, Cooke C, Gardner D, Kisely S, Tett SE. A comparison of antidepressant use in Nova Scotia, Canada and Australia. Pharmacoepidemiol Drug Saf. 2008;17(7):697–706.
3. Schildkraut JJ, Gordon EK, Durell J. Catecholamine metabolism in affective disorders. I. Normetanephrine and VMA excretion in depressed patients treated with imipramine. J Psychiatr Res. 1965;3(4):213–28.
4. Michel TM, Frangou S, Thiemeyer D, Camara S, Jecel J, Nara K, Brunklaus A, Zoechling R, Riederer P. Evidence for oxidative stress in the frontal cortex in patients with recurrent depressive disorder—a postmortem study. Psychiatry Res. 2007;151(1–2):145–50.
5. Cryan JF, Lucki I. Antidepressant like behavioral effects mediated by hydroxy tryptamine receptors. The Journal of Pharmacology experimental Therapeutics. 2000;295:1120–6.
6. Dhingra D, Sharma A. Review on antidepressant plants. Natural Products Radiance. 2005:144–52.
7. Zhang J, Wu J, Fujita Y, Yao W, Ren Q, Yang C, Li S, Shirayama Y, Hashimoto K. Antidepressant effects of TrkB ligands on depression-like behaviour and dendritic changes in mice after inflammation. Int J Neuropsychopharmacol. 2015:1–12.
8. Ghani A. Medicinal plants of Bangladesh. The Asiatic Society of Bangladesh: Dhaka; 1998.
9. Akobundu IO, Agyakwa C. A handbook of west African weeds. Ibadan (Nigeria): International institute of tropical agriculture; 1987.
10. Burkill HM. The useful plants of west tropical Africa. Edition Royal Botonaic Gardens Kew: London. 1985:431–2.
11. David BLAc. Medicine at your feet: Healing plants of the Hawaiian Kingdom *Commelina diffusa* (Honohono); 1998. http://www.medicineatyourfeet.com/
12. Leonard DB. Medicine at your feet: Healing plants of the Hawaiian Kingdom. 2012;1. http://www.medicineatyourfeet.com/
13. Seaforth CE, Adams CD, Sylvester Y. A guide to the medicinal plants of Trinidad and Tobago. Commonwealth Science Council, Commonwealth Secretariat, London, UK. 1983; p.222.
14. Beira A, Leon MC, Iglesias E, Ferrandiz D, Herrera R, Volpato G, Godinez D, Guimarais M. Alvarez R. Estudios etnobotanicos sobre plantas medicinales en la provincia de Camaguey (Cuba) Anales del Jardín Botánico de Madrid. 2004;61(2):185–203.
15. Khan MAA, Islam MT, Sadhu SK. Evaluation of phytochemical and antimicrobial properties of *Commelina diffusa* Burm. f. Orient Pharm Exp Med 2011;11 (4):235–241.
16. Mensah AY, Houghton PJ, Dickson RA, Fleischer TC, Heinrich M, Bremner P. In vitro evaluation of effects of two Ghanaian plants relevant to wound healing. Phytother Res. 20(11):941–4.
17. Houghton PJ, Hylands PJ, Mensah AY, Hensel A, Deters AM. In vitro tests and ethnopharmacological investigations: wound healing as an example. J Ethnopharmacol. 2005;100(1):100–7.

18. Plants HJL. Used against cancer. A survey. Lloydia. 1969;32:247–96.

19. Youn JY, Park HY, Cho HK. Anti-hyperglycemic activity of *Commelina communis* L.: inhibition of α-glucosidase. Diabetes Res Clin Pract. 2004;66:149–55.

20. Oudhia, P. Kaua-kaini (*Commelina benghalensis* Linn.) Society for Parthenium Management(SOPAM) 28-A, Greeta Nagar, Raipur – 492001 India.2004.

21. Walker CIB, Trevisan G, Rossato MF, Franciscato C, Pereira ME, Ferreira J, Manfron MP. Antinociceptive activity of Mirabilis jalapa in mice. J Ethnopharmacol. 2008;120:169–75.

22. Ghani A. Medicinal plants of Bangladesh with chemical constituents and uses. 2nd ed. Dhaka, Bangladesh: The Asiatic Society of Bangladesh; 2003. p. 331–2.

23. Gupta BD, Dandiya PC, Gupta ML. A psychopharmacological analysis of behavior in rat. Japan J Pharm. 1971;21:293–8.

24. Takagi K, Watanabe M, Saito H. Studies on the spontaneous movement of animalsby the hole cross test: effect of 2-dimethylaminoethane. Its acylates on the central nervoussystem. Jpn J Pharmacol. 1971;21:797–810.

25. Porsolt RD, Bertin A, Behavioural JM. Despair in mice: a primary screening test for antidepressants. Archives Internationales de Pharmacodynamie et de Therapie. 1977;229:327–36.

26. Steru L, Chermat R, Thierry B, Simon P. The tail suspension test: a new method for screening antidepressants in mice. Psychopharmacology. 1985; 85:367–70.

27. Hossain MM, Hasan SMR, Akter R, Islam MN, Saha MR, Rashid MJ, Saha MR, Mazumder MEH, Rana S. Evaluation of analgesic and neuropharmacological properties of the aerial part of *Tinospora cordifolia* miers.In mice. Stam J Pharma Scis. 2009;2:31–7.

28. Protapaditya D, Sangita C, Priyanka C, Sanjib B. Neuropharmacological properties of *Mikania scandens* (L.) Willd. (Asteraceae). Journal of Advanced Pharmaceutical Technology and Research. 2011;2(4):255–9.

29. Mansur R, Martz W, Effects CE. Of acute and chronic administration of Cannabis Satis and (–) 9-transtetrahydrocannabinaol on the behaviour of rats in open field arena. Psychopharmacol. 1980;2:5–7.

30. Rakotonirina VS, Bum EN, Rakotonirina A, Bopelet M. Sedative properties of the decoction of the rhizome of *Cyperus articulatus*. Fitoterapia. 2001;72:22–9.

31. Kavita G, Vijay KL, Shivesh J. Anticonvulsant potential of ethanol extracts and their solvent partitioned fractions from *Flemingia strobilifera* root. Pharm Res. 2013;5(4):265–70.

32. Kumar K, Sharma S, Kumar P, Deshmukh R. Therapeutic potential of GABA(B) receptor ligands in drug addiction, anxiety, depression and other CNS disorders. Pharmacol Biochem Behav. 2013;110:174–84.

33. Uma AB, Radha Y, Prachi DP, Mandar RZ, Rahul SS. Study of central nervous system depressant and behavioral activity of an ethanol extract of *Achyranthes aspera*(Agadha) in different animal models. International Journal of Applied and Basic Medical Research. 2011;1(2):104–8.

34. Shans-Ud-Doha KM, Zobaer AM, Sitesh CB, Nazmul Q. Antinociceptive, anti-inflammatory, antimicrobialand central nervous system depressant activities of ethanolic extract of leaves and roots of *Gomphostemma parviflorum* var. parviflorum wall. Pharm Res. 2013;5(4):233–40.

35. Subarnas A, Tadano T, Nakahata N, Arai Y, Kinemuchi H, Oshima Y, Kisara K, Ohizumi Y. A possible mechanism of antidepressant activity of beta-amyrin palmitate isolated from *Lobelia inflates* leaves in the forced swimming test. Life Sci. 1993;52:289–96.

36. Dhingra D, Sharma A. Evaluation of antidepressant-like activity of glycyrrhizin in mice. Indian J Pharmacol. 2005;37(6):390–4.

37. Protapaditya D, Sangita C, Priyanka C, Sanjib B. Neuropharmacological properties of Mikania Scandens (L.) Willd. (Asteraceae). Journal of Advanced Pharmaceutical Technology and Research. 2011;2(4):255–9.

38. Kumaresan PT, Asish T, Vijaya C. Neuropharmacological activity of *Lippia nodiflora* Linn. Pharm Res. 2011;3(3):194–200.

39. Khatoon MM, Khatun MH, Islam ME, Parvin MS. Analgesic, antibacterial and central nervous system depressant activities of Albizia proceraleaves. Asian Pacific Journal of Tropical Biomedicine. 2014;4(4):279–84.

40. Huang F, Xiong Y, Xu L, Ma S, Dou C. Sedative and hypnotic activities of the ethanol fraction from Fructus schisandrae in mice and rats. J Ethnopharmacol. 2007;110:471–5.

# 3

# Mitigative effects of *Moringa oleifera* against liver injury induced by artesunate-amodiaquine antimalarial combination in *wistar* rats

Mitchel Otieno Okumu[1*], Francis Okumu Ochola[2], James Mucunu Mbaria[1], Laetitia Wakonyu Kanja[1], Daniel Waweru Gakuya[3], Alice Wairimu Kinyua[3], Paul Onyango Okumu[4] and Stephen Gitahi Kiama[5]

## Abstract

**Background:** Artesunate-amodiaquine (AS-AQ) is an antimalarial drug. It is associated with improved cure rates, accelerated response to therapy and delayed development of resistance. However, liver damage, neurotoxicity and agranulocytosis have been reported as adverse effects whose origins have been linked to free radicals generated by the drug. According to native *materia medica*, *Moringa oleifera (MO)* has wide utility in ethnomedicine. However, there is paucity of information on the hepatoprotective efficacy of this plant. The present study evaluated the mitigative effects of *MO* leaf extracts against liver injury induced by AS-AQ combination in female *Wistar* rats.

**Methods:** Dry leaf powder of *MO* was extracted with water and a 20:80 *v/v* mixture of water and methanol to give aqueous (AQ) and aqueous-methanol (AQ-ME) *MO* leaf extracts respectively. In vitro hydroxyl free radical scavenging activity of serial dilutions (10–100 μg/ml) of each of the extracts was then evaluated using an assay model where butylated hydroxytoluene (BHT) served as a reference standard. The extract with better free radical scavenging activity was then evaluated for hepatoprotective effects against AS-AQ intoxication in female *Wistar* rats based on the Acute Toxic Class method (OECD 2000). Serum asparate amino transferase (AST), alanine amino transferase (ALT), total bilirubin and histological examination of rat liver sections were used to evaluate the hepatoprotective activity of the selected *MO* leaf extract. Siliphos® (standard hepatoprotectant) was used for comparison.

**Results:** There was a concentration dependent increase in the hydroxyl free radical scavenging activity of *MO* leaf extracts and standard (BHT) with values ranging from 46.36–66.36% for the AQ extract, 41.04–60.95% for the AQ-ME extract and 44.93–65.23% for BHT with corresponding $IC_{50}$ values of 26.84 μg/ml, 51.88 μg/ml and 32.58 μg/ml respectively. A 1000 mg/kg dose of the AQ-ME *MO* leaf extract significantly ($p < 0.05$) lowered AST values of AS-AQ intoxicated rats to a level comparable to the standard hepatoprotectant; Siliphos®. Serum ALT and TB were also lowered but this was not statistically significant ($p > 0.05$). The 1000 mg/kg dose also reduced hepatocyte degeneration in rats treated with four times the clinical dose of AS-AQ. This study suggests that the hepatoprotective activity of the leaves of *MO* may have some relation to its free radical scavenging properties. These leaves may thus be useful in mitigating free radical initiated disease conditions.

**Conclusion:** The aqueous-methanol *Moringa oleifera* leaf extract exhibits free radical scavenging and hepatoprotective properties. Further investigations on the structural identity of the phytoconstituents and their mechanisms of action should be performed to facilitate the development of a potent medicinal agent.

**Keywords:** *Moringa oleifera*, Artesunate-amodiaquine, Hepatoprotective activity, *Wistar* rats

* Correspondence: mytchan88@gmail.com
[1]Department of Public Health, Pharmacology and Toxicology, Faculty of Veterinary Medicine, University of Nairobi, P.O BOX 29053-00625, Nairobi, Kenya
Full list of author information is available at the end of the article

## Background

Intimate proximity of the liver to the small intestines and blood circulation exposes it to many foreign substances or their metabolites which may induce injury [1]. Access to antimalarials in the African region is unabated resulting in unwarranted self-medication practices whose net result may be untoward effects such as toxicity [2, 3]. Artesunate-amodiaquine is a fixed dose combination currently in use for the treatment of uncomplicated malaria [4]. At high doses, the drug causes liver damage, neurotoxicity and agranulocytosis associated to free radicals generated by the drug [5, 6]. Siliphos˙ is an antioxidant substance made up of a complex of silybin (a flavonoid) and phosphatidylcholine (a phospholipid). This complex has been reported to have good hepatoprotective activity [7]. MO is a plant associated with antioxidant properties [8]. Positive correlations have been made between the antioxidant and hepatoprotective properties of other plants such as *Acacia catechu*, *Camellia sinensis*, *Magnifera indica*, *Punica granatum* and *Phyllanthus emblica* [9]. However, there is paucity of information on the antioxidant and hepatoprotective effects of MO. The present study aims to determine the antioxidant and protective effects of leaves of MO on the liver of artesunate-amodiaquine intoxicated female *Wistar* rats.

## Methods
### Chemicals

Pure artesunate drug powder (SIGMA A3731), pure amodiaquine drug powder (FLUKA A2799) and phosphate buffer saline (PBS) tablets were purchased from Sigma-Aldrich chemical company (St. Louis, MO). Siliphos˙ was purchased from iherb, California USA and diagnostic kits (MIND-RAY) were purchased from SHENZEN MINDRAY Biomedical electronics, Shenzen, China. All other reagents were analytical grade and of high purity.

### Collection and identification of plant material

Fresh aerial plant material of MO was collected from Kibwezi, Makueni county in Kenya (2°25S'37°58′E) (Fig. 1). The leaves were carefully seperated from the

plant, duplicate samples prepared and authenticated by a botanist at the National Museums Herbarium. A voucher specimen number (NMK/BOT/CTX/1/2) was assigned to the specimen for future reference.

### Preparation of extracts

Leaves of MO were air-dried under shade for 1 week and powdered using an electric mill. A slightly modified method of Anwar et al., [10] was used to prepare water and aqueous-methanol extracts. For the aqueous extract, one hundred grams of dry MO leaf powder was weighed and poured into a 500 ml volumetric flask wrapped in tin foil. Water was gradually added to this flask and the flask gently shaken until a slurry of uniform consistency was formed. The contents were then stirred by use of a magnetic stirrer for 48 h and subsequently centrifuged at 3000 RPM for 10 min. The supernatant was collected into amber coloured plastic bottles and freeze dried to obtain a dry lyophilized powder which was weighed and kept in air-tight containers awaiting further work.

Similarly, the aqueous-methanolic extract was prepared by weighing one hundred grams of dry MO leaf powder into a 500 ml volumetric flask wrapped in tin foil. A mixture of water and methanol (20:80 *v*/v) was gradually added to this flask and the flask gently shaken until a slurry of uniform consistency was formed. The contents were then stirred using a magnetic stirrer for 48 h and subsequently centrifuged at 3000 RPM for 10 min, supernatant collected and poured into a round bottomed flask. Owing to the different boiling points of water and methanol, the round bottomed flask was then attached to a rotary evaporator whose operating temperature was then set at 40 °C. The setup was allowed to run for 6 h to remove methanol after which the semisolid mass was transferred to a 40 °C sand bath and left overnight. The resulting solid mass was then collected and stored in air-tight containers awaiting further work.

### Determination of hydroxyl radical scavenging activity

The method of Klein et al., [11] was used. Briefly, extract concentrations (10–100 µg/ml) were added to a 3 ml mixture containing 1.5 mM Ferrous sulphate, 6 mM

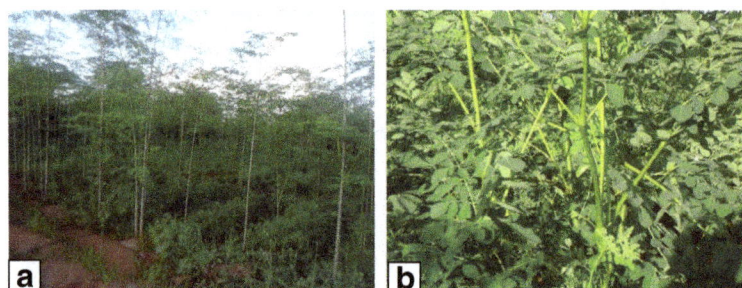

**Fig. 1 a** *Moringa oleifera* whole plant **b** aerial parts of *Moringa oleifera*

hydrogen peroxide and 20 mM sodium salicylate. The resulting solution was then incubated at 37 °C for 1 h. The intensity of the colour developed was measured at 532 nm using a Spectronic 21D Milton Roy UV-VIS Spectrophotometer (USA). The capacity of the samples to scavenge hydroxyl free radicals was calculated using the formula as described by Singh et al., [12].

%Scavenging capacity of sample extracts on hydroxyl radicals

$$= \frac{A_{Control} - A_{Sample}}{A_{Control}} \times 100$$

Where;

A $_{Control}$ = Absorbance of the control (Ferrous sulphate, hydrogen peroxide and sodium salicylate).

A $_{Sample}$ = Absorbance of the sample (Ferrous sulphate, hydrogen peroxide, sodium salicylate and varied concentrations of leaf extracts of MO.

The concentration of the extracts which inhibited 50% of hydroxyl radicals was calculated using regression analysis in MS Excel 2007.

## Ethical considerations

Before commencing in vivo studies in Wistar rats, ethical clearance was sought from the biosafety, animal use and ethics committee of the University of Nairobi. A reference number was given for future reference BAUEC/J56/76385/2014.

## Occupational health and personal protective equipment (PPE)

Established protocols [13] for handling laboratory animals were followed throughout the study. Latex hand gloves and protective masks were used at all times. In addition, anti-tetanus and anti-rabies vaccines were made available and stored under refrigeration.

## Preparation of animals

Thirty-six healthy, 8–10 week old female Wistar rats weighing 180–200 g were used for the study. The animals were nulliparious and non-pregnant and were purchased from the animal holding unit of the Department of Public Health, Pharmacology and Toxicology of the University of Nairobi. They were then housed in polypropylene cages measuring 35 (L) × 25 (W) × 18 (H) and lined with wood shavings. Temperature of the animal house was maintained at 25 ± 3 °C and 50–60% relative humidity for a period of 10 days to enable the animals to acclimate to the laboratory conditions. A 12-h light and dark cycle was maintained and the animals were sustained on water ad libitum and standard rat pellets from a commercial feed supplier (Unga feeds, Kenya Limited).

## Experimental design

From our previous studies on acute oral toxicity of MO [14], a 1000 mg/kg dose of the aqueous-methanol MO leaf extract was used in evaluating hepatoprotective activity against AS-AQ intoxication. Thirty six rats were randomly assigned to 12 groups (each 3 animals) based on the Acute Toxic Class method [15]. The animals were labelled to enable identification. All test substances; Siliphos*, MO, AS-AQ were dissolved in physiological buffer saline (PBS) for administration to rats by oral gavage over a 5-day period as follows;

Group I- Orally received 2 ml of PBS once daily.
Group II- Orally received a 1000 mg/kg dose of MO leaf extract once daily.
Group III- Orally received 200 mg/kg of Siliphos* once daily.
Group IV-Orally received 4, 2, 2, 2,2 mg/kg of artesunate (AS) and 10.8, 5.4, 5.4, 5.4 and 5.4 mg/kg dose of amodiaquine (AQ). This is equivalent to the clinical dose of AS-AQ for the treatment of uncomplicated malaria [16, 17] and is referred to in this experiment as clinical dose of AS-AQ.
Group V-Orally received 8,4,4,4 and 4 mg/kg dose of artesunate (AS) and 21.6, 10.8, 10.8, 10.8 and 10.8 mg/kg dose of amodiaquine (AQ). This is equivalent to double the clinical dose of AS-AQ (2 × clinical dose of AS-AQ).
Group VI- Orally received 16, 8, 8, 8 and 8 mg/kg of artesunate (AS) and 43.2, 21.6, 21.6, 21.6 and 21.6 mg/kg of amodiaquine (AQ). This is equivalent to four times the clinical dose of AS-AQ (4 × clinical dose of AS-AQ).
Group VII-Rats were first orally pre-treated with a 200 mg/kg dose of the standard hepatoprotectant (Siliphos*) followed an hour later by treatment with the clinical dose of AS-AQ as previously described.
Group VIII- Rats were orally pre-treated with a 200 mg/kg dose of the standard hepatoprotectant (Siliphos*) followed an hour later by treatment with 2 × clinical dose of AS-AQ as previously described.
Group IX- Rats were first orally pre-treated with a 200 mg/kg dose of the standard hepatoprotectant (Siliphos*) followed an hour later by treatment with 4 × clinical dose of AS-AQ as previously described.
Group X- Rats were first orally pre-treated with a 1000 mg/kg dose of MO leaf extract followed an hour later by treatment with the clinical dose of AS-AQ as previously described.
Group XI- Rats were first orally pre-treated with a 1000 mg/kg dose of MO leaf extract followed an hour later by treatment with 2 × clinical dose of AS-AQ as previously described.
Group XII- Rats were first orally pre-treated with a 1000 mg/kg dose of MO leaf extract followed an hour later by treatment with 4 × clinical dose of AS-AQ as previously described.

### Blood collection, necropsy and disposal of rat carcasses

Twenty-four hours after administration of the last treatment, individual animals were held with a warm cloth to dilate the blood vessels. The lateral tail vein was then gently punctured using a 21-gauge hypodermic needle attached to a 2 ml syringe. One ml of blood was allowed to collect in the syringe and then transferred to vacutainers lined with a clot activator. The clotted blood was then centrifuged at 3000 RPM for 10 min and serum collected by use of micropipettes into cryo-vials which were capped and stored at 4 °C awaiting biochemical analysis. The levels of serum aspartate aminotransferase (AST), alanine amino transferase (ALT) and total bilirubin (TB) in the different treatment groups were assayed using standard protocols of MIND-RAY commercial kits [18]. Animals were then humanely euthanized by use of a 150 mg/kg dose of intravenous sodium pentobarbital injection. Livers were harvested, weighed and preserved in 10% neutral buffered formalin solution for 24 h awaiting histological examination. Rodent carcasses were then placed in zip locked non-polyvinylchloride (non-PVC) transparent plastic bags and incinerated.

### Histological examination

A slightly modified method of Palipoch and Punsawad [19] was used. Formalin preserved liver tissues were washed with 70% ethanol. The tissues were then placed in metallic caskets, stirred by use of a stirrer followed by dehydration in graded ethanol (70–100%) and embedded in paraffin wax by use of an embedding machine. The paraffinized blocks were then sectioned using a rotatory ultra microtome, transferred to glass slides and allowed to dry overnight. The slides were then stained by haemotoxylin and eosin (H&E) dye and mounted on a light microscope for observation.

### Statistical analysis

Results of the analysis of the hepatospecific markers of liver injury were expressed as mean ± SEM and analyzed using one-way analysis of variance (ANOVA) followed by least significant difference as post hoc test using Gen Stat Statistical Software 4th edition. ($p \leq 0.05$) was considered significant.

## Results

### Hydroxyl radical scavenging capacity of *Moringa oleifera* leaf extracts

It was shown on Fig. 2 that there was a concentration dependent increase in the in vitro hydroxyl radical scavenging activity of *MO* extracts and butylated hydroxyl toluene (BHT). The scavenging activity of the AQ extract was in the range 46.36–66.36% compared to 41.04–60.95% of the AQ-ME extract and 44.93–65.23% of BHT. However, the ability of the AQ extract to

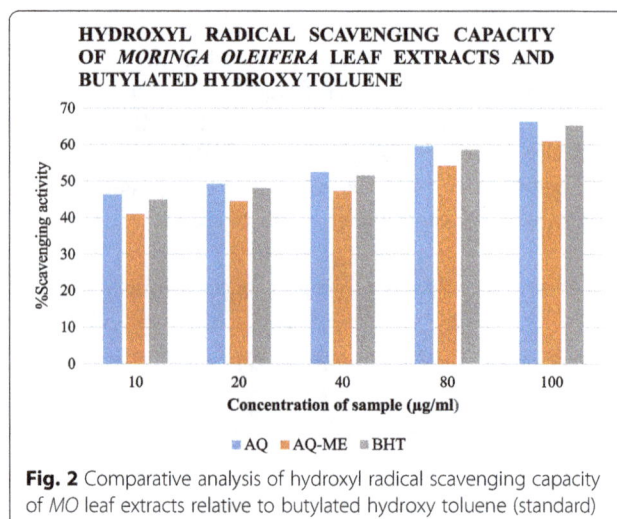

**Fig. 2** Comparative analysis of hydroxyl radical scavenging capacity of *MO* leaf extracts relative to butylated hydroxy toluene (standard)

scavenge these free radicals (66.36%) was found to be higher than both the AQ-ME extract (60.95%) and BHT (65.23%). Regression analysis in MS excel established the concentration of the extracts and standard necessary to inhibit 50% of the hydroxyl radicals ($IC_{50}$) Table 1.

### Changes in serum liver markers

It was shown on Table 2, that there was a dose-dependent increase in the levels of AST, ALT and TB following treatment with the AS-AQ antimalarial combination. Moreover, pre-treatment with Siliphos* (200 mg/kg body weight per oral) and AQ-ME leaf extract of *MO* at a dose of 1000 mg/kg body weight per oral significantly reduced the levels of serum AST but non-significantly reduced the levels of ALT and TB when compared to the AS-AQ intoxicated groups.

### Histological examination of rat liver sections

It was shown on Fig. 3 that the administration of four times the clinical dose of AS-AQ resulted in vacuolation and necrosis of hepatocytes.

It was shown on Fig. 4 that pre-treatment of rats with a 1000 mg/kg dose of *MO* before administration of four times the clinical dose of AS-AQ resulted in mild improvement in the degree of vacuolation and hepatic congestion.

**Table 1** $IC_{50}$ values of *MO* leaf extracts and butylated hydroxy tolune (BHT) against hydroxyl free radicals

| Sample | OH radical scavenging activity (µg/ml) |
|---|---|
| Water (AQ) extract | 26.84 |
| Aqueous-methanol (AQ-ME) extract | 51.88 |
| Butylated hydroxyl toluene (BHT) | 32.58 |

**Table 2** Evaluation of the effect of *MO* leaf extract on AS-AQ intoxicated *Wistar* rats by using biomarkers of liver injury

| Group | Treatment code (n = 3) | AST (IU/L) | ALT (IU/L) | TB (mg/dl) |
|---|---|---|---|---|
| 1 | PBS only | 122.37 ± 13.73 | 65.18 ± 20.08 | 0.83 ± 0.67 |
| 2 | SCG | 127.67 ± 25.07 | 78.95 ± 24.11 | 3.08 ± 1.30 |
| 3 | MCG | 113.93 ± 5.46* | 80.73 ± 21.65 | 1.69 ± 0.38 |
| 4 | CD-ASAQ | 138.97 ± 13.14 | 76.44 ± 0.85 | 2.92 ± 2.06 |
| 5 | 2 × CD-ASAQ | 158.8 ± 20.08 | 85.70 ± 17.55 | 1.19 ± 0.94 |
| 6 | 4 × CD-ASAQ | 220.33 ± 53.97* | 90.39 ± 13.62 | 2.70 ± 0.96 |
| 7 | S + CD-ASAQ | 130.97 ± 16.61 | 58.01 ± 20.16 | 1.15 ± 0.57 |
| 8 | S + 2CD-ASAQ | 125.74 ± 45.13 | 64.47 ± 23.65 | 2.00 ± 2.07 |
| 9 | S + 4CD-ASAQ | 184.00 ± 23.60 | 68.00 ± 28.83 | 2.93 ± 2.32 |
| 10 | M + CD-ASAQ | 138.77 ± 24.33 | 66.37 ± 13.29 | 0.53 ± 0.35 |
| 11 | M + 2CD-ASAQ | 171.13 ± 52.88 | 80.38 ± 21.56 | 1.61 ± 0.80 |
| 12 | M + 4CD-ASAQ | 140.03 ± 24.45* | 76.77 ± 14.61 | 1.17 ± 0.66 |

Values are expressed as mean ± SEM (n = 3) significantly different at *$p \leq 0.05$

*PBS* physiological buffer saline, *SCG* siliphos\* control group, *MCG* moringa control group, *CD-ASAQ* clinical dose of artesunate-amodiaquine, *2 × CD-AS-AQ* double the clinical dose of artesunate-amodiaquine, *4 × CD-ASAQ* four times the clinical dose of artesunate-amodiaquine, *S + CD-ASAQ* pre-treatment with Siliphos\*followed an hour later by treatment with a clinical dose of artesunate-amodiaquine, *S + 2\* CD-ASAQ* pre-treatment with Siliphos\* followed an hour later by treatment with double the clinical dose of ASAQ, *S + 4 × CD-ASAQ* pre-treatment with Siliphos\* followed an hour later by treatment with four times the clinical dose of ASAQ, *M + CD-ASAQ* pre-treatment with the aqueous-methanol *MO* leaf extract followed an hour later by treatment with the clinical dose of AS-AQ, *M + 2 × CD: ASAQ* pre-treatment with the aqueous-methanol *MO* leaf extract followed an hour later by treatment with double the clinical dose of ASAQ, *M + 4 × CD-ASAQ* pre-treatment with the aqueous-methanol *MO* leaf extract followed an hour later by treatment with four times the clinical dose of AS-AQ

## Discussion

The hydroxyl free radical is one of the most potent reactive oxygen species in biological systems [20, 21]. It undergoes chemical reactions with many components of biological cells such as amino acids, sugars, lipids and nucleotides which may result in cell damage [20, 21]. Within biological systems, hydroxyl free radicals may be generated from the catalytic degradation of hydrogen peroxide [22]. In the in vitro context, the hydroxyl free radical may be generated by the Fenton reaction which involves the interaction of transition metals such as Iron II ($Fe^{2+}$) and hydrogen peroxide [23]. From the present study, we established a concentration dependent increase

in the in vitro hydroxyl free radical scavenging effect of *MO* leaf extracts. This observation is in agreement with the work of other authors [21, 22, 24]. Moreover, butylated hydroxy toluene (standard antioxidant) showed better scavenging capacity than both the aqueous and the aqueous-methanolic *MO* leaf extracts. Based on the work of other workers [25–27], butylated hydroxytoluene is a synthetic compound made up of polyphenolics with marked antioxidant activity.

The inhibitory concentration value at 50% ($IC_{50}$) refers to the concentration of the antioxidant substance sufficient to inhibit free radical activity by 50% [22]. The lower this value, the higher the antioxidant capacity of medicinal

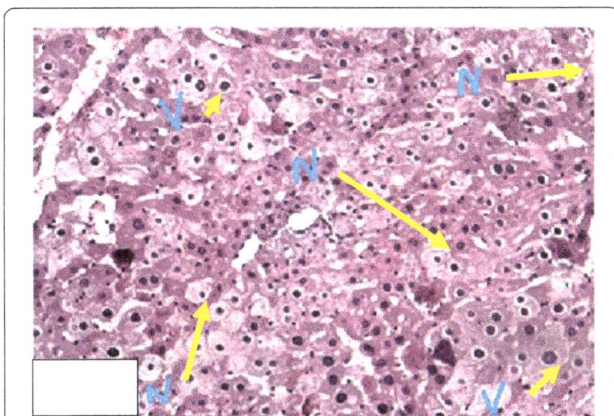

**Fig. 3** Photomicrograph of liver section from a rat treated with four times the clinical dose of AS-AQ. (Magnification ×400). V = Hepatic vacuolation, N = Hepatic cell necrosis

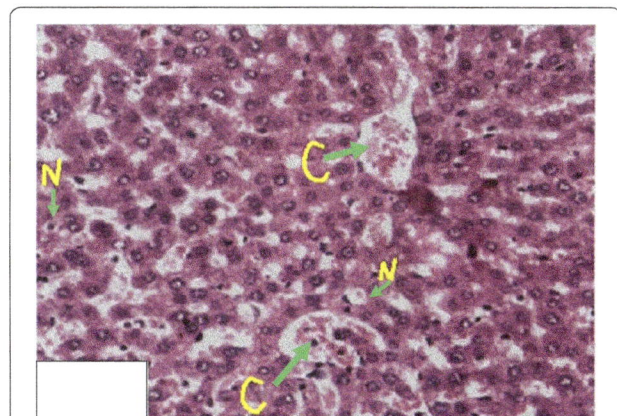

**Fig. 4** Photomicrograph of liver section from a rat pre-treated with a 1000 mg/kg dose of aqueous-methanolic *MO* leaf extract and four times the clinical dose of ASAQ. (Magnification ×400). C = Hepatic vein congestion, N = Hepatic cell necrosis

plants [22, 24]. The aqueous *MO* leaf extract had a lower $IC_{50}$ value than both the aqueous-methanolic *MO* leaf extract and butylated hydroxytoluene. This may imply that the AQ *MO* leaf may have better antioxidant properties than the AQ-ME *MO* leaf extract. However, according to Moon and Shibamoto [28], at least two antioxidant assays should be used to evaluate the antioxidant properties of medicinal plants.

In our previous work [29], we reported the total phenolic, flavonoid and ascorbic acid contents of *MO* leaf extracts. It is on the backdrop of these results that the aqueous-methanolic *MO* leaf extract was selected for evaluation of hepatoprotective activity in *Wistar* rats.

There is a large body of literature available on the hepatoprotective activity of medicinal plants against carbon tetrachloride, ethanol or paracetamol toxicity [30–33]. However, the level of exposure of these chemicals to man may be very low. To the best of our knowledge, this is the first report of the protective effects of the aqueous-methanolic *MO* leaf extract against AS-AQ induced liver injury in *Wistar* rats. This report is based on evidence of biochemical and histologic findings. Similar effects of liver protection were also observed in rats dosed with Siliphos*, which was used as a positive control.

Siliphos* is a complex of silybin and phosphatidylcholine [7]. The former is a flavonoid produced from the fruit of the milk thistle, *Silybum marianum* while the latter is a lipid-soluble derivative of soy. Given that silybin is lipid-incompatible, the combination with phosphatidylcholine facilitates passage of the flavonoid through biological membranes [7]. Some workers have reported on the protective effect of Siliphos* against carbon tetrachloride, acetaminophen, alcohol and mushroom poisoning [7, 34–36].

Artesunate-amodiaquine is an antimalarial agent. It comprises of artesunate and amodiaquine. The former is a potent and rapidly acting blood schizontocide while the latter is used in prophylaxis and treatment of malaria [37, 38]. The drug is safe at therapeutic doses but high doses of artesunate causes congestion and dilation of hepatic sinudoids, vacuolation as well as necrosis [37]. A cytotoxic mechanism characterized by protein carbonylation, formation of reactive oxygen species and lipid peroxidation has been associated with the clinical use of amodiaquine [38].

In the present study, liver injury due to AS-AQ intoxication was observed as elevated levels of hepatospecific parameters like AST, ALT and TB. Studies on the histopathology of liver sections from rats treated with high doses of AS-AQ also corroborate findings of biochemical analysis. Hepatocytes carry out a host of metabolic activities under the influence of enzymes [39]. AST and ALT are found in higher concentrations in the cytoplasm. High levels of these enzymes in the serum may be indicative of loss of the functional integrity of hepatocytes and subsequent leakage of cell contents [40]. Group 6 rats (4 × AS-AQ dose) registered the highest elevation of these enzymes. However, since AST is also present in the kidney and cardiac muscles [40], it may be suggested that AS-AQ may have some toxic effects on these organs as well. Pre-treatment with 1000 mg/kg of the *MO* leaf extract (group 12) significantly lowered the elevated levels of AST. This reduction was comparable to the control (group 3) and the hepatotoxic agent (group 6).

Bilirubin is a principle indicator of cholestatic liver injury [41]. In the present study, AS-AQ intoxicated rats were characterized by high serum bilirubin activity (group 4 and 6). However, the levels were not significantly different from the control group. This observation may suggest that AS-AQ may not be associated with cholestatic liver injury.

Histological examination of the liver sections of ASAQ intoxicated rats (group 6) showed significant hepatotoxicity characterized by vacuolation, necrosis of hepatocytes and congestion of central veins (Fig. 3). However, animals pre-treated with the aqueous alcoholic extract of *MO* (group 12), the extent of hepatic distortion was decreased relative to the damage observed in the ASAQ intoxicated group (Fig. 4).

In our previous work on the aqueous methanolic extract of *MO* leaf extract, we identified flavonoids, phenolics and ascorbic acid as phytoconstituents [29]. These secondary plant metabolites have been identified as natural antioxidants [23]. Thus, the observed free radical scavenging and hepatoprotective activities of the aqueous-methanolic *MO* leaf extract may be attributable to the antioxidant phytoconstituents.

Discussions are still ongoing as to what effect is produced when AS-AQ and the *MO* leaf extract are concurrently used in a *Plasmodium falciparum* infected animal model. Some published works [42, 43] have reported on the effectiveness of *MO* seeds on *Plasmodium falciparum* and *Schistosoma cercariae*. Nonetheless, similar activity is yet to be reported on the leaves. Other authors have suggested that antioxidants and supplements of herbal origin (grape fruit juice, orange fruit juice, ascorbic acid) may alter the efficacy of antimalarial drugs in clearing parasitaemia [44–46].

## Conclusion

Based on our preliminary investigations it can be concluded that the aqueous-methanol *Moringa oleifera* leaf extract exhibits free radical scavenging and hepatoprotective properties. However, in a bid to develop a potent medicinal agent, further investigations on the structural identity of the phytoconstituents as well as the mechanism behind the observed effects should be performed.

## Acknowledgments
The authors would like to express their gratitude to Dr. Joshua Onono and Dr. Florence Mutua of the Department of Public Health, Pharmacology and Toxicology for providing assistance on statistical work. This work was financially supported by the Carnegie corporation of New York through Regional Initiative in Science and Education-African Natural Product Network (RISE-AFFNET).

## Authors' contributions
MOO, AWK, POO participated in the conduction of experiments. FOO, JMM, LWK and DWG made substantial contributions to concept design and conduction of research. Data analysis and interpretation was done by MOO and POO. MOO, FOO, JMM and DWG participated in drafting the manuscript and LWK, SGK, POO, DWG revised the manuscript critically for intellectual content. MOO and AWK made the necessary corrections in the write up and JMM, DWG and SGK gave final approval for the submission of revised version. All authors read and approved the final manuscript.

## Competing interests
The authors declare that they have no competing interest.

## Author details
[1]Department of Public Health, Pharmacology and Toxicology, Faculty of Veterinary Medicine, University of Nairobi, P.O BOX 29053-00625, Nairobi, Kenya. [2]Department of Pharmacology and Toxicology, Faculty of Medicine, Moi University, P.O BOX 3900-30100, Eldoret, Kenya. [3]Department of Clinical Studies, Faculty of Veterinary Medicine, University of Nairobi, P.O BOX 29053-00625, Nairobi, Kenya. [4]Department of Veterinary Pathology, Microbiology and Parasitology, Faculty of Veterinary Medicine, University of Nairobi, P.O BOX 29053-00625, Nairobi, Kenya. [5]Department of Veterinary Anatomy and Physiology, Faculty of Veterinary Medicine, University of Nairobi, P.O BOX 29053-00625, Nairobi, Kenya.

## References
1. Roy S, Bhattacharya S. Arsenic-induced histopathology and synthesis of stress proteins in liver and kidney of Channa Punctatus. Ecotoxicol Environ Saf. 2006;65(2):218–29.
2. Ruebush TK, Kern MK, Campbell CC, Oloo AJ. Self-treatment of malaria in rural areas of western Kenya. Bull World Health Organ. 1995;73(2):229–36.
3. Breman JG. The ears of the hippopotamus; manifestations and estimates of the malaria burden. Am J Trop Med Hyg. 2001;64(1-2):1–11.
4. Nosten F. White NJ Artemisinin-based combination treatment of falciparum malaria. Am J Trop Med Hyg. 2007;77(6):181–92.
5. Schramm B, Valeh P, Baudin E, Mazinda S, Smith R, Pinoges L, Sunday gar T, Zolla YM, Jones JJ, Conte E, Bruneel A, Branger M, Jullien V, Carn G, Kiechel JR, Ashley EA, Geurin PJ. Tolerability and safety of artesunate-amodiaquine and artemether-lumefantrine fixed dose combinations for the treatment of uncomplicated plasmodium falciparum malaria: two open-label, randomized trials in Nimba county, Liberia. Malar J. 2013;12:250.
6. Davis TM, Binh TQ, Ilet KF, Batty KT, Phuong HL, Chiswell GM, Phuong VD, Agus C. Penetration of dihydroartemisinin into cerebrospinal fluid after administration of intravenous artesunate in severe falciparum malaria. Antimicrob Agents Chemother. 2003;47(1):368–70.
7. Kidd P, Head K. A review of the bioavailability and clinical efficacy of milk thistle phytosome: a silybin-phosphatidylcholine complex (Siliphos). Altern Med Rev. 2005;10(3):193–203.
8. Santos AF, Argolo AC, Paiva AC, Coelho LC. Antioxidant activity of Moringa Oleifera tissue extracts. Phytother Res. 2012;26(9):1366–70.
9. Hiraganahalli BD, Chinampudur VC, Dethe S, Mundkinajeddu D, Pandre MK, Balachandran J, Agarwal A. Hepatoprotective and antioxidant activity of standardized herbal extracts. Pharmacogn Mag. 2012;8(30):116–23.
10. Anwar F, Kalsoom U, Sultana B, Mushtaq M, Mehmood T, Arshad HA. Effect of drying method on the total phenolics and antioxidant activity of cauliflower (Brassica oleraceae. L) extracts. Int Food Res J. 2013;20(2):653–9.
11. Klein SM, Cohen G, Cederbaum AI. Production of formaldehyde during metabolism of dimethyl sulfoxide by hydroxyl radical generating system. Biochemist. 1981;20(21):6006–12.
12. Singh R, Singh N, Saini BS, Rao HS. In vitro antioxidant activity of pet ether extract of black pepper. Indian J Pharmacol. 2008;40(4):147–51.
13. OECD. (2000). Guidance document on the recognition, assessment and use of clinical signs as humane endpoints for experimental animals used in safety evaluation. Series on testing and assessment.
14. Okumu MO, Mbaria JM, Kanja LW, Gakuya DW, Kiama SG, Ochola FO, Okumu PO. Acute toxicity of the aqueous-methanolic Moringa Oleifera (lam) leaf extract on female Wistar albino rats. Int J of Basic Clin Pharmacol. 2016;5(5):1856–61.
15. OECD. (2001).Test guideline 423: acute oral toxicity-acute toxic class method. OECD guidelines for the testing of chemicals.
16. Angus BJ, Thaiaporn I, Chanthapadith K, Suputtamongkol Y, White NJ. Oral artesunate dose-response relationship in acute falciparum malaria. Antimicrob Agents Chemother. 2002;46(3):778–82.
17. Obianime AW, Aprioku JS. Mechanism of action of artemisinins on biochemical, hematological and reproductive parameters in male guinea pigs. Int J Pharmacol. 2011;7(1):84–95.
18. Schumann G, Bonora R, Ceriotti F, Ferard G, Ferrero CA, PFH F, Gella FJ, Hoelzel W, Jorgensen PJ, Kanno T, Kessner A, Klauke A, Kristiansen N, Lessinger JM, TPJ L, Misaki H, Panteghini M, Pauwels J, Schiele F, Schimmel HG, Weidemann G, Siekmann L. IFCC primary reference procedures for the measurement of catalytic activity concentrations of enzymes at 37°C. Part 5. Reference procedure for the measurement of catalytic concentration of aspartate aminotransferase. Clin Chem Lab Med. 2002;40(7):725–33.
19. Palipoch S, Punsawad C. Biochemical and histological study of rat liver and kidney injury induced by Cisplatin. J Toxicol Pathol. 2013;26(3):293–9.
20. Alam MN, Bristi NJ, Rafiquzzaman M. Review on in vivo and in vitro methods evaluation of antioxidant activity. Saudi Pharm J. 2013;21(2):143–52.
21. Sowndhararajan K, Kang SC. Free radical scavenging activity from different extracts of leaves of Bauhinia Vahlii Wight & Arn. Saudi J Biol Sci. 2013;20(4):319–25.
22. Adjimani JP, Asare P. Antioxidant and free radical scavenging activity of iron chelators. Toxicol Rep. 2015;2:721–8.
23. Duan X, Wu G, Jiang Y. Evaluation of the antioxidant properties of litchi fruit phenolics in relation to pericarp browning prevention. Molecules. 2007;12(4):759–71.
24. Wang H, Gao XD, Zhou GC, Cai L, Yao WB. In vitro and in vivo antioxidant activity of aqueous extract from Choerospondias Axillaris fruit. Food Chem. 2008;106(3):888–95.
25. Habu JB, Ibeh BO. In vitro antioxidant capacity and free radical scavenging evaluation of active metabolite constituents of Newbouldia laevis ethanolic leaf extract. Biol Res. 2015;48(1):16.
26. Bjorkhem I, Henriksson-Freyschuss A, Breuer O, Diczfalusy U, Berglund L, Henriksson P. The antioxidant butylated hydroxytoluene protects against atherosclerosis. Arterioscler Thromb. 1991;11:15–22.
27. Sharma OP, Bhat TK. DPHH antioxidant assay revisited. Food Chem. 2009; 113(4):1202–5.
28. Moon JK, Shibamoto T. Antioxidant assays for plant and food components. J Agric Food Chem. 2009;57(5):1655–66.
29. Okumu MO, Mbaria JM, Kanja LW, Gakuya DW, Kiama SG, Ochola FO. Phytochemical profile and antioxidant capacity of leaves of Moringa oleifera (lam) extracted using different solvent systems. JPharmacognPhytochem. 2016;5(4):302–8.
30. Nirmala M, Girija K, Lakshman K, Divya T. Hepatoprotective activity of Musa Paradisiaca on experimental animal models. Asian Pac J Tropic Biomed. 2012;2(1):5–11.
31. Kumar KE, Harsha KN, Sudheer V, Babu NG. In vitro antioxidant activity and in vivo hepatoprotective activity of the aqueous extract of Allium Cepa bulb in ethanol induced liver damage in rats. Food Sci Human Wellness. 2013; 2(3-4):132–8.
32. Krithika R, Verma RJ. Mitigation of carbon tetrachloride-induced damage by Phyllanthus Amarus in liver of mice. Acta Pol Pharm. 2009;66(4):439–44.
33. Senthilkumar R, Chandran R, Parimelazhagan T. Hepatoprotective effect of Rhodiola Imbricata rhizome against paracetamol-induced liver toxicity in rats. Saudi J Biol Sci. 2014;21(5):409–46.
34. Hikino H, Kiso Y, Wagner H, Fiebig M. Antihepatotoxic actions of flavonolignans from Silybum Marianum fruits. Planta Med. 1984;50:248–50.
35. Conti M, Malandrino S, Magistretti MJ. Protective activity of silipide on liver damage in rodents. Jpn J Pharmacol. 1992;60(4):315–21.

36. Enjalbert F, Rapior S, Nouguier-Soule J, Guillon S, Amouroux N, Cabot C. Treatment of amatoxin poisoning:20-year retrospective analysis. J Toxicol Clin Toxicol. 2002;40(6):715–57.

37. Alyousif MS, Saifi MA, Ahmed M, Alouysif SM. Histopathological changes induced by artesunate in liver of Wistar rat. Int J Pharmacol. 2017;13(1):104–8.

38. Heidari R, Babaei H, Eghbal MA. Amodiaquine-induced toxicity in isolated rat hepatocytes and the cytoprotective effects of taurine and/or N-acetyl cysteine. ResPharmSci. 2014;9(2):97–105.

39. Aneja S, Vats M, Aggarwal S, Sardana S. Phytochemistry and hepatoprotective activity of the aqueous extract of Amaranthus Tricolor Linn. Roots. J.Ayurveda.Integr. Med. 2013;4(4):211–5.

40. Drotman RB, Lawhorn GT. Serum enzymes as indicators of chemically induced liver damage. Drug Chem Toxicol. 1978;1(2):163–71.

41. Achliya GS, Wadodkar SG, Dorle AK. Evaluation of hepatoprotective effect of *Amalkadi ghrita* against carbon tetrachloride induced hepatic damage in rats. JEthnopharmacol. 2004;90(2-3):229–32.

42. Gbeassor M, Kedjagni AY, Koumaglo K, De Souza C, Agho K, Aklikokou K, Amegho KA. *In vitro* antimalarial activity of six medicinal plants. Phytother Res. 1990;4(3):115–7.

43. Olsen A. Low technology water purification by bentonite clay and *Moringa oleifera* seed flocculation as performed in sudanese villages: effects on Schistosoma Mansoni cercariae. Water Res. 1987;21(5):517–22.

44. Talman AM, Dormarle O, McKenzie FE, Ariey F, Robert V. Gametocytogenesis: the puberty of plasmodium falciparum. Malar J. 2004;3:24.

45. Bledsoe GH. Malaria primer for clinicians in the United States. South Med J. 2005;98(12):1197–204.

46. Owira PM, Ojewole JA. The grapefruit: an old wine in a new glass? Metabolic and cardiovascular perspectives. Cardiovasc J Afric. 2010;21(5):280–5.

# 4

# Improved micropropagation of *Bacopa monnieri* (L.) Wettst. (Plantaginaceae) and antimicrobial activity of in vitro and ex vitro raised plants against multidrug-resistant clinical isolates of urinary tract infecting (UTI) and respiratory tract infecting (RTI) bacteria

Sk Moquammel Haque[1], Avijit Chakraborty[1], Diganta Dey[2], Swapna Mukherjee[3], Sanghamitra Nayak[4] and Biswajit Ghosh[1*]

## Abstract

**Background:** Nowadays the multidrug-resistant (MDR) bacterial pathogens are a major concern of the medical science. Medicinal plants may be considered as new sources for producing antibacterial agents. The present study aimed to standardize an improved method for micropropagation and in vitro biomass production of *Bacopa monnieri*. Second aim is to evaluate the antimicrobial potency of in vitro cultured and ex vitro field grown micropropagated plants against different MDR clinical isolates of human urinary tract infecting (UTI) and respiratory tract infecting (RTI) pathogens.

**Methods:** Micropropagation of *B. monnieri* were performed following standard tissue culture method. The role of 6-benzylaminopurine (BAP), kinetin and spermidine on multiple shoot induction were evaluated. Antimicrobial activity of ethanol, methanol and acetone extract of in vitro and ex vitro plants of *B. monnieri* were screened by agar cup method against five MDR-UTI bacteria, four MDR-RTI bacteria and three microbial type culture collection (MTCC) bacteria and two fungi. Minimum inhibitory concentration (MIC), minimum bactericidal concentration (MBC) and minimum fungicidal concentration (MFC) were also determined.

**Results:** Synergistic effect of BAP and spermidine had improved shoot induction with a maximum of 123.8 shoot-buds per explant. Optimum micropropagation with 34.9 elongated shoots per explant was recorded in Murashige and Skoog medium containing 1.5 mg/L BAP and 2.0 mM spermidine. Methanolic extract of ex vitro plants showed maximum activity against MDR-UTI strain of *Escherichia coli* (sample-9) [ZI 18 ± 0.68 mm, MIC 2.5 μg/mL, MBC 5.0 μg/mL]. Acetone extract of ex vitro plant exhibited maximum inhibition against MDR-RTI strain of *Klebsiella pneumoniae* (sample-38) [ZI 14 ± 0.22 mm, MIC 5.0 μg/mL, MBC 7.5 μg/mL]. The extracts of *B. monnieri* were bactericidal rather than bacteriostatic against all UTI and RTI bacteria tested.

(Continued on next page)

* Correspondence: ghosh_b2000@yahoo.co.in
[1]Plant Biotechnology Laboratory, Post Graduate Department of Botany, Ramakrishna Mission Vivekananda Centenary College, Rahara, Kolkata 700118, India
Full list of author information is available at the end of the article

(Continued from previous page)

**Conclusions:** The present manuscript demonstrated an efficient in vitro method for large scale biomass production of *B. monnieri*. Furthermore, the methanolic extract of *B. monnieri* have potential antimicrobial activity against clinical isolates of MDR-UTI and MDR-RTI bacterial strains. Hence this plant may further use to treat these infectious diseases. The comparative results show ex vitro grown plants have slightly better antimicrobial activities as compared to the in vitro plants.

**Keywords:** *Bacopa monnieri*, Clinical isolates, Micropropagation, Multidrug-resistant, RTI bacteria, Spermidine, UTI bacteria,

## Background

In more than 80% of developed countries, plants have been traditionally used as remedy because they are the actual good source of different pharmacologically active compounds [1]. *Bacopa monnieri* (L.) Wettst. (family Plantaginaceae) is an important medicinal plant grown throughout the Indian subcontinent and traditionally been used in Ayurvedic system of medicine [2, 3]. This species is one of the best versatile 'tonic herbs' stimulates brain, heart, liver, and kidney health. It also used as a revitaliser of sensory organs, water retention and blood cleaning, relaxant, neuroprotective as well as in the treatment of allergic disorders of skin, snake bite, enlargement of the spleen, rheumatism, leprosy, epilepsy, asthma, hoarseness and anxiety. *Bacopa monnieri* extract has proven sedative, anti-inflammatory and antipyretic, anti-cancer, anti-oxidant, immuno-modulatory, antiulcerogenic, antistress, anti-leishmanial, antipyretic, analgesic and anti-aging properties [4–9]. Kishore [6] had designated *B. monnieri* as a "complete herbal medicine" due to multipurpose usage of

this wonder medicinal plant. The antimicrobial property of *B. monnieri* was previously screened by few scientists, but majority of this reports are against standard bacterial strains [10–12]. Although one report are available where clinical isolates of human pathogenic strains are tested, but these are not multidrug-resistant (MDR) strains [13]. Antibacterial resistance has become one of the grave public health concerns, globally, over the last two decades [14, 15]. In modern years, there has been a rising interest in investigating and evolving new antimicrobial agents from various sources to combat microbial resistance [16]. The MDR microbial pathogens imply a most important threat to human health. The worldwide surge in MDR bacteria and the proximity of urinary tract infectious and respiratory tract infectious disease demand alternative curative approaches to supplement the existing medications.

*Bacopa monnieri* was positioned second in a priority list of the most significant medicinal plants, assessed on the basis of their medical reputation, commercial value, and potential for advance research and development by the

**Table 1** Antimicrobial activities of nine clinical isolates of the human UTI and RTI bacteria against 15 well known drugs

| Antibiotics | UTI Pathogens | | | | | RTI Pathogens | | | |
|---|---|---|---|---|---|---|---|---|---|
| | Sample 5 (*Escherichia coli*) | Sample 9 (*Escherichia coli*) | Sample 11 (*Escherichia coli*) | Sample 19 (*Klebsiella pneumoniae*) | Sample 26 (*Klebsiella pneumoniae*) | Sample 31 (*Klebsiella pneumoniae*) | Sample 35 (*Klebsiella pneumoniae*) | Sample 36 (*Klebsiella pneumoniae*) | Sample 38 (*Klebsiella pneumoniae*) |
| Amoxiline | R | S | S | R | R | R | R | R | R |
| Amikacin | S | S | S | R | R | S | S | R | R |
| Aztreonam | R | R | R | R | R | NT | R | NT | NT |
| Ceftriaxone | R | R | S | R | R | R | R | R | S |
| Cefuroxime | R | R | S | R | I | R | R | R | R |
| Ciprofloxacin | R | NT | I | I | I | R | R | R | R |
| Piperacillin | S | S | S | R | S | S | NT | R | NT |
| Cefoperazone | R | NT | S | R | R | S | S | R | R |
| Ceftazidime | R | R | S | R | R | NT | NT | R | R |
| Ofloxacin | R | R | R | I | S | NT | NT | NT | NT |
| Sulbactum | S | R | S | R | S | R | R | S | NT |
| Nitrofurantoin | S | R | S | NT | S | R | R | S | S |
| Meropenum | S | NT | NT | I | R | S | R | R | R |
| Doxycycline | S | R | S | S | S | NT | S | S | R |
| Norfloxacin | R | S | S | I | S | R | R | R | R |

*R* resistant, *S* sensitive, *I* intermediate, *NT* not tested

Improved micropropagation of Bacopa monnieri (L.) Wettst. (Plantaginaceae) and antimicrobial activity...

23

National Medicinal Plants Board of India (2004) [17]. Due to illegal over-collection of the pharmaceutical companies, it has now been depleted from its natural habitat and recognized as an endangered plant of India [3, 18]. In this circumstances, the demand for good quality planting material of this wonder curative herb is increasing day-after-day, which necessitate the improvement of the existing micropropagation methods for rapid and constant supply of planting materials round the year. On other hand, land is not available for medicinal plant cultivation as compare to crop plants [19], so in vitro biomass production is alternative option to produce huge amounts of pharmaceutically active compounds round the year without any cultivation land. Although micropropagation of *B. monnieri* has been studied by several group of researchers for more than four decades [2, 3], yet based on their

wonder medicinal properties, the additional research is much needed for further improvement of the micropropagation protocol. The present study was thus aimed to the—(1) development of high frequency micropropagation method, (2) screening of the antimicrobial activities of different solvent-extracts of *B. monnieri* against various pathogenic strains of MDR bacteria and standard laboratory strains (MTCC) of bacteria and fungi.

## Methods

### Surface sterilization and initial culture establishment

Shoot tips (8–10 mm) of *Bacopa monnieri* (L.) Wettst. (family Plantaginaceae) were collected from the healthy plants grown in an experimental garden of our college and were washed with 2.5% (*w/v*) systematic fungicide (Bavistin) for 15 min followed by 2.5% liquid detergent

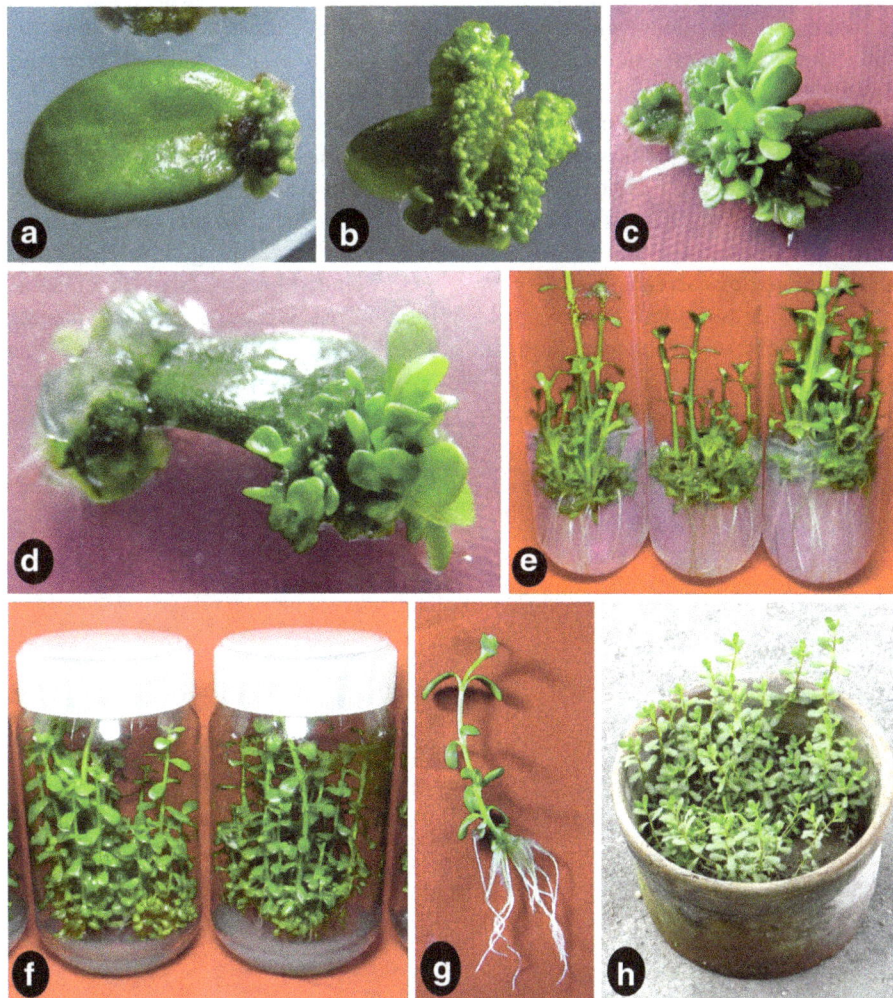

**Fig. 1** Different stages of micropropagation of *Bacopa monnieri*. **a** Induction of shoot buds from the cut edges of leaf after 8 days of inoculation in medium containing 0.5 mg/L KIN. **b** Shoot buds induced in medium containing 1.5 mg/L BAP after 12 days of inoculation. **c** & **d** Shoot buds start to elongate in medium containing 1.5 mg/L BAP and 2.0 mM spermidine after 21 days of inoculation. **e** Elongated shoots after 42 days of inoculation. **f** Plants grown in half strength MS medium without any PGR. **g** A complete plantlets with well developed root system ready for field transfer. **h** Tissue culture derived ex vitro field grown micropropagated plants

(Tween-20) solution for 2 min. Finally, the explants were surface-disinfected with mercuric chloride (HgCl$_2$) solution (0.1%, $w/v$) for 8 min and rinsed 3 times with sterile distilled water. Then all the explants were implanted on Murashige and Skoog (MS) [20] basal medium without any plant growth regulator (PGR) for the establishment of an initial sterile culture.

## Micropropagation

The mature leaves (12–15 mm) were cut from the in vitro established infection-free plants and were used as initial explants for micropropagation purpose. Two different cytokinins viz. 6-Benzylaminopurine (BAP) and Kinetin (KIN) are tested in six different concentrations (0.5, 1.0, 1.5, 2.0, 2.5, 3.0 mg/L). The effect of Spermidine (1.0, 1.5, 2.0, 2.5 mM) in combination with optimum cytokinin was also evaluated for better results. After 3 weeks, all the explants were subcultured to their respective fresh medium for the elongation of the adventitious shoots. After another 3 weeks, all cultures were transferred to half-strength MS medium without any PGR for further elongation and in vitro rooting. Ultimately, the micropropagated plants with well developed root systems, were acclimatized and transferred to the field conditions following the methods previously standardized by us [21].

## Extract preparation for antimicrobial screening

Fresh leaves of both in vitro cultured and ex vitro, field grown micropropagated plants were collected and air dried in closed and dark environment at 40 °C for 7 days. Dry leaves were powdered in mixture grinder and kept at 4 °C for further use. The powdered plant material was extracted in three different solvent (methanol, ethanol, acetone) for 12 h with the help of Soxlet apparatus. Then the extracts were air dried for 24 h and finally dissolved in dimethyl sulfoxide (DMSO) to prepare dilution for further study.

## Collection and maintenance of test organisms

A total of 14 microorganisms (9 pathogenic and 5 standard laboratory microorganisms) were used in this experiment. The pathogenic organisms are MDR clinical isolates of human UTI and RTI bacteria (Table 1). The microbial type culture collection (MTCC) strains of three bacteria and two fungi were used as standard test organisms. Different pathogenic and standard bacterial strains of gram negative namely *Klebsiella pneumoniae*, *Escherichia coli*, gram positive *Bacillus subtilis*, *Staphylococcus aureus* and two standard fungal stains of *Aspergillus fumigatus*, *Candida albicans* were tested.

## Antimicrobial screening by agar cup method

The antimicrobial activity was screened by agar well diffusion method. Saborouds dextrose agar was used as the culture media for fungi and Muller Hinton agar medium was used for bacteria. The inoculums were prepared in fresh nutrient broth from well-maintained slant culture. The inoculums were standardized following McFarland

**Table 2** Effect of two different cytokinins supplemented with MS basal medium and culture duration (i.e., regeneration cycles) on adventitious shoot induction from leaf explant of *Bacopa monnieri*

| Concentration of plant growth regulators | | | Response (%) | Number of shoot buds induced per leaf explant (after 12 d of implantation) | No. of elongated (≥ 1 cm) shoot buds per leaf explant (after 42 d of implantation) |
|---|---|---|---|---|---|
| BAP (mg/L) | KIN (mg/L) | Spermidine (mM) | | | |
| – | – | – | 0 | 0$^a$ | 0$^a$ |
| 0.5 | – | – | 96.7 | 53.5 ± 1.7$^{cd}$ | 11.7 ± 0.3$^c$ |
| 1.0 | – | – | 100 | 76.7 ± 1.2$^{de}$ | 16.1 ± 0.2$^d$ |
| 1.5 | – | – | 100 | 92.4 ± 3.7$^{ef}$ | 22.5 ± 0.4$^{ef}$ |
| 2.0 | – | – | 100 | 84.1 ± 3.2$^e$ | 19.2 ± 0.5$^e$ |
| 2.5 | – | – | 100 | 78.2 ± 2.4$^e$ | 13.8 ± 0.2$^{cd}$ |
| – | 0.5 | – | 90.0 | 45.0 ± 1.3$^{bcd}$ | 9.5 ± 0.6$^c$ |
| – | 1.0 | – | 93.3 | 62.8 ± 1.9$^d$ | 13.6 ± 0.7$^{cd}$ |
| – | 1.5 | – | 100 | 73.5 ± 2.2$^{de}$ | 16.0 ± 0.3$^d$ |
| – | 2.0 | – | 100 | 81.3 ± 2.5$^e$ | 18.2 ± 1.0$^{de}$ |
| – | 2.5 | – | 100 | 75.4 ± 1.9$^{def}$ | 15.4 ± 0.8$^d$ |
| 1.5 | – | 1.0 | 100 | 106.0 ± 3.2$^f$ | 27.3 ± 0.7$^{fg}$ |
| 1.5 | – | 1.5 | 100 | 114.2 ± 2.6$^{fg}$ | 30.7 ± 0.9$^g$ |
| 1.5 | – | 2.0 | 100 | 123.8 ± 3.4$^g$ | 34.9 ± 1.2$^h$ |
| 1.5 | – | 2.5 | 100 | 117.6 ± 3.1$^{fg}$ | 31.4 ± 1.1$^{gh}$ |

Each value represents the mean ± standard error, $n = 30$ (3 set, 10 samples in each set). Mean followed by the same letters in each column are not significantly different at $P < 0.05$ according to Tukey's multiple range test. *BAP* 6-Benzylaminopurine, *KIN* Kinetin

**Table 3** Antimicrobial activities of the three different solvent extracts of ex vitro Bacopa monnieri plants

| Solvent | Extract conc. (mg/cup) | Zone of Inhibition (mm) | | | | | | | | | | | | | |
| | | MDR-UTI bacteria | | | | | MDR-RTI bacteria | | | | MTCC bacteria | | | MTCC fungus | |
| | | Sample 5 | Sample 9 | Sample 11 | Sample 19 | Sample 26 | Sample 31 | Sample 35 | Sample 36 | Sample 38 | MTCC 109 | MTCC 441 | MTCC 3160 | MTCC 870 | MTCC 1637 |
|---|---|---|---|---|---|---|---|---|---|---|---|---|---|---|---|
| Acetone | 0.75 | – | 12 ± 0.11 | – | R | 12 ± 0.22 | – | 9 ± 0.28 | – | – | – | – | – | 8 ± 0.08 | – |
| | 1.5 | 11 ± 0.11 | 13 ± 0.26 | – | R | 14 ± 0.32 | – | 11 ± 0.58 | 10 ± 0.56 | – | – | 8 ± 0.36 | 8 ± 0.33 | 10 ± 0.38 | 12 ± 0.22 |
| | 3.0 | 13 ± 0.24 | 15 ± 0.66 | – | R | 15 ± 0.36 | 9 ± 0.22 | 12 ± 0.11 | 11 ± 0.32 | 8 ± 0.11 | 12 ± 0.11 | 11 ± 0.32 | 12 ± 0.48 | 11 ± 0.28 | 14 ± 0.18 |
| | 4.5 | 15 ± 0.36 | 16 ± 0.33 | 11 ± 0.11 | R | 16 ± 0.14 | 11 ± 0.11 | 12 ± 0.56 | 13 ± 0.88 | 9 ± 0.28 | 14 ± 0.26 | 13 ± 0.44 | 14 ± 0.55 | 12 ± 0.56 | 16 ± 0.38 |
| | 6.0 | 15 ± 0.22 | 16 ± 0.48 | 13 ± 0.24 | R | 16 ± 0.18 | 11 ± 0.58 | 12 ± 0.22 | 13 ± 0.44 | 9 ± 0.22 | 14 ± 0.44 | 15 ± 0.48 | 14 ± 0.58 | 12 ± 0.88 | 19 ± 0.12 |
| Ethanol | 0.75 | – | 14 ± 0.18 | – | R | – | – | – | – | – | – | – | – | – | – |
| | 1.5 | – | 16 ± 0.38 | – | R | – | 8 ± 0.28 | 9 ± 0.48 | – | 10 ± 0.21 | 11 ± 0.32 | – | – | – | 10 ± 0.26 |
| | 3.0 | – | 17 ± 0.22 | 12 ± 0.32 | R | – | 9 ± 0.44 | 10 ± 0.22 | – | 11 ± 0.44 | 13 ± 0.22 | 8 ± 0.38 | 10 ± 0.22 | 10 ± 0.21 | 14 ± 0.46 |
| | 4.5 | 11 ± 0.18 | 17 ± 0.18 | 14 ± 0.11 | R | – | 11 ± 0.22 | 11 ± 0.48 | 8 ± 0.32 | 11 ± 0.22 | 15 ± 0.48 | 10 ± 0.22 | 13 ± 0.33 | 11 ± 0.26 | 18 ± 0.55 |
| | 6.0 | 13 ± 0.22 | 17 ± 0.66 | 14 ± 0.62 | R | 10 ± 0.11 | 11 ± 0.22 | 12 ± 0.56 | 10 ± 0.44 | 10 ± 0.28 | – | 12 ± 0.22 | 16 ± 0.48 | 11 ± 0.18 | 21 ± 0.38 |
| Methanol | 0.75 | 11 ± 0.26 | 13 ± 0.78 | – | R | 8 ± 0.33 | 7 ± 0.56 | – | – | 10 ± 0.28 | 11 ± 0.48 | – | 10 ± 0.22 | 12 ± 0.18 | 12 ± 0.18 |
| | 1.5 | 12 ± 0.88 | 16 ± 0.18 | – | R | 10 ± 0.24 | 9 ± 0.88 | – | 9 ± 0.88 | 12 ± 0.32 | 13 ± 0.66 | – | 12 ± 0.48 | 14 ± 0.11 | 16 ± 0.77 |
| | 3.0 | 13 ± 0.48 | 18 ± 0.11 | – | R | 11 ± 0.18 | 11 ± 0.22 | 8 ± 0.11 | 11 ± 0.88 | 13 ± 0.12 | 13 ± 0.78 | 9 ± 0.48 | 14 ± 0.55 | 16 ± 0.22 | 18 ± 0.34 |
| | 4.5 | 14 ± 0.54 | 18 ± 0.66 | 10 ± 0.24 | R | 12 ± 0.38 | 12 ± 0.38 | 8 ± 0.88 | 12 ± 0.48 | 13 ± 0.21 | 13 ± 0.48 | 10 ± 0.52 | 14 ± 0.33 | 16 ± 0.38 | 18 ± 0.72 |
| | 6.0 | 14 ± 0.22 | 18 ± 0.68 | 13 ± 0.34 | R | 13 ± 0.62 | 13 ± 0.62 | 9 ± 0.32 | 12 ± 0.48 | 14 ± 0.22 | 13 ± 0.28 | 12 ± 0.66 | 14 ± 0.68 | 16 ± 0.18 | 18 ± 0.38 |

Each value represents the mean ± standard error. R Resistant, Sample 5, 9, 11 – Escherichia coli, Sample 19, 26, 31, 35, 36, 38 – Klebsiella pneumoniae, MTCC 109 – Klebsiella pneumoniae, MTCC 441 – Bacillus subtilis, MTCC 3160 – Staphylococcus aureus, MTCC 870 – Aspergillus fumigatus, MTCC 1637 – Candida albicans

standards by regulating the turbidity of the broth culture by adding sterile broth. Petri dishes were spread with the inoculums and holes (8 mm) were punctured using sterile cork-borer. The plant extracts of different solvents were dissolved in DMSO and were added to the respective holes. DMSO being the negative control exhibited no zone of inhibition against any of the tested microorganisms. Experimental cultures were incubated for 24 h at 37 °C (for bacteria) and 72 h at 26 °C (for fungi). After incubation, the zones of inhibition (ZI) were measured and photographed with Canon 'PowerShot SX700 HS' camera.

### Minimum inhibitory concentration (MIC)

The MIC was determined by two fold broth dilution method [22] for showing antimicrobial activity of the plant extract against all the test organisms. The dried plant extracts were resuspended in DMSO to make 100 mg/mL concentration, then added to broth media using serial dilution. Thereafter 100 µl inoculum was added to every tube and incubated at 26 °C for 72 h (for fungi) or 37 °C for 24 h (for bacteria). The MIC value of both fungi and bacteria was taken as the lowermost concentration of the plant extracts in the tube that exhibited no turbidity following incubation.

### Minimum bactericidal and fungicidal concentration (MBC and MFC)

The minimum bactericidal and fungicidal concentration (MBC and MFC) was determined by the viable cell count method [23] by subculturing 50 µl of each dilution used in MIC experiment. Minimum concentration of plant extract, showing no visible growth on subculturing, was taken as MBC or MFC.

### Statistical analysis

In present experimental design, each treatment of micropropagation was repeated thrice with 10 explants per treatment. All data were subjected to one-way analysis of variance (ANOVA) with the help of SPSS software (IBM® SPSS, version 21.0, Chicago, IL). After conducting an ANOVA, the means were further separated using Tukey's test at $P \leq 0.05$ [24]. All types of antimicrobial tests are also repeated three times.

### Results
#### Micropropagation

The effect of different concentrations (ranging from 0.5 mg/L to 2.5 mg/L) of BAP and KIN alone on in vitro adventitious shoot multiplication from leaf explants, was investigated (Fig. 1 a–d). The adventitious shoot-buds

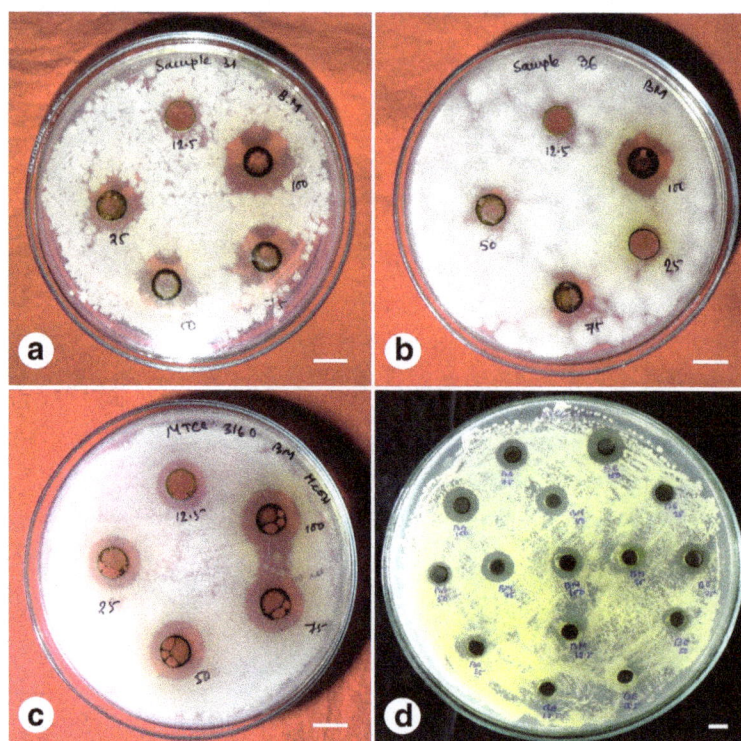

**Fig. 2** Antimicrobial activities of *Bacopa monnieri* [bar = 10 mm]. **a** Activities of methanol extract against MDR-RTI clinical strain *Klebsiella pneumoniae* [Sample 31], (**b**) Activities of methanol extract against MDR-RTI clinical strain *Klebsiella pneumoniae* [Sample 36], (**c**) Activities of methanol extract against standard bacterial strain *Staphylococcus aureus* [MTCC 3160], (**d**) Activities of ethanol, methanol, and acetone extracts against standard fungal strain *Candida albicans* [MTCC 1637]

were induced from the cut edges within 6 to 7 days of implantation, followed by swelling at the cut edges. A total of 92.4 shoot buds were induced after 12 days of culture in MS basal medium containing 1.5 mg/L BAP, whereas maximum of 81.3 shoot buds were induced in the presence of KIN (2.0 mg/L) after same duration (Table 2). Greater concentration of cytokinin is not only abridged the quantity of shoot buds, but also suppressed the growth of the multiplied shoots. Spermidine in combination with the optimum concentration of BAP (1.5 mg/L) significantly increased the rate of shoot induction. MS basal medium supplemented with 1.5 mg/L BAP and 2.0 mM spermidine was found to be the best combination of growth regulators with a maximum of 123.8 shoot buds per leaf explant, after 12 days of culture.

Although the huge numbers of shoot buds were induced, the elongation of these newly induced buds was a real problem and few of them had elongated at a time in presence of cytokinin only. Spermidine had played an affirmative role on shoot bud elongation in B. monnieri. Only 22.5 shoot buds are elongated in the presence of 1.5 mg/L BAP alone, but this numbers increased up to 34.9 when supplemented with 2.0 mM spermidine along with 1.5 mg/L BAP (Fig. 1e). Further elongation and in vitro rooting was achieved in half strength of MS medium without any PGR (Fig. 1f). A maximum of 13.2 roots per shoot with a length of 4.5 cm was noted within 18 day of implantation (Fig. 1g). In vitro derived plantlets were successfully acclimatized with a survival rate of 96.7%. All the plants were grown healthily with a morphology alike to that of the source plants (Fig. 1h).

**Table 4** MIC and MBC/MFC (mg/mL) of the three different solvents of ex vitro plants of *Bacopa monnieri*

| Microorganisms | | | Inhibition type | Inhibiting/cidal concentrations (mg/mL) of different solvent extracts | | |
|---|---|---|---|---|---|---|
| Type | Bacteria / fungi | Strain | | Acetone | Ethanol | Methanol |
| Pathogenic | MDR-UTI bacterial strains | Sample 5 | MIC | 5.0 | 7.5 | 5.0 |
| | | | MBC | 10.0 | 12.5 | 12.5 |
| | | Sample 9 | MIC | 5.0 | 2.5 | 2.5 |
| | | | MBC | 10.0 | 5.0 | 5.0 |
| | | Sample 11 | MIC | 5.0 | 5.0 | 7.5 |
| | | | MBC | 12.5 | 10.0 | 12.5 |
| | | Sample 19 | MIC | R | R | R |
| | | | MBC | R | R | R |
| | | Sample 26 | MIC | 2.5 | 25.0 | 10.0 |
| | | | MBC | 5.0 | 30.5 | 17.5 |
| | MDR-RTI bacterial strains | Sample 31 | MIC | 7.5 | 7.5 | 10.0 |
| | | | MBC | 10.0 | 12.5 | 15.0 |
| | | Sample 35 | MIC | 7.5 | 5.0 | 15.0 |
| | | | MBC | 12.5 | 7.5 | 17.5 |
| | | Sample 36 | MIC | 5.0 | 10.0 | 7.5 |
| | | | MBC | 10.0 | 15.0 | 15.0 |
| | | Sample 38 | MIC | 15.0 | 12.5 | 5.0 |
| | | | MBC | 17.5 | 17.5 | 7.5 |
| Standard | MTCC bacterial strains | MTCC 109 | MIC | 5.0 | 5.0 | 7.5 |
| | | | MBC | 12.5 | 12.5 | 12.5 |
| | | MTCC 441 | MIC | 7.5 | 12.5 | 10.0 |
| | | | MBC | 10.0 | 17.5 | 15.0 |
| | | MTCC 3160 | MIC | 10.0 | 15.0 | 2.5 |
| | | | MBC | 12.5 | 22.5 | 7.5 |
| | MTCC fungal strains | MTCC 870 | MIC | 2.5 | 10.0 | 2.5 |
| | | | MFC | 7.5 | 12.5 | 5.0 |
| | | MTCC 1637 | MIC | 7.5 | 7.5 | 1.25 |
| | | | MFC | 12.5 | 12.5 | 5.0 |

*R* Resistant, Sample 5, 9, 11 – *Escherichia coli*, Sample 19, 26, 31, 35, 36, 38 – *Klebsiella pneumoniae*, MTCC 109 – *Klebsiella pneumoniae*, MTCC 441 – *Bacillus subtilis*, MTCC 3160 – *Staphylococcus aureus*, MTCC 870 – *Aspergillus fumigatus*, MTCC 1637 – *Candida albicans*

## Antimicrobial activity

In the present study, all UTI and RTI strains, collected from the patients, were routinely categorized in our laboratory, and examined individually for the resistance pattern against multidrug (Table 1). Result in the present study revealed that all the extracts (ethanol, methanol and acetone) of *B. monnieri* were more or less effective against all the test organisms except one (Sample 19) (Table 3). Overall, methanolic extract proved more effective than other two extracts with very clear ZI (Fig. 2a–c). In case of MDR-UTI strain of *E. coli* (Sample 9) methanolic extract exhibited maximum inhibition (ZI 18 mm), whereas another strain of *E. coli* (Sample 5) and *K. pneumoniae* (Sample 26) showed maximum inhibition (ZI 15 mm and 16 mm respectively) with acetone extract. For MDR-RTI bacteria, methanol extract showed maximum inhibition (ZI 14 mm) against *K. pneumoniae* (Sample 38). In case of all three MTCC bacteria, the maximum inhibition was noted with acetone extract. The fungal strain of *C. albicans* (MTCC 1637) showed maximum inhibition (ZI 21 mm) with ethanolic extract (Fig. 2d).

All the three types of extracts of *B. monnieri* were found to show potential anti-UTI and anti-RTI activity with MIC values ranging between 2.5–25.0 mg/mL. The MIC range was noted to be comparatively lower (1.25–10.0 mg/mL) against two fungal strains. In case of UTI and RTI bacteria, all the extracts exhibited MBC/MIC ratio less than "32", which indicated that the test extracts of *B. monnieri* were bactericidal rather than bacteriostatic. Methanol was found to be the most potent (MIC 2.5–15.0 mg/mL), while acetone and ethanol showed more or less similar inhibitory activity (MIC 2.5–25.0 mg/mL and 2.5–30.0 mg/mL respectively) against all the microorganisms tested including MDR-UTI and MDR-RTI pathogens. Therefore, among all the test extracts, methanol was most potent against both bacteria and fungi (Table 4).

The antibacterial and antifungal activity of ex vitro plants is slightly better compared to the in vitro plants; however, the potency of the in vitro plants is not also negligible (Fig. 3).

## Discussion

The cytokinin BAP or KIN alone was sufficient for induction of adventitious shoot buds from the leaf explants of *B. monnieri*. Higher concentration of cytokinin had reduced the number of shoots, a finding similar to that noted in *Tylophora indica* [19]. BAP was found to be more effective than KIN for adventitious shoot induction in *B. monnieri*. Similar results were reported in *Capsicum frutescens* where BAP proved to be the best among four of the cytokinins tested [25]. Micropropagation methods of *B. monnieri* have been studied by many groups for more than four decades

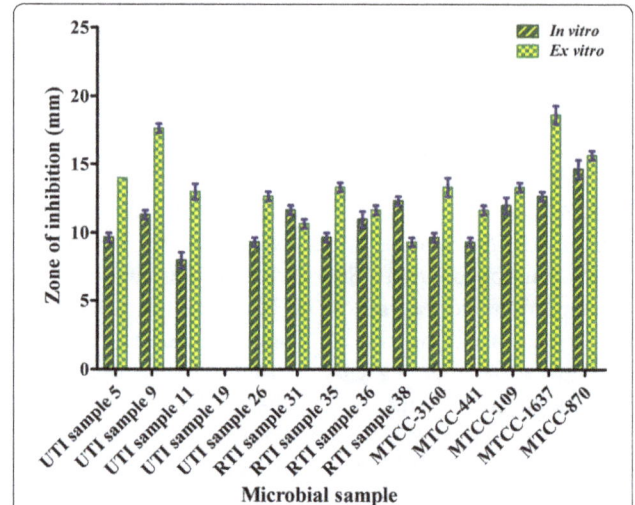

**Fig. 3** Antimicrobial activities of the methanolic extracts of in vitro and ex vitro raised plants of *Bacopa monnieri*. (Sample 5, 9, 11, 19, 26, 31, 35, 36, and 38 are clinical isolates of MDR human UTI and RTI bacteria; MTCC 109, 441 and 3160 are standard bacterial strains and MTCC 870 and 1637 are standard fungal strains of microbial type culture collection (MTCC)

and till the research is continuing for improvement of these protocols [2, 3, 26–30]. So far, to our present knowledge, the present manuscript is the first report describing the promoting role of spermidine on micropropagation of *B. monnieri*. The addition of spermidine along with the optimum concentration of BAP has proven helpful in increasing the adventitious shoot bud induction rate of *B. monnieri*. Chi et al. [31] had also described the enhancing role polyamines in the shoot regeneration of *Brassica campestris*. Polyamines have been found to act as a growth stimulant and sometimes as the enhancer of the action of PGRs [32]. Polyamines play crucial role in the growth and development of higher plants by influencing cell division, stem elongation, root growth and many other functions [33]. Present findings showed the exogenous application of spermidine had not only enhanced the shoot induction rate, but also had significantly improved the growth and elongation of the adventitious shoots in *B. monnieri*. The similar optimistic role of polyamines, especially spermidine, on the growth and development of plants was previously reported by several authors [25, 34].

The antimicrobial property of *B. monnieri* was previously reported by few researchers against several standard bacterial strains [10–12, 35]. Only Hema et al. [13] had described the antimicrobial property of *B. monnieri* against clinical isolates of human pathogenic strains, but these are not MDR strains. Antibacterial resistance has become one of the grave public health concerns, globally, over the last two decades [14, 15]. Particularly, MDR is a major concern in present day medical science.

In this study standard laboratory microorganisms as well as MDR-UTI and MDR-RTI pathogens are found to be susceptible to various extracts of *B. monnieri*. The wonder plant *B. monnieri* is pharmaceutically very significant as it contains many secondary metabolites viz. alkaloids, flavonoid, phenolic, glycosides, and other substances like stigmastanol, stigmasterol and β-sitosterol, triterpene oligoglycosides, bacomosaponins A and B, bacomosides A, B1, and B2 [4, 9]. A group of secondary metabolite compounds has effective antimicrobial properties [36]. Mainly, methanol extract contains more antioxidant as because of this it might be used as folk medicide [37]. It was also reported that the methanol extract of *B. monnieri* exhibited the more significant inhibitory effect against *Klebsiella pneumoniae*, *Staphylococcus aureus* which corroborates with our findings [38, 39]. Similar to our findings against *Candida albicans* Canli et al. [40] also reported that the ethanolic extract exhibited best anti-fungal activity among all other solvent extracts against *Lycoperdon lividum*.

The study of in vitro and ex vitro plants exhibited the antimicrobial activity was better in ex vitro field grown plants than in vitro plants (Fig. 3). With a similar approach, a comparative study was conducted by few researchers in recent past [41–44]. Some of them reported the in vitro plants exhibited more antimicrobial activity as compared to ex vitro plants [42, 43], whereas the majority of them reported ex vitro plants are superior or more or less comparable as compare to in vitro plants [41, 44]. The in vitro plants, producing secondary metabolites at a primary stage of growth, provides an opportunity for fast production of pharmacologically important compounds that can be utilized for medicinal purposes [41].

Bacterial resistance against existing drugs has directed to severe health concerns all over the world [45]. Our present findings confirm that *B. monnieri* is very effective against MDR-UTI and RTI clinical isolates, where majority of the commercially available antibiotics are unable to treat those. Similarly, in very recent times few researchers had reported that *B. monnieri* proved to be effective against clinical isolates of *Escherichia coli*, *Klebsiella pneumoniae* [13] and *Staphylococcus aureus* [46]; although their pathogens are not MDR strains. Because of *B. monnieri* contains many bioactive metabolite, the crude extract shows more effectiveness rather than commercial antibiotics. In addition, the herbal formulation have no side effect, which is an important advantage over commercial antibiotics. The determination of minimum lethal concentration (MLC), also known as the MBC or MFC, is the most common estimation of bactericidal or fungicidal activity [16]. Overall, present study exhibited a substantial bactericidal activity of the tested extracts of *B. monnieri* against the clinical isolates of MDR-UTI and RTI strains as indicated by the MBC/MIC ratio less than "32" [47].

## Conclusion

The present manuscript described a very reliable method for large scale multiplication of *B. monnieri*. In addition, present findings show the methanolic extract of *B. monneari* have potential antimicrobial activity against clinical isolates of MDR-UTI and MDR-RTI bacterial strains. In future this plant may be used to treat these infectious diseases. Though in vitro plants show slightly lesser antimicrobial potency as compared to ex vitro plants, they can be produced in large quantities using very little space throughout the year. Present protocol can be commercially implemented by pharmaceutical industries to address cumulative market demand of *B. monnieri*.

### Acknowledgements

SMH acknowledges the Ministry of Minority Affairs and University Grant Commission for providing the Maulana Azad National Fellowship. SMH, AC and BG thankful to Swami Kamalasthananda, Principal, Ramakrishna Mission Vivekananda Centenary College, Rahara, Kolkata (India), for the facilities provided for the present study. DD acknowledges technical and management support provided by Ashok Laboratory Clinical Testing Centre. Private Limited, Kolkata.

### Authors' contributions

SMH performed all the plant tissue culture related experiments and write up a part of manuscript. AC screened the antimicrobial activities of plant extracts and write up a part of manuscript. DD collected the clinical isolates and checked their response against multidrug. SM and SN was involved in result interpretation and made necessary correction in the write up. Critical revision of the article was done by SM, SN and BG. Conception, experiment design, overall monitoring and final approval of the article was done by BG. All authors read and approved the final manuscript.

### Competing interests

All authors declare that they have no competing interests.

### Author details

[1]Plant Biotechnology Laboratory, Post Graduate Department of Botany, Ramakrishna Mission Vivekananda Centenary College, Rahara, Kolkata 700118, India. [2]Department of Microbiology, Ashok Laboratory Clinical Testing Centre Private Limited, Kolkata 700068, India. [3]Department of Microbiology, Dinabandhu Andrews College, Garia, Kolkata 700084, India. [4]Centre of Biotechnology, Siksha O Anusandhan University, Bhubaneswar 751030, India.

### References

1. Gobalakrishnan R, Kulandaivelu M, Bhuvaneswari R, Kandavel D, Kannan L. Screening of wild plant species for antibacterial activity and phytochemical analysis of *Tragia involucrata* L. J Pharm Anal. 2013;3:460–5.
2. Tiwari V, Tiwari KN, Singh BD. Shoot bud regeneration from different explants of *Bacopa monniera* (L.) Wettst by trimethoprim and bavistin. Plant Cell Rep. 2006;25:629–35.
3. Ramesh M, Vijayakumar KP, Karthikeyan A, Pandian SK. RAPD based genetic stability analysis among micropropagated, synthetic seed derived and hardened plants of *Bacopa monnieri* (L.): a threatened Indian medicinal herb. Acta Physiol Plant. 2011;33:163–71.
4. Zhou Y, Shen YH, Zhang C, Zhang WD. Chemical constituents of *Bacopa monnieri*. Chem Nat Compd. 2007;43:355–7.
5. Rajani M. *Bacopa monnieri*, a nootropic drug. In: Ramawat KG, Mérillon JM, editors. Bioactive molecules and medicinal plants. New York: Springer; 2008. p. 175–95.

6. Kishore K. Brahmi: a complete herbal medicine. J Pharm Res. 2012;5:3139–42.

7. Al-Snafi AE. The pharmacology of *Bacopa monniera*. A review, Int J Pharma Sci Res. 2013;4:154–9.

8. Aguiar S, Borowski T. Neuropharmacological review of the nootropic herb *Bacopa monnieri*. Rejuvenation Res. 2013;16:313–26.

9. Ohta T, Nakamura S, Nakashima S, Oda Y, Matsumoto T, Fukaya M, Yano M, Yoshikawa M, Matsuda H. Chemical structures of constituents from the whole plant of *Bacopa monniera*. J Nat Med. 2016;70:404–11.

10. Sampathkumar P, Dheeba B, Venkatasubramanian V, Arulprakash T, Vinothkannan R. Potential antimicrobial activity of various extracts of *Bacopa monnieri* (Linn.). Int J of Pharmacol. 2008;4:230–2.

11. Alam K, Parvez N, Yadav S, Molvi K, Hwisa N, Sharif SMA, Pathak D, Murti Y, Zafar R. Antimicrobial activity of leaf callus of *Bacopa monnieri* L. Pharm Lett. 2011;3:287–91.

12. Joshi BB, Patel MGH, Dabhi B, Mistry KN. In vitro phytochemical analysis and anti-microbial activity of crude extract of *Bacopa monniera*. Bull Pharma Med Sci. 2013;1:128–31.

13. Hema TA, Arya AS, Subha S, John CRK, Divya PV. Antimicrobial activity of five South Indian medicinal plants against clinical pathogens. Int J Pharm Bio Sci. 2013;4:70–80.

14. Dey D, Ray R, Hazra B. Antimicrobial activity of pomegranate fruit constituents against drug-resistant *Mycobacterium tuberculosis* and β-lactamase producing *Klebsiella pneumoniae*. Pharm Biol. 2015;53:1474–80.

15. Dey D, Ray R, Hazra B. Antitubercular and antibacterial activity of quinonoid natural products against multi-drug resistant clinical isolates. Phytother Res. 2014;28:1014–21.

16. Balouiri M, Sadiki M, Ibnsouda SK. Methods for in vitro evaluating antimicrobial activity:A review. J Pharm Anal. 2016;6:71–9.

17. National Medicinal Plants Board. Thirty two prioritized medicinal plants, National Informatics Centre, Ministry of Health and Family Welfare, Department of Ayush, Government of India. 2004.

18. Karthikeyan A, Madhanraj A, Pandian SK, et al. Genetic variation among highly endangered *Bacopa monnieri* (L.) Pennell from Southern India as detected using RAPD analysis. Genet Resour Crop Evol. 2011;58:769–82.

19. Haque SM, Ghosh B. Field evaluation and genetic stability assessment of regenerated plants produced via direct shoot organogenesis from leaf explant of an endangered "Asthma plant" (*Tylophora indica*) along with their in vitro conservation. Natl Acad Sci Lett. 2013;36:551–62.

20. Murashige T, Skoog F. A revised medium for rapid growth and bioassays with tobacco tissue culture. Physiol Plant. 1962;15:473–97.

21. Haque SM, Ghosh B. Micropropagation, in vitro flowering and cytological studies of *Bacopa chamaedryoides*, an ethno-medicinal plant. Environ Exp Biol. 2013;11:59–68.

22. Wiegand I, Hilpert K, Hancock REW. Agar and broth dilution methods to determine the minimal inhibitory concentration (MIC) of antimicrobial substances. Nat Protoc. 2008;3:163–75.

23. Toda M, Okubo S, Hiyoshi R, Shimamura T. The bactericidal activity of tea and coffee. Lett Appl Microbiol. 1989;8:123–5.

24. Haynes W, Tukey's test, In: Encyclopedia of systems biology. Dubitzky W, Wolkenhauer O, Cho K-H, et al. editors. New York: Springer; 2013. p. 2303–2304.

25. Kumar V, Sharma A, Prasad BCN, Gururaj HB, Giridhar P, Ravishankar GA. Direct shoot bud induction and plant regeneration in *Capsicum frutescens* Mill.: influence of polyamines and polarity. Acta Physiol Plant. 2007;29:11–8.

26. Thakur S, Ganpathy PS, Johri BN. Differentiation of abnormal plantlets in *Bacopa monnieri*. Phytomorphology. 1976;26:422–4.

27. Banerjee M, Shrivastava S. An improved protocol for in vitro multiplication of *Bacopa monnieri* (L.). World J Microbiol Biotechnol. 2008;24:1355–9.

28. Ceasar SA, Maxwell SLPKB, Karthigan M, Ignacimuthu S. Highly efficient shoot regeneration of *Bacopa monnieri* (L.) using a two-stage culture procedure and assessment of genetic integrity of micropropagated plants by RAPD. Acta Physiol Plant. 2010;32:443–52.

29. Kumari U, Vishwakarma RK, Gupta N, Ruby SMV, Khan BM. Efficient shoots regeneration and genetic transformation of Bacopa monniera. Physiol Mol Biol Plants. 2015;21:261–7.

30. Largia MJV, Shilpha J, Pothiraj G, Ramesh M. Analysis of nuclear DNA content, genetic stability, Bacoside A quantity and antioxidant potential of long term in vitro grown germplasm lines of *Bacopa monnieri* (L.). Plant Cell Tissue Organ Cult. 2015;120:399–406.

31. Chi CL, Lin WS, Lee JEE, Pua EC. Role of polyamines on de novo shoot morphogenesis from cotyledons of *Brassica campestris* ssp. pekinensis (Lour) Olsson in vitro. Plant Cell Rep. 1994;13:323–9.

32. Moshkov IE, Novikova GV, Hall MA, George EF. Plant growth regulators III: ethylene, abscisic acid, their analogues and inhibitors, miscellaneous compounds. In: George EF, Hall MA, de Klerk GJ, editors. Plant propagation by tissue culture. 3rd ed. Netherlands: Springer; 2008. p. 227–82.

33. Podwyszyn' ska M, Kosson R, Treder J. Polyamines and methyl jasmonate in bulb formation of in vitro propagated tulips. Plant Cell Tissue Organ Cult. 2015;123:591–605.

34. Satish L, Rency AS, Rathinapriya P, Ceasar SA, Pandian S, Rameshkumar R, Rao TB, Balachandran SM, Ramesh M. Influence of plant growth regulators and spermidine on somatic embryogenesis and plant regeneration in four Indian genotypes of finger millet (*Eleusine coracana* L. Gaertn). Plant Cell Tissue Organ Cult. 2016;124:15–31.

35. Ghosh T, Maity TK, Bose A, Dash GK, Das M. Antimicrobial activity of various fractions of ethanol extract of *Bacopa monnieri* Linn. aerial parts. Indian J Pharm Sci. 2007;69:312–4.

36. Banasiuk R, Kawiak A, Krolicka A. In vitro cultures of carnivorous plants from the *Drosera* and *Dionaea* genus for the production of biologically active secondary metabolites. Bio Technologia. 2012;93:87–96.

37. Hossain MS, Rahman MS, Imon AHMR, Zaman S, ASMBA S, Mondal M, SarwarA HTB, Adhikary BC, Begum T, Tabassum A, Alam S, Begum MM. Ethnopharmacological investigations of methanolic extract of *Pouzolzia Zeylanica* (L.) Benn. Clin Phytosci. 2016;2:10.

38. Rajashekharappa S, Krishna V, Sathyanarayana BN, Gowdar HB. Antibacterial activity of bacoside-A- an active constituent isolated of *Bacopa monnieri* (L.) Wettest. Pharmacologyonline. 2008;2:517–28.

39. Mathur A, Verma SK, Purohit R, Singh SK, Mathur D, Prasad GBKS, Dua VK. Pharmacological investigation of *Bacopa monnieri* on the basis of antioxidant, antimicrobial and anti-inflammatory properties. J Chem Pharm Res. 2010;2:191–8.

40. Canli K, Altuner EM, Akata I, Turkmen Y, Uzek U. In vitro antimicrobial screening of *Lycoperdon lividum* and determination of the ethanol extract composition by gas chromatography/mass spectrometry. Bangladesh J Pharmacol. 2016;11:389–94.

41. Ncube B, Ngunge VNP, Finnie JF, Van Staden J. A comparative study of the antimicrobial and phytochemical properties between outdoor grown and micropropagated *Tulbaghia violacea* Harv. plants. J Ethnopharmacol. 2011; 134:775–80.

42. Kumari A, Baskaran P, Van Staden J. In vitro propagation and antibacterial activity in *Cotyledon orbiculata*: a valuable medicinal plant. Plant Cell Tissue Organ Cult. 2016;124:97–104.

43. Baskaran P, Singh S, Van Staden J. In vitro propagation, proscillaridin A production and antibacterial activity in *Drimia robusta*. Plant Cell Tissue Organ Cult. 2013;114:259–67.

44. Khateeb WA, Hussein E, Qouta L, Datt MA, Shara BA, Abu-zaiton A. In vitro propagation and characterization of phenolic content along with antioxidant and antimicrobial activities of Cichorium pumilum Jacq. Plant Cell Tissue Organ Cult. 2012;110:103–110.

45. Phull A-R, Abbas Q, Ali A, Raza H, Kim S-J, Zia M, Haq IU. Antioxidant, cytotoxic and antimicrobial activities of green synthesized silver nanoparticles from crude extract of *Bergenia ciliate*. Future J Pharma Sci. 2016;2:31–6.

46. Emran TB, Rahman MA, Uddin MMN, Dash R, Hossen MF, Mohiuddin M, Alam MR. Molecular docking and inhibition studies on the interactions of *Bacopa monnieri*'s potent phytochemicals against pathogenic *Staphylococcus aureus*. DARU J Pharma Sci. 2015;23:26.

47. Cockerill FR. Conventional and genetic laboratory tests used to guide antimicrobial therapy. Mayo Clin Proc. 1998;73:1007–21.

# 5

# Evaluation of the efficacy of *Acalypha wilkesiana* leaves in managing cardiovascular disease risk factors in rabbits exposed to salt-loaded diets

Kingsley Omage[1]* (iD), Marshall A. Azeke[2] and Sylvia O. Omage[3]

## Abstract

**Background:** This study was conducted to evaluate the therapeutic benefits of oral administration of extracts of *Acalypha wilkesiana* leaves on some serum parameters that are indicators or risk factors of cardiovascular diseases, in salt loaded rabbits.

**Method:** Thirty experimental rabbits used for this study were randomized into five groups (A to E) of six rabbits. Rabbits in groups A to D were given salt loaded diets. Groups B and C animals were also treated with aqueous and ethanol extracts of *Acalypha wilkesiana* leaves respectively while rabbits in group E served as control.

**Results:** Salt loading resulted in a significantly ($P < 0.05$) higher serum albumin, cholesterol, LDL-cholesterol and lower serum globulin, HDL-cholesterol, triglycerides, as compared with the control. Treatment with *Acalypha wilkesiana* leaf extracts (aqueous or ethanol), at a dose of 300 mg/kg body weight, resulted in a significantly ($P < 0.05$) higher serum triglycerides, HDL-cholesterol, globulin, and lower serum total protein, albumin, LDL-cholesterol, cholesterol, as compared with the control, in the salt loaded rabbits.

**Conclusion:** *Acalypha wilkesiana* may be useful in the management of risk factors of cardiovascular diseases.

**Keywords:** *Acalypha wilkesiana*, Salt loaded diet, Ethanol extract, Aqueous extract, Cholesterol

## Background

Sodium, an essential nutrient, is the principal cation of extracellular fluid and a major determinant of intravascular fluid volume. There are considerable human and animal experimental studies implicating excessive dietary salt intake in cardiovascular diseases especially hypertension [1, 2]. Increase in blood pressure leads to damages to the kidney, heart, blood vessels, brain and the eyes. Major risk factors are; age, elevated LDL-cholesterol level, low HDL-cholesterol, microalbuminuria. Analysis of blood samples also show abnormalities in plasma fasting blood glucose, total cholesterol and HDL-cholesterol, etc. These deleterious effects of excess salt can be managed with the use of medications or medicinal herbs.

Medicinal herbs are plants which contain substances that can be used for therapeutic purposes, of which are precursors for the synthesis of drugs [3]. *Acalypha wilkesiana*, commonly called Irish petticoat, Jacob's coat and Copper leaf (local name), belongs to the family Euphorbiaceae, subfamily Acalyphoideae, tribe Acalypheae. The plant is native to the south pacific islands (Bismarck Islands, Fiji, Vanuatu). The plant has been reported to contain sesquiterpenes, monoterpenes, triterpenoids and polyphenols [4]. The leaves reportedly contain saponins, tannins, anthraquinones and glycosides [5]. Characterization of *A. wilkesiana* leaf extracts by gas chromatograhy-mass spectrometry (GC-MS) indicated that glycoside, terpenes, and alkaloid were present while the major components detected from the isolated yellow oil of *A. wilkesiana* were 15-hydroxy pentadecanoic acid, 2-ethyl – 2-methyl tridecanol, pentadecanal, n-decanoic acid and cholesterol [6]. GC-MS chromatogram of the aqueous leaf extract of *A. wilkesiana muell*

* Correspondence: omagekingsley@yahoo.com
[1]Department of Biochemistry, College of Basic Medical Sciences, Igbinedion University, Okada, Edo State, Nigeria
Full list of author information is available at the end of the article

*arg* indicated the presence of nine compounds (mostly straight chain alkanes) which includes iminostilbene, 5-acetyl-2-amino-4-methyl thiazole, pentadecane, octadecane, eicosane, heptadecane, nonadecane, tetratriacontane, 2-decyldodecylcyclohexane and 2-methyltricosane, as well as carboxylic acids [7]. These alkanes have been reported to possess a good antimicrobial effect especially on *Enterococcus faecalis* and *Staphylococcus aureus* [7].

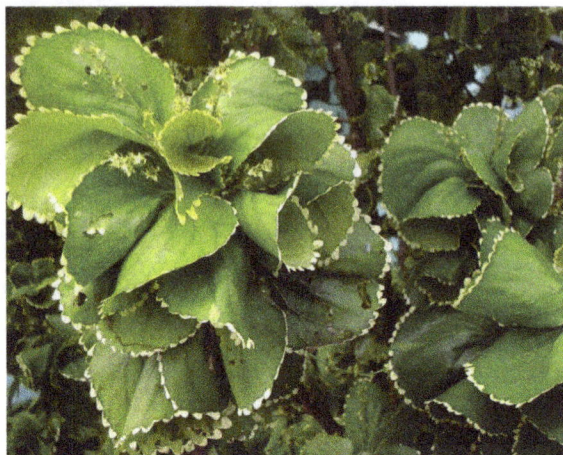

The plant has antimicrobial and antifungal properties and in traditional medicine, the leaves are eaten as vegetables in the management of hypertension, a risk factor for cardiovascular diseases, being a diuretic plant. However, the scientific basis for its use in the management of risk factors of cardiovascular diseases has not been rationalized. Thus, the aim of this study was to evaluate the effects of oral administration of extracts of *Acalypha wilkesiana* leaves on some serum parameters that are indicators or risk factors of cardiovascular diseases, with a view to ascertaining its therapeutic benefits, using salt loaded experimental rabbits.

## Methods

### Plant materials

*Acalypha wilkesiana* leaves were purchased from gardens within Benin City and authenticated at the Department of Plant Biology and Biotechnology, University of Benin, Benin City. The leaves were properly selected to remove unwanted materials and then air dried. The dried leaves were then pulverized into fine powder and weighed.

### Preparation of ethanol extract

Two hundred grams of the pulverized leaves was soaked in 800 ml of ethanol (95%) for 72 h (3 days). The mixture was occasionally stirred using a magnetic stirrer to ensure proper mixture of the vessel content. The content was then filtered using a sintered funnel, (which is equivalent

to four folds of bandage or sheet of cheese cloth). The extract (filtrate) was then concentrated using rotary evaporator and weighed [4].

### Preparation of aqueous extract

Two hundred grams of the pulverized leaves was soaked in 800 ml of distilled water for 72 h (3 days), and treated as described above for ethanol extract [4].

### Preparation of salt-loaded diet (feed)

The salt-loaded diet (8% NaCl and 92% feed) used for this study was prepared by mixing eight (8) grams of analytical NaCl (from BDH Chemicals, England) with ninety-two (92) grams of the feed. The mixture was fed to the experimental rabbits, ad libitum [8], as described in the experimental design below.

### Experimental animals

Thirty adult male rabbits of the New Zealand strain, weighing between 1.0–1.6 kg, were used for this study. The experimental rabbits were obtained from local breeders within Benin City. The rabbits were kept in the animal house of the Department of Biochemistry, University of Benin and maintained on a 12-h light and dark cycle in clean disinfected cages. They were allowed free access to feed (standard pelletized growers feed from UAC- Vital Feed, Jos, Plateau State) and water throughout the duration of the experiment. Prior to the commencement of the study, the animals were allowed to adjust and adapt to the new environment for a period of 3 weeks [9]. The experimental procedures performed on the animals were approved by the Animal Ethics Committee of the Faculty of Life Sciences, University of Benin, Nigeria. The use of rabbits for the study was also according to the Ethical Guidelines Involving Whole Animal Testing of the Animal Ethics Committee, Faculty of Life Sciences, University of Benin. After 3 weeks of acclimatization, the experimental rabbits were then randomized into five groups (A to E) of six (6) rabbits each.

### Experimental design

The rabbits in the groups, A, B, C, D and E were treated as follows;

Group A rabbits: were given continuous salt-loaded diet.

Group B rabbits: were given salt-loaded diet and treated with aqueous extract.

Group C rabbits: were given salt-loaded diet and treated with ethanol extract.

Group D rabbits: were given salt-loaded diet and not treated with the extract.

Group E rabbits: were neither given salt loaded diet nor treated with the extract (Control).

Groups A, B, C and D rabbits were fed with the salt-loaded diet for a period of seventy (70) days. After the 70th day, group A animals were maintained on the salt loaded diet till the 77th day while groups B and C animals were discontinued on the salt loaded diet (after the 70th day) and treated with aqueous and ethanol extracts of *Acalypha wilkesiana* leaves respectively, till the 77th day (i.e. for a period of 7 days). Also, after the 70th day, group D animals were discontinued on the salt-loaded diet and given normal diet till the 77th day, while group E animals were neither given salt-loaded diets nor treated with the extract throughout the duration of the experiment (i.e. it served as control) [8].

### Administration of Extracts

Five grams of the concentrated extracts were suspended in distilled water for administration to the experimental animals. The extracts (aqueous or ethanol) were administered orally at a dose of 300 mg/kg body weight for a period of 7 days [8].

### Collection of blood

After 70 days of salt loaded diets and prior to treatment (i.e. Day 71) with the extracts, blood samples were collected from the veins located on the dorsal side of the ear lobes of the experimental animals (rabbits), using sterilized hypodermic needles. Also, on the 78th day, after treatment with the extracts for a period of 7 days, blood samples were collected from the animals. Blood samples were collected into plane sterile universal tubes immersed in ice. The tubes were centrifuged at 3500 rpm for 10 min and clear serum obtained which were used for further analysis [8].

### Assay methods

Triacylglycerol (TG) and Total Cholesterol (Chol) were determined by the method of Neetu and Neelima, (2013) [10]. HDL – Cholesterol (HDL) was determined

by the method of Leticia, (2014) [11]. LDL – Cholesterol (LDL) was by the equation of Friedwald [12]. (LDL-cholesterol (mg/dl) = Total Cholesterol −TG/5 − HDL-cholesterol). Glucose was determined by the methods of Basul et al. [13] and Renjie et al. [14]. Total Protein (TP) was determined by the method of Dipali et al. [15], (Biuret method). Albumin (ALB) was by dye binding method [16]. The amount of Globulin (GLB) was calculated as a difference between total serum proteins and serum albumin. All reagents were purchased from RANDOX DIAGNOSTIC, UK.

### Statistical analysis

Data are represented as Mean ± S.E.M ($n = 6$). Significance of difference was tested by Student t-Test, ANOVA and Turkey-Kramer test, using the GraphPad Instat Version 3 (GraphPad Software Inc. San Diego, California U.S.A.). Statistical Significance was set at $P < 0.05$.

### Results

The effects of oral administration of extracts (aqueous and ethanol) of *Acalypha wilkesiana* leaves on some serum parameters in salt loaded experimental rabbits, are as described below.

Table 1 shows the effect of salt loading for 70 days on the mean serum cholesterol, triglycerides, HDL-cholesterol and LDL-cholesterol levels (mg/dl) of normal rabbits. All the groups given salt load (groups A, B, C and D) showed significantly ($P < 0.05$) higher levels of cholesterol, LDL-cholesterol and lower levels of triglycerides, HDL-cholesterol as compared with the control (group E), after 70 days of salt loading. Administration of the extracts (aqueous or ethanol) of *Acalypha wilkesiana* leaves, at a dose of 300 mg/kg body weight for a period of 1 week, resulted in significantly ($P > 0.05$) lower levels of cholesterol, LDL-cholesterol and higher triglycerides, HDL-cholesterol levels.

**Table 1** Serum Cholesterol, Triglycerides, HDL-Cholesterol, LDL-Cholesterol (mg/dl) of salt-loaded rabbits; treated with aqueous (B) and ethanol (C) extracts of *Acalypha wilkesiana* leaves, continuous salt loading (A), salt loaded and non-treated (D), non-loaded and non-treated (E)

| SERUM | DAY | GROUP A (Cont. Salt) | B (Salt + Aq. Ext) | C (Salt +Et. Ext) | D (Salt + No Ext) | E (Control) |
|---|---|---|---|---|---|---|
| CHOL (mg/dl) | 71 | 94.69 ± 8.06 | 93.09 ± 6.03[*] | 96.93 ± 8.57[*] | 91.51 ± 3.36 | 59.04 ± 6.83 |
|  | 78 | 99.96 ± 5.36 | 70.18 ± 3.92[**] | 64.32 ± 7.00[**] | 86.92 ± 6.05 | 60.27 ± 5.61 |
| TG (mg/dl) | 71 | 77.47 ± 8.46 | 75.28 ± 7.94[*] | 73.09 ± 8.3[*] | 73.76 ± 9.34 | 118.22 ± 9.32 |
|  | 78 | 70.53 ± 4.63 | 84.64 ± 4.06[**] | 89.32 ± 5.29[**] | 76.45 ± 3.84 | 118.40 ± 8.97 |
| HDL (mg/dl) | 71 | 48.41 ± 2.87 | 46.84 ± 5.73[*] | 46.98 ± 6.78[*] | 45.95 ± 2.94 | 86.32 ± 5.92 |
|  | 78 | 43.25 ± 5.18 | 67.73 ± 7.85[**] | 65.77 ± 3.73[**] | 49.66 ± 8.90 | 85.47 ± 8.81 |
| LDL (mg/dl) | 71 | 14.65 ± 8.47 | 13.40 ± 4.28[*] | 12.96 ± 5.82[*] | 14.12 ± 5.50 | −12.04 ± 4.18 |
|  | 78 | 17.24 ± 6.97 | 6.09 ± 5.38[**] | 4.08 ± 9.64[**] | 12.04 ± 4.12 | −11.31 ± 3.05 |

Data represent Means ± S.E.M ($n = 6$). For each serum parameter, Means with different symbol [*], [**] along columns, are significantly different ($p < 0.05$)

Table 2 shows the effect of salt loading for 70 days on the mean plasma glucose, serum albumin, globulin and total protein levels (mg/dl) of normal rabbits. All the groups given salt load (groups A, B, C and D) showed significantly ($P < 0.05$) higher levels of albumin and significantly lower levels of globulin, as compared with the control (group E), after 70 days of salt loading. Administration of the extracts (aqueous or ethanol) of *Acalypha wilkesiana* leaves, at a dose of 300 mg/kg body weight for a period of 1 week, resulted in significantly ($P > 0.05$) lower levels of albumin, total protein and significantly higher levels of globulin.

## Discussion

Hypertriglyceridemia is a recognized risk factor for coronary heart disease [17]. High triglyceride (TG) is a trait common in many conditions, including insulin resistance, hypertension, and centrally mediated obesity [18], and in lipase deficiency [19, 20]. Increased risk is thought to be manifested largely through a reduction in HDL cholesterol [17]. However, since elevated triglycerides result in significantly altered composition of all plasma lipoproteins, the contribution of other pathways to this increased pathology is possible.

As with the effect of salt load on plasma glucose levels of the experimental animals, the serum triglyceride also decreased due to salt loading. This may signify increased energy metabolism in the animals. Increased sodium also stimulated increased lipolysis and glycogenesis. This may be responsible for the decreases in the levels of glucose and triglycerides. Treatment with the extracts resulted in further decreases in the plasma glucose levels and significantly higher serum triglycerides, as compared with the untreated group. This may suggest a sparing effect of the plant on the triglycerides breakdown with consequent increase in glucose utilization. Thus, salt loading

tends to increase the breakdown of triglycerides or increase the rate of lipolysis.

The liver both produces and breaks down cholesterol, as needed. Broken down cholesterol is normally excreted into the bile, but with chronic hepatitis C, there is sometimes a blockage of bile flow either inside the liver (due to cirrhosis) or outside the liver (most often due to gallstones), as a result of which blood cholesterol rises. The more the bile flow is obstructed, the more elevated the cholesterol will become. The increase in total cholesterol may be due to cirrhosis or gallstones, since it is significant. The significantly lower cholesterol levels after treatment with the extract may be possibly due to the steroids (phytosterols) constituent of the plant leaves [4], as reported in our previous study of the plant, which is higher in the ethanol extract. The plasma cholesterol-lowering properties of plant sterols have been known since the 1950s [21]. The composition of plant sterols and plant stanols lowers blood cholesterol levels by inhibiting the absorption of dietary and endogenously produced cholesterol from the small intestine and the plant sterols/stanols are only poorly absorbed themselves.

Cholesterol contained in HDL particles is considered beneficial for the cardiovascular health, in contrast to "bad" LDL cholesterol [22]. HDL serves to remove cholesterol from peripheral cells to the liver, where the cholesterol is converted to bile acids and excreted into the intestine [23]. This function may be affected by salt load as it resulted in lower serum HDL-cholesterol levels of the experimental animals. After 1 week of treatment with the extracts (aqueous or ethanol) of *Acalypha wilkesiana* leaves, the HDL-cholesterol levels were seen to be significantly higher in the treated groups, when compared with the untreated group (D). This indicates the possible protective or beneficial effect of the plant with respect to cardiovascular health. An inverse relationship between HDL-cholesterol levels in serum and the

**Table 2** Plasma Glucose (mg/dl) and serum Albumin, Globulin, Total Protein (g/dl) of salt-loaded rabbits; treated with aqueous (B) and ethanol (C) extracts of *Acalypha wilkesiana* leaves, continuous salt loading (A), salt loaded and non-treated (D), non-loaded and non-treated (E)

|  | DAY | GROUPS | | | | |
|---|---|---|---|---|---|---|
|  |  | A (Cont. Salt) | B (Salt + Aq.Ext) | C (Salt + Et.Ext) | D (Salt + NoExt) | E (Control) |
| PLASMA GLUCOSE (mg/dl) | 71 | 74.13 ± 8.82 | 73.33 ± 8.11 | 77.47 ± 6.85 | 76.53 ± 6.33 | 94.80 ± 5.05 |
|  | 78 | 72.75 ± 2.79 | 66.75 ± 0.82 | 67.26 ± 0.83 | 80.23 ± 4.67 | 95.30 ± 4.52 |
| SERUM ALBUMIN (g/dl) | 71 | 6.33 ± 0.74 | 6.15 ± 1.08* | 5.87 ± 0.43* | 5.60 ± 0.54 | 2.92 ± 0.18 |
|  | 78 | 7.08 ± 0.09 | 3.58 ± 0.42** | 2.70 ± 0.32** | 4.57 ± 0.39 | 2.85 ± 0.26 |
| SERUM GLOBULIN (g/dl) | 71 | 1.16 ± 0.83 | 1.08 ± 0.29* | 1.15 ± 1.05* | 1.07 ± 0.15 | 3.67 ± 1.29 |
|  | 78 | 1.02 ± 0.35 | 1.95 ± 0.94* | 2.03 ± 0.22* | 1.56 ± 0.54 | 3.71 ± 0.68 |
| SERUM TOTAL PROTEIN (g/dl) | 71 | 6.48 ± 0.17 | 6.66 ± 0.10* | 6.89 ± 1.57* | 6.28 ± 0.06 | 7.39 ± 1.01 |
|  | 78 | 6.11 ± 0.24 | 4.02 ± 0.35** | 4.79 ± 0.17** | 6.62 ± 0.38 | 7.59 ± 0.85 |

Data represent Means ± S.E.M ($n = 6$). For each serum parameter, Means with different symbol *, ** along columns, for each parameter, are significantly different ($p < 0.05$)

incidence or prevalence of coronary heart disease (CHD) has been demonstrated in a number of epidemiological studies. The importance of HDL-cholesterol as a risk factor for CHD is however recognized [24].

Studies have repeatedly demonstrated a strong association between both total and LDL-cholesterol concentration and coronary heart risk. There is a strong link between mean fat consumption, mean serum cholesterol concentration and the prevalence of coronary heart disease. The exception is where cardiovascular risk is only moderate-perhaps owing to high alcohol consumption [25]. In recent times, there has been a decline in the prevalence of atherosclerosis and atherosclerosis –related deaths possibly due to effective management of the risk factors that predispose to this disorder. The major identified risk factors are elevated LDL-cholesterol, reduced HDL-cholesterol [26] hypertension and non-insulin dependent diabetes mellitus [27]. Lowering of serum lipid concentrations, particularly LDL and VLDL fractions is therefore considered as one of the strategies that can delay the on-set of chronic disorders associated with hyperlipidemia in humans. The plant (*A. wilkesiana*) may be beneficial in this respect, since treatment with the extracts of the leaves resulted in decreases in the serum levels of LDL-cholesterol and corresponding increases in the serum levels of HDL-cholesterol.

According to the low-density-lipoprotein (LDL) receptor hypothesis, development of atherosclerosis is caused by a high concentration of LDL-cholesterol in the blood. Lowering LDL-cholesterol concentration therefore reverses, or at least retards the onset of atherosclerosis, thus preventing cardiovascular disease. Research findings have proved that lowering the concentrations of plasma lipids could diminish the complications of atherosclerosis and hypertension thereby prolonging life [28, 29].

The observations that salt increases glycaemic response attracted considerable attention in the light of the observed association between hypertension and diabetes [30, 31]. Reports by Yang et al. [32], Idowu et al. [33] and Ma et al. [34] had further highlighted some of the severe complications associated with both diseases. However, the plant may be a potential hypoglycemic or anti-diabetic agent, since it had a reducing effect on the plasma glucose levels.

Total protein, a measurement of all the proteins in the blood (many of which are produced by the liver), is a test of the functional status of the liver. Salt loading had no effect on serum total protein (g/dl) of the experimental animals. However, administration of the extracts resulted in significant decreases in the levels of total protein. This may be connected with the protein content of the leave which is lower in the aqueous extract and higher in the ethanol extract, comparatively [3], as our previous study showed. Proteins demonstrate numerous

biological functions such as enzymes, regulator of metabolism, as antibodies and component of complement system. Plasma proteins maintain the osmotic pressure of plasma. They transport hormones, vitamins, metals and drugs often serving as reservoirs for their use. Most plasma proteins are synthesized in the liver, and are of relevance to the clinical laboratory. The most common changes in the protein concentration in disease result from the acute phase reaction proteins. Examples of such proteins are $X_1$-antitrypsin, $\alpha$-acid glycoprotein, ceruloplasmin, Albumin, transferin hepaloglobin etc. [35]

Salt loading resulted in significantly higher serum albumin (g/dl) in all the groups given salt load. Albumin is essential for maintaining the oncotic pressure in the vascular system. The increase in albumin levels due to salt loading may be an attempt by the homeostatic mechanism of the animals to balance the effect of increased oncotic pressure due to salt load. Albumin helps in transporting small molecules through the blood, including bilirubin, calcium, progesterone, and medications [36], and plays an important role in keeping the fluid from the blood from leaking out into the tissues. However, administration of the extracts resulted in significant decreases in the serum albumin levels of the treated groups. Since sustained increase in sodium and chloride ions (occasioned by salt loading) expands asymptotically the extracellular fluid space by inducing thirst and water drinking and causing, through its osmotic action, an internal redistribution of fluid from the intra- to extracellular compartment, the liver possibly up-regulated the synthesis of albumin to balance the oncotic pressure to ensure normal physiology. This however, may be countered by the effect of the plant as occasioned by the decrease in albumin levels after treatment with the extracts (aqueous or ethanol). In those with ascites, a complication of liver cirrhosis that results in an abnormal accumulation of fluid in the abdomen, there may also be up-regulated albumin synthesis, but blood levels will be low due to the larger volume of distribution.

Salt loading resulted in significantly lower levels of serum globulin. The globulins perform a number of enzymatic functions in the plasma, but equally important, they are principally responsible for the body's both natural and acquired immunity against invading organisms [37]. High salinity tends to decrease or depress the normal synthesis of globulin in the experimental animals, which was relieved at cessation of salt load, as indicated in the untreated group. Administration of the extracts however, also resulted in an increase in the globulin levels, with the aqueous extract shown to be significantly higher. This may be connected with the actions of some of the phytochemical constituents of this plant like the flavonoids, saponins and anthraquinones [5], which are related to immune functions.

## Conclusion

Salt loading resulted in; increased LDL-cholesterol, total cholesterol, albumin and decreased triglycerides, HDL-cholesterol, globulin, which are risk factors for cardio-vascular diseases. But treatment with *Acalypha wilkesiana* leave extracts (aqueous or ethanol) had a reducing effect on the serum LDL-cholesterol, total cholesterol, albumin, total protein and an increasing effect on HDL-cholesterol, globulin, which is beneficial in the management of cardiovascular diseases. Thus, *Acalypha wilkesiana* may be useful, as claimed in traditional medicine, in the management of cardiovascular diseases.

### Abbreviations

ALB: Albumin; Aq.: Aqueous; BCG: Bromocresol green; CHD: Coronary Heart Disease; CHOL: Cholesterol; CVD: Cardiovascular Diseases; Et.: Ethanol; Ext.: Extract; GLOB: Globulin; HDL: High Density Lipoprotein; LDL: Low Density Lipoprotein; S.E.M: Standard Error of Mean; TG: Triglycerides; TP: Total Protein; VLDL: Very Low Density Lipoprotein

### Acknowledgments

The Authors are grateful to the authorities of Department of Biochemistry, University of Benin (Edo State, Nigeria) for providing the necessary laboratory facilities.

### Authors' contributions

OK: Concepts, Design, Experimental Studies, Data acquisition and Analysis, Manuscript preparation, Statistical Analysis. AAM: Concepts, Design, Experimental Studies, Data acquisition and Analysis. IOS: Design, Experimental Studies, Data acquisition and Analysis. All authors read and approved the final manuscript.

### Competing interests

The authors wish to state that there are no competing interests associated with this publication and there has been no significant financial support for this work that could have influenced its outcome.

### Author details

[1]Department of Biochemistry, College of Basic Medical Sciences, Igbinedion University, Okada, Edo State, Nigeria. [2]Department of Biochemistry, Faculty of Natural Sciences, Ambrose Alli University, Ekpoma, Edo State, Nigeria. [3]Department of Biochemistry, Faculty of Life Sciences, University of Benin, Benin, Edo State, Nigeria.

### References

1. Jody LG, Jennifer JD, Shannon LL, Paul WS, David GE, William BF. Dietary sodium loading impairs microvascular function independent of blood pressure in humans: role of oxidative stress. J Physiol. 2012;590:5519–28.
2. Joe B, Shapiro JI. Molecular mechanisms of experimental salt-sensitive hypertension. JAHA. 2012;1:3.
3. Omage K, Azeke AM, Ihimire II, Idagan AM. Phytochemical, proximate and elemental analysis of Acalypha Wilkesiana leaves. Scientific Journal of Pure and Applied Sciences. 2013;2(9):323–31.
4. Omage K, Azeke AM. Medicinal potential of *Acalypha wilkesiana* leaves. Advances in Research (AIR). 2014b;2(11):655–65.
5. Enwa FO. A preliminary study on antibacterial efficacy of the Methanolic extract of *Acalypha wilkesiana* leaves against selected clinical isolates. Adv Life Sci Technol. 2014;18:72–6.
6. Iyekowa O, Oviawe AP, Ndiribe JO. Antimicrobial activities of *Acalypha Wilkesiana* (red Acalypha) extracts in some selected skin pathogens Zimbabwe. J Sci Technol. 2016;11:48–57.
7. Akinloye DI, Osatuyi OA, Musibau OG, Yusuf AA, Adewuyi S. In vitro antioxidant activities, elemental analysis and some bioactive constituents of *Acalypha wilkesiana* Muell Arg and *Acalypha wilkesiana* java white leaf extracts. J Chem Soc Nigeria. 2016;41(2):150–7.
8. Omage K, Azeke AM. Serum Aminotransferase activities and Bilirubin levels in salt loaded experimental rabbits treated with aqueous and ethanol extracts of *Acalypha wilkesiana* leave. Nigeria Journal of Experimental and Clinical Biosciences. 2014a;2(1):37–41.
9. Omage K, Azeke AM, Orhue NEJ. Implications of oral administration of extracts of *Acalypha wilkesiana* leave on serum electrolytes, urea and creatinine in normal experimental rabbits. Biokemistri. 2015;27(2):56–62.
10. Neetu M, Neelima S. Blood viscosity, lipid profile and lipid peroxidation in Type-1 diabetic patients with good and poor Glycemic control. N Am J Med Sci. 2013;5(9):562–6.
11. Leticia O, Alberto D, George G, Nina V, Jorge M, Hirian A. Diets Containing Sea cucumber (Isostichopus badionotus) meals are Hypocholesterolemic in young rats. PLoS One. 2014;
12. Seth SM, Micheal JB, Mohamed BE, Eliot AB, Peter PT, John WM. Friedewald-estimated versus directly measured low-density lipoprotein cholesterol and treatment implications. J Am Coll Cardiol. 2013;62(8):732–9.
13. Basu S, Yoffe P, Hills N, Lustig RH. The relationship of sugar to population-level diabetes prevalence: an econometric analysis of repeated cross-sectional data. PLoS One. 2013;8(2):e57873.
14. Renjie Q, Yongxu C, Xuxiong H, Xugan W, Xiaozhen Y, Rui T. Effect of hypoxia on immunological, physiological response, and Hepatopancreatic metabolism of juvenile Chinese mitten crab Eriocheir Sinensis. Aquac Int. 2011;19(2):283–99.
15. Dipali JS, Hitesh AV, Mahesh KV, Ashok BK, Ravishankar BA. Comparative study on chronic Administration of go Ghrita (cow ghee) and Avika Ghrita (ewe ghee) in albino rats. Ayu. 2012;33(3):435–40.
16. Bates RG, Paabo M. Measurement of ph. In: Lundblad RL, editor. Handbook of biochemistry and molecular biology. 4th ed. Boca Raton: F. MacDonald Press; 2010. p. 709–13.
17. Paul SJ, Donald AS, Adi EM, Om G, Yehuda H, Helena WR, Mark DS, John AS. America Association of Clinical Endocrinologists' guidelines for Management of Dyslipidemia and Prevention of atherosclerosis. Endocr Pract. 2012;18(1):1–78.
18. Michael M, Neil JS, Christie B, Vera B, Michael HC, Henry NG. Triglycerides and cardiovascular disease: a scientific statement from the America heart association. Circulation. 2011;123:2292–333.
19. Elizabeth KY, Cynthia C, Daniel LS. HDL-ApoE content regulates the displacement of hepatic lipase from cell surface Proteoglycans. Am J Pathol. 2009;175(1):448–57.
20. Iseghohi SO, Orhue NEJ, Omage K. Pre-exposure to *Dennettia tripetala* Ethanolic fruit extract prevents biochemical alterations in rats subsequently exposed to a single dose of carbon tetrachloride. Int J Pharmacol Phytochem Ethnomed. 6:8–16.
21. Zoe H, Julian SB. Plant sterols lower cholesterol, but increase risk for coronary heart disease. Online J Biol Sci. 2014;14(3):167–9.
22. Emma L. Cholesterol. Lipidomics Gateway. 2009;22:55–81.
23. Erifeta OG, Omage K, Uhumwangho SE, Njoya KH, Amegor OF, Okonkwo CA. Comparative evaluation of antioxidant effects of watermelon and Orange, and their effects on some serum lipid profile of Wistar albino rats. Int J of Nutri and Metab. 2011;3(8):97–102.
24. Erifeta OG, Omage K, Waliu AO. Comparative study on effects of water melon and Orange on Glycemic index, histopathology and body weight changes in Wistar albino rats following consumption. Asian J of Appl Sci. 2013;1(4):108–12.
25. Douglas BK. Iron behaving badly: inappropriate iron Chelation as a major contributor to the Aetiology of vascular and other progressive inflammatory degenerative diseases. BMC Med Genet. 2009;2:2.
26. Ime FA, Item JA, Edisua HI, Mary AI, Essien UE. Effect of traditional diets on oxidative stress and lipid profile of Alloxan induced diabetic rats. Afr J Food Sci. 2011;5(3):143–7.
27. Rama N, Reddy A. Antidiabetic activity of 2-amino-(5-Fluoro-2-Oxoindolin-3-ylidene) Benzoxazole-5-Carbohydrazide in rats. J Biomed Pharmaceut Res. 2014;3(6):78–81.

28. Enechi OC, Manyawo NL, Ugwu PCO. Effects of ethanol seed extract of Buccholzia coriacea (wonderful kola) on the lipid profile of albino rats. Afr J Biotechnol. 2013;12(32):5075–9.

29. Kevin CM, Andrea LL, Mathew SR, Mary RD, Belinda HJ, Shneyvas ED, James RB. Lipid-altering effects of a dietary supplement tablet containing free plant sterols and Stanols in men and women with primary Hypercholesterolaemia: a randomized placebo-controlled crossover trial. Int J Food Sci Nutr. 2012;63(4):476–82.

30. Ebadollah H, Samaz NP, Jahanbaksh S, Rasoul A, Kamran S. Association between diabetic retinopathy and left ventricular dysfunction in diabetic patients with unstable angina. J Cardiovasc Thoraxic Res. 2012;4(4):113–7.

31. Masaaki M, Machiko I, Kazuo I, Kimihiko A. Impaired fasting glucose as an independent risk factor for hypertension among healthy middle-aged Japanese subjects with optimal blood pressure: the Yuport medical checkup Centre retrospective cohort study. Diabetol Metab Syndr. 2013;5:81.

32. Yang H, Wang Q, Zhu D. Influence of Euonymus Alatus Sied extracts on MDCK proliferation and high concentration of glucose induced cell injury. Life Sci J. 2008;5(4):41–6.

33. Idowu AT, Peter GCO, Liasu AO, Reuben O. Influence of acute intake of cooking salt and laboratory salt on Glyceamic response to glucose loading in rats. Nat Sci. 2009;7(11):70–3.

34. Ma H, Yang Y, Cheng S. Transforming growth factor in diabetes and renal disease. Nat Sci. 2009;7(1):91–5.

35. Aghagboren CO, Uadia OP, Omage K. Comparative Hypoglyceamic properties of Scoparia Dulcis and Loranthus begwensis as well as their effects on some biochemical parameters in normal and Alloxan-induced diabetic rats. J Pharmaceut Biol. 2014;4(1):31–40.

36. Pratt DS. Liver chemistry and function tests. In: Feldman M, Friedman LS, Brandt LJ, editors. Sleisenger and Fordtran's gastrointestinal and liver disease. 9th ed. Philadelphia: Saunders Elsevier; 2010. chap 73.

37. Bruning A, Gingelmaier A, Friese K, Mylonas I. New prospects for nelfinavir in non-HIV related diseases. Curr Mol Pharmacol. 2010;3P:91–7.

# 6

# Bioactivities of *Bruguiera gymnorrhiza* and profiling of its bioactive polyphenols by HPLC-DAD

Imtiaz Mahmud, Md. Nazmul Hasan Zilani, Nripendra Nath Biswas and Bishwajit Bokshi[*]

## Abstract

**Background:** In folk medicine leaves and stem of *Bruguiera gymnorrhiza* (L.) are commonly used to treat diarrhea, fever, diabetes, pain and a number of ailments. The present study was carried out to explore antioxidant, analgesic and antidiarrhoeal activities of ethanol extract of leaves and stem of *B. gymnorrhiza* and also to analyze its major bioactive natural polyphenols by HPLC-DAD.

**Methods:** Total polyphenol content was spectrophotometrically determined using Folin Chiocalteu's reagent while the flavonoids by aluminum chloride colorimetric assay. Antioxidant activity was determined by DPPH free radical scavenging, reducing power, nitric oxide and hydrogen peroxide scavenging assays. Identification and quantification of bioactive polyphenols were done by HPLC-DAD method. Antidiarrhoeal activity of the extracts was evaluated using experimentally castor oil induced diarrhea in mice. Acetic acid induced writhing method was used to evaluate the analgesic activity. Acute oral toxicity and brine shrimp lethality assay were performed to check the cytotoxic potential.

**Results:** Both the leave and stem extracts contain significant amount of phenolic and flvonoid content. Extracts showed DPPH radical scavenging, nitric oxide, hydrogen peroxide scavenging and also concentration dependent reducing power activity. HPLC analysis of both extract indicated the presence of significant amount of vanillic acid along with other phenolic constituents. Both extracts showed significant ($P < 0.01$) analgesic and antidiarrhoeal activity. Furthermore, extracts showed negligible toxic effect.

**Conclusion:** Along with other phenolic compounds, vanillic acid present in the extract may be responsible for antioxidant, analgesic and antidiarrhoeal activities. Altogether these results rationalize the use of this plant in traditional medicine.

**Keywords:** Polyphenol, HPLC, Vanillic acid, Analgesic activity, Antidiarrhoeal activity

## Background

Natural products are supposed to be an important source of new chemical substances with potential therapeutic applications. The medicinal value of the plants lies in some chemical active substances that produce a definite pharmacological action on biological system. The most important of these chemically active constituents of plants are alkaloid, tannin, flavonoid and phenolic compounds [1, 2]. Since antiquity many plants are used as folk medicine to treat infectious diseases such as urinary tract infections, diarrhoea, cutaneous abscesses, bronchitis and parasitic diseases [3]. In the last few years, a number of studies have been conducted in different medicinal plants in different countries to prove the medicinal efficiency [4, 5]. Bangladesh owing to its favorable climatic influences has been blessed with massive natural resources including explored and unexplored medicinal plants [6, 7]. Several plant species of Bangladesh are traditionally used to treat different ailments. Some of them are also used to treat pain and diarrhea.

*Bruguiera gymnorrhiza* (L.) (Rhizophoraceae) is an evergreen mangrove tree, widely distributed in tropical and subtropical coastlines. In Bangladesh it is mainly found in the Sundarbans. In folk medicine fruits, barks

* Correspondence: bokshi06@yahoo.com
Pharmacy Discipline, Life Science School, Khulna University, Khulna 9208, Bangladesh

and leaves are commonly used to treat diarrhea, fever, diabetes, pain, burns, intestinal worms, and liver disorders [8]. Previous investigations on this plant have shown the presence of Brugunin A; Bruguierol D; Bruguierols A, B, C; Aminopyrine; 7,3′,4′,5′-tetrahydroxy-5-methoxyflavone; 3-β-(Z)-coumaroyllupeol; Menisdaurillide; Vomifoliol; Bruguiesulfurol; Apiculol; Steviol [9–11].

To the best of our knowledge, very few pharmacological studies have been reported so far on *B. gymnorrhiza*, the medicinal plant of the Sundarbans. As a part of the continuation of our research on bioactivity screening of Bangladeshi medicinal plants, present study was carried out to assess antioxidant, analgesic, antidiarrhoeal, activities and HPLC profiling of leaves and stem extracts of *B. gymnorrhiza* in order to scientifically evaluate the claimed biological activities.

## Methods

### Chemicals and reagents
2, 2-Diphenyl-1-picryldydrazyl (DPPH·), ascorbic acid, arbutin (AR), gallic acid (GA), hydroquinone (HR), (+)-catechin (CH), vanillic acid (VA), caffeic acid (CA), syringic acid (SA), (−)-epicatechin (EC), vanillin (VL), *p*-coumaric acid (PCA), *trans*-ferulic acid (TFA), rutin hydrate (RH), ellagic acid (EA), benzoic acid (BA), rosmarinic acid (RA), myricetin (MC), quercetin (QU), *trans*-cinnamic acid (TCA), kaempferol (KF) and butylated hydroxy toluene (BHT) were purchased from Sigma–Aldrich (St. Louis, MO, USA). Ethanol and HPLC grade acetonitrile, methanol, acetic acid were obtained from Merck (Darmstadt, Germany). Standard drug diclofenac sodium, loperamide hydrochloride and vincristine sulfate were purchased from Square Pharmaceuticals Ltd. and Beacon Pharmaceuticals Ltd. Bangladesh respectively.

### Plant materials and extraction
For the present investigation the leaf and stem of *Bruguiera gymnorrhiza* were collected from the Sundarban of Khulna, Bangladesh area in April 2015 and were identified by expert at the Bangladesh National Herbarium (Accession no.: DACB-41874), Dhaka, Bangladesh. The shade dried plant parts were ground into a coarse powder with the help of a suitable grinder (Capacitor start motor, Wuhu motor factory, China). About 150 gm powder of stem and 250 gm of leaf were macerated in 800 ml and 1000 ml of 95% ethanol of about twelve days. After filtration and evaporation of solvent the yield of the stem and leaf extract was 2.8 and 6.7% w/w respectively and it was stored at 4 °C until analysis commenced.

### Experimental animals
Young Swiss-albino mice aged 4–5 weeks, average weight 18–25 g were used for the experiment. The mice were purchased from the Animal Research Branch of the International Centre for Diarrhoeal Disease and Research, Bangladesh (ICDDR, B). They were kept in standard environmental condition (Temperature of 24 ± 1 °C; 12 h light and dark cycle with controlled humidity) for one week for adaptation after purchase and fed standard pellet diet and water *ad libitum* properly.

### Phytochemical screening
Qualitative phytochemical tests were carried out for the identification of alkaloids, glycosides, flavonoids, saponins, tannin, gums, and terpenoids in the samples [12]. Alkaloids were detected using the Dragendroff's, Mayer's, Hager's and Wagner's tests. Lead acetate, alkaline reagent, ferric chloride and ammonia tests were used for detection of flavonoids. Legal's test, Molisch, Keller-Kiliani and Borntrager's tests were performed to identify glycosides. For identification of tannin potassium dichromate test, ferric chloride, potassium hydroxide and lead acetate tests were followed. Salkowski test and froth test were used to detect the presence of terpenoids and for saponins respectively. Molisch test was performed for detecting the existence of gum in the samples.

### Total phenolic content
The total phenolic content of the extracts of *B. gymnorrhiza* was determined by the modified Folin-Ciocalteu method [13]. In 0.5 ml extract (1 mg/ml), 5 ml of 10% (v/v) Folin-Ciocalteu reagent and 4 ml of sodium carbonate (75 g/L) solution were added. The mixture was vortexed for 15 s and allowed to incubate at 40 °C for 30 min. The absorbance of the resultant mixture was measured at 765 nm against the suitable blank by using Shimadzu UV-visible spectrophotometer (Model 1800, Japan). The standard curve was prepared using different concentration (0.1 to 0.5 mg/mL) of gallic acid.. Based on the measured absorbance of the extracts, total phenolic content of both extracts was calculated and expressed in terms of milligram of gallic acid equivalent (GAE) per gram of dry extract.

### Total flavonoid content
The total flavonoid content of the extracts was determined according to aluminum chloride colorimetric method [14]. In 1 ml extract solution (1 mg/ml), 4 ml distilled water and 0.3 ml sodium nitrate (50 g/L) were successively mixed. Five minutes later, 0.3 ml aluminum chloride (100 g/L) was added to the mixture with constant shaking. At the sixth minute 2 ml of 1 M sodium hydroxide was added and the volume was adjusted to 10 ml. Then absorbance was measured at 510 nm. For this assay quercetin was used as standard. Based on the measured absorbance of the extracts, Quercetin

Equivalent (QE) was calculated from the calibration line and then total flavonoid content (TFC) in plant extract was expressed in terms of milligram of quercetin equivalent (QE) per gram of dry extract.

### DPPH radical scavenging assay

Quantitative measurements of radical scavenging assay were carried out according to the method described by Khirul *et al.* [15]. The reaction mixture contained 2 ml of extract at concentration ranging from 1 to 512 µg/ml and 6 ml of a 0.04% (w/v) solution of DPPH in methanol. The commercial known antioxidant, ascorbic acid was used for comparison. Discolouration was measured at 517 nm by using spectrophotometer after incubation of 30 min in the darkroom. Measurement was performed at least in triplicate. The percentage of the DPPH free radical was calculated using the following equation:

$$\text{DPPH scavenging effect } (\%) = ((A_0 - A_1)/A_0) \times 100$$

Where, $A_0$ was the absorbance of the control and $A_1$ was the absorbance in the presence of the extract. The $IC_{50}$ (concentration providing 50% inhibition) values were calculated using the dose inhibition curve in linear range by plotting the extract concentration versus the corresponding scavenging effect.

### Reducing power assay

The reducing power was determined according to the method of Sanjib *et al.* [16]. An alequite of 1 ml of various concentrations of extracts (10-100 µg/ml) were mixed with 2.5 ml of 200 mmol/l sodium phosphate buffer (pH 6.6) and 2.5 ml of 1% potassium ferricyanide. The mixture was incubated at 50 °C for 20 min. After 2.5 ml of 10% trichloroacetic acid was being added, the mixture was centrifuged at 3000 rpm for 10 min. 5 mL of this mixture was mixed with 5 mL of deionised water and 1 ml of 0.1% of ferric chloride, and ten minutes later the absorbance was measured at 700 nm. The assays were carried out in triplicate and the results were expressed as mean values ± standard deviations. Ascorbic acid was used as standard.

### Hydrogen peroxide scavenging assay

The scavenging capacity for hydrogen peroxide was measured according to the method of Rahmat *et al.* [17]. A solution of hydrogen peroxide (2 mM) was prepared in 50 mM phosphate buffer (pH 7.4). Hydrogen peroxide concentration was determined spectrophotometrically at 230 nm absorption using the molar extinction coefficient for hydrogen peroxide of 81 $M^{-1}cm^{-1}$. Then 1 ml of various concentrations (25–250 µg/ml) of extracts, ascorbic acid was transferred into the test tubes and their volumes were made up to 4 ml with 50 mM phosphate buffer (pH 7.4) or solvent (methanol). After addition of 6 ml hydrogen peroxide solution, tubes were vortexed and absorbance of the hydrogen peroxide at 230 nm was determined after 10 min, against a suitable blank. 50 mM phosphate buffer without hydrogen peroxide was used as blank. Hydrogen peroxide scavenging ability (in triplicate) was calculated by the formula:

$$\% \text{ scavenging } = (1 - A_e/A_o) \times 100$$

Where, $A_o$ is the absorbance without sample, and $A_e$ is absorbance with sample.

### Nitric oxide scavenging assay

Nitric oxide scavenging activity was measured spectrophotometrically according to Usha and Suriyavathana [18]. Three millilitres of 10 mM Sodium nitroprusside in 0.2 M phosphate buffered saline (pH 7.4) was mixed with different concentrations (5–100 µg/ml) of extracts and incubated at room temperature for 150 min. After incubation time, 0.5 ml of Griess reagent (1% sulfanilamide, 0.1% naphthylethylene diamine dihydrochloride in 2% $H_3PO_4$) was added. The absorbance of the chromophore formed during diazotization of the nitrite with sulphanilamide and subsequent coupling with naphthylethylenediaminedihydrochloride was read at 546 nm. Ascorbic acid was used as standard in this study. Percentage radical scavenging activity of the sample was calculated as follows: % NO radical scavenging activity = (control OD- sample OD/control OD) × 100. The analysis was performed in triplicate. The sample concentration providing 50% inhibition ($IC_{50}$) under the assay condition was calculated from the graph of inhibition percentage against sample concentration.

### HPLC detection and quantification of polyphenolic compounds

Chromatographic analyses were carried out on a Thermo Scientific DionexUltiMate 3000 Rapid Separation LC (RSLC) systems (Thermo Fisher Scientific Inc., MA, USA), coupled to a quaternary rapid separation pump (LPG-3400RS), Ultimate 3000RS autosampler (WPS-3000) and rapid separation diode array detector (DAD-3000RS). Phenolic compounds were separated on Acclaim® C18 (4.6 × 250 mm; 5 µm) column (Dionix, USA) which was controlled at 30 °C using a temperature controlled column compartment (TCC-3000).

The phenolic composition of the leaves & stem extract of *B. gymnorrhiza* was determined by HPLC, as described by Sarunya & Sukon with some modifications [18]. The mobile phase consisted of acetonitrile (solvent A), acetic acid solution pH 3.0 (solvent B), and methanol (solvent C). The system was run with the following gradient elution program: 0 min, 5% A/95%B; 10 min, 10% A/80% B/10%C; 20 min, 20% A/60% B/20%C and 30 min, 100%A. There was a 5 min post run at initial conditions for equilibration of the column. The flow rate was kept constant throughout the analysis at 1 ml/min and the injection volume was 20 µl. For UV detection, the wavelength program was optimized to monitor phenolic compounds at their respective maximum absorbance wavelengths as follows: λ 280 nm held for 18.0 min, changed to λ 320 nm and held for 6 min, and finally changed to λ 380 nm and held for the rest of the analysis and the diode array detector was set at an acquisition range from 200 nm to 700 nm. The detection and quantification of GA, CH, VA, CA, and EC was done at 280 nm, of PCA, RH, and EA at 320 nm, and of MC, QU, and KF at 380 nm, respectively.

A stock standard solution (100 µg/ml) of each phenolic compound was prepared in methanol by weighing out approximately 0.0050 g of the analyte into 50 ml volumetric flask. The mixed standard solution was prepared by diluting the mixed stock standard solutions in methanol to give a concentration of 5 µg/ml for each polyphenols except (+)-catechin hydrate, caffeic acid, rutin hydrate (4 µg/ml) and quercetin (3 µg/ml). All standard solutions were stored in the dark at 5 °C and were stable for at least three months. The calibration curves of the standards were made by a dilution of the stock standards (five set of standard dilutions) with methanol to yield 1.0–5.0 µg/ml for GA, CH, VA, EC, PCA, EA, MC, KF; 0.5–4.0 µg/ml for CH, CA, RH, and 0.25–3.0 µg/ml for QU. The calibration curves were constructed from chromatograms as peak area vs. concentration of standard.

Solution of ethanol extracts (leaves & stem) of *B. gymnorrhiza* at a concentration of 10 mg/ml was prepared in ethanol by vortex mixing (Branson, USA) for 30 min. The samples were stored in the dark at low temperature (5 °C). Spiking the sample solution with phenolic standards was done for additional identification of individual polyphenols. Prior to HPLC analysis, all solutions (mixed standards, sample, and spiked solutions were filtered through 0.20 µm nylon syringe filter (Sartorius, Germany) and then degassed in an ultrasonic bath (Hwashin, Korea) for 15 min [19].

## Analgesic activity

Analgesic activity of the extracts was tested using the model of acetic acid induced writhing in mice [20]. The experimental laboratory mice were arbitrarily divided in six groups each containing six mice. The first group, treated as control group, was administered orally with 1% (v/v) Tween-80 in distilled water at the dose of 10 ml/kg body weight. The second group received standard diclofenac sodium (25 mg/kg). Third to sixth groups were treated with the extract at the doses of 250 and 500 mg/kg body weight. Experimental samples, standard drug and control vehicle were administered orally 30 min prior to intraperitoneal administration of 0.7% of acetic acid. After an interval of 5 min, the number of writhes was counted for a period of 15 min. The number of writhes in the second, third, fourth, fifth and sixth groups were compared to that of the control group to calculate the percent inhibition of writhing calculated using the formula: % Inhibition of writhing $= (1 - W_0/W_1) \times 100$; Where, $W_1$ and $W_0$ represent the mean writhing of the control and standard or sample groups, respectively.

## Antidiarrhoeal activity

Antidiarrhoeal activity of the extracts was assessed according to Bokshi *et al.* [21]. The mice were all screened initially by giving 0.3 ml of castor oil and only those showing diarrhoea were selected for the final experiment. The test animals were randomly chosen and divided into six groups having six mice in each; they were accurately weighed & properly marked of the experimental groups, group-I or the control received only distilled water containing 1% Tween-80. Group-II or standard received standard antimotility drug, Loperamide at a dose of 3 mg/kg-body weight as oral suspension. The test groups (III, IV, Vand VI) were treated with suspension of leaf and stem extracts at the oral dose of 250 & 500 mg/kg-body weight. Test samples, control and loperamide were given orally by means of a feeding needle. Individual animals of each group were placed in separate cages having adsorbent paper beneath and examined for the presence of diarrhoea every hour in four hours of experimental period. Number of stools or any fluid material that stained the adsorbent paper were counted at each successive hour during the 4 h period and were noted for each mouse. The latent period of each mouse also counted. At the beginning of each hour new papers were placed for the old ones. During an observation period of 4 h, the total number of fecal output including diarrheic feces excreted by the animals was recorded. A numerical score based on stool consistency was assigned as normal stool (1) and watery stool (2).

## Acute toxicity test

Acute oral toxicity of the extracts was assessed in mice according to the guidelines of the Organization for Economic Cooperation and Development [22]. The mice were fasted overnight (16 h), divided into 10 groups (n = 5) and the extracts were orally administered at the dose of 100, 200,400, 800 and 1000 mg/kg body weight. The control group received distilled water. Then individual observations for lethality and any physical sign of toxicity of mice were started during the first two hours continuously and then at six hours interval for 24 h time period and finally after every 24 h up to 14 days.

## Cytotoxic activity

Cytotoxic activity of extracts was carried out according to the Meyer method [23]. *Artemia salina* leach (brine shrimp eggs) was used as the test organism. It was hatched in simulated sea water. Two days were allowed to hatch the shrimp and to be matured as nauplii. Constant oxygen supply was carried out through the hatching time. For the experiment, 50 mg of the extracts was dissolved in dimethylsulfoxide (DMSO) and solutions of varying concentrations (400, 200, 100, 50, 25, 12.5, 6.25, 3.125, 1.563, 0.781 µg/ml) were prepared using simulated seawater. The concentration of DMSO in these test tubes did not exceed 10 µl/ml. The solutions were then added to the pre-marked vials containing 10 live brine shrimp nauplii in 5 ml simulated seawater. After 24 h, the vials were inspected and the number of survived nauplii in each vial was counted. From this data, the percent of lethality of the brine shrimp nauplii for each concentration of extracts and control was calculated. The lethal concentration $LC_{50}$ of the test samples after 24 h was obtained by a plot of percentage of the shrimps killed against the sample concentration (toxicant concentration) and the best fit line was obtained from the curve data by means of regression analysis. In this assay vincristin sulfate was used as standard.

## Statistical analysis

One-way ANOVA followed by Dunnett's test were performed and the results were considered statistically significant when $p < 0.05$. Data acquisition, peak integration, and calibrations in HPLC were performed with Dionix Chromeleon software (Version 6.80 RS 10).

## Results

In the phytochemical screening the extracts revealed the presence of some of the therapeutically active phytochemicals. Leaves extract showed the presence of anthraquinone glycosides, flavonoids, alkaloids, tannin, saponins and absence of terpenoid and gum. One the other hand, anthraquinone glycosides, flavonoids, alkaloids, tannin, saponins and gum were present and terpenoid was absent in the stem extract.

The absorbance values of different concentrations of gallic acid were plotted and a standard calibration curve (y = 8.8234x + 0.1616; $R^2$ = 0.9933) was found. The total polyphenol content of the stem and leaf extract was calculated using the equation and was found to be 40 mg and 33 mg GAE/g of dry extract respectively. Standard quercetin calibration curve (y = 0.5034x + 0.0075; $R^2$ = 0.9816) was used to estimate the total flavonoid content. And it was found to be 23 and 17 milligram quercetin equivalents per gram of the dry weight of stem and leaf extract respectively.

Identification and quantification of individual phenolic compounds in the extracts were analysed by HPLC. The chromatographic separations of polyphenols in standard and leaf and stem extract were shown in Figs. 1, 2 and 3 respectively. The content of each phenolic compound found in the leaf and stem extracts was calculated from the corresponding calibration curve and presented as the mean of five determinations as shown in Tables 1 and 2. The experimental results indicated that leaf extract contained gallic acid, vanillic acid, vanillin and ellagic acid whereas stem extract contained gallic acid, (+)-catechin, vanillic acid, vanillin, ellagic acid and

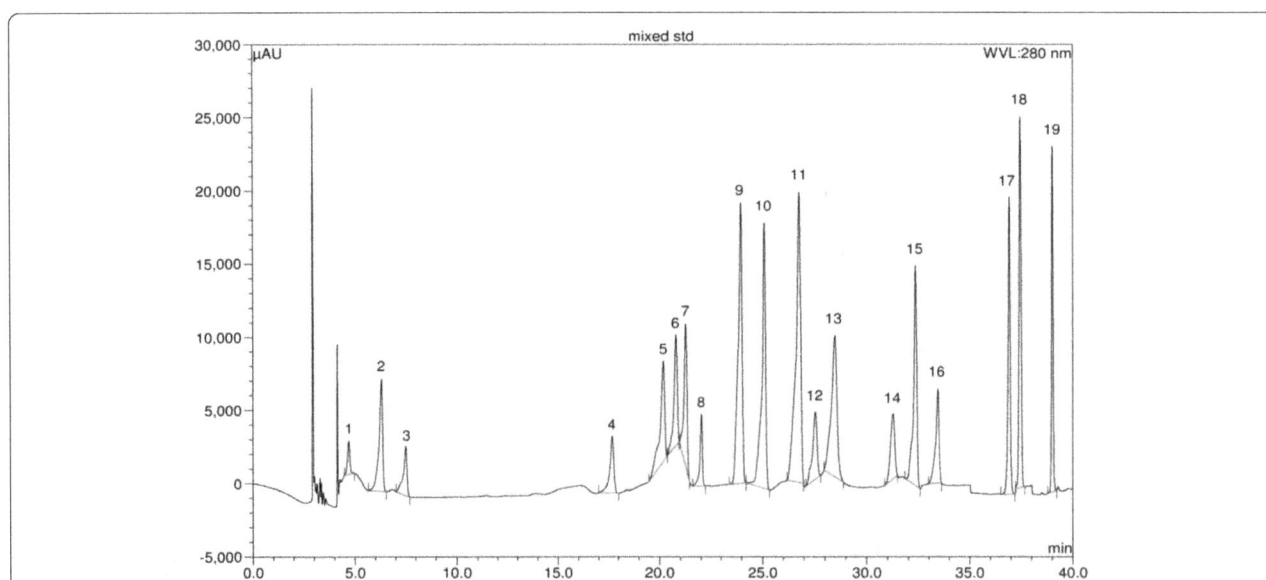

**Fig. 1** HPLC chromatogram of a standard mixture of polyphenolic compounds. (Peaks: 1: arbutin; 2: gallic acid; 3: hydroquinone; 4: (+)-catechin; 5: vanillic acid; 6: caffeic acid; 7: syringic acid; 8: (−)-epicatechin; 9: vanillin; 10: *p*-coumaric acid; 11: *trans*-ferulic acid; 12: rutin hydrate; 13: ellagic acid; 14: benzoic acid; 15: rosmarinic acid; 16: myricetin; 17: quercetin; 18: *trans*-cinnamic acid; 19: kaempferol)

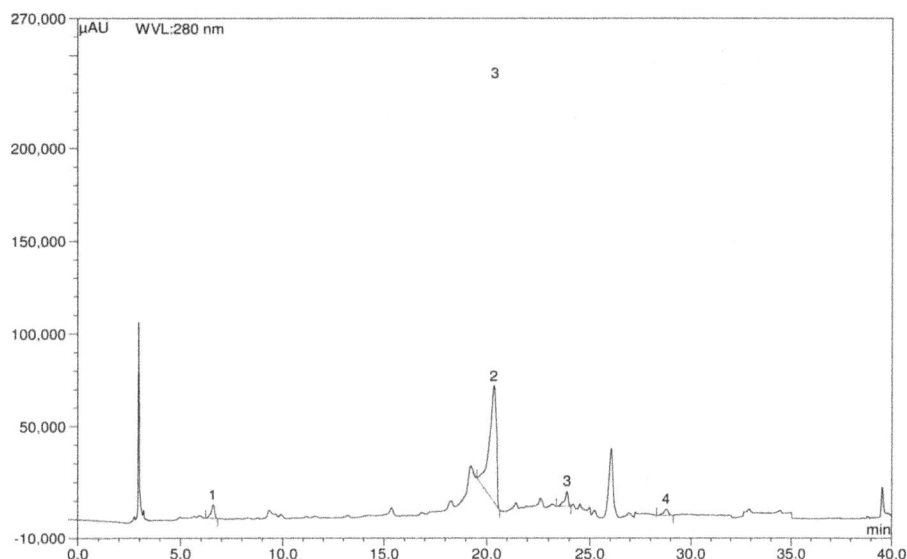

**Fig. 2** HPLC chromatogram of leaf extract. (Peaks: 1: gallic acid; 2: vanillic acid; 3: vanillin; 4: ellagic acid)

benzoic acid. Among these compounds vanillic acid was found the highest in both extracts.

### DPPH radical scavenging assay

In the DPPH free radical scavenging assay the $IC_{50}$ values of leaf and stem were found to be ~73 & ~62 µg/ml respectively that were comparable to standard ascorbic acid ($IC_{50} = $ ~14 µg/ml).

### Hydrogen peroxide scavenging assay

In the hydrogen peroxide scavenging assay the $IC_{50}$ value of ascorbic acid, leaf and stem were found to be ~45, ~174 & ~130 µg/ml respectively.

### Nitric oxide scavenging activity

In the nitric oxide scavenging assay the $IC_{50}$ value of ascorbic acid, leaf and stem were found to be ~17, ~97 & ~57 µg/ml respectively.

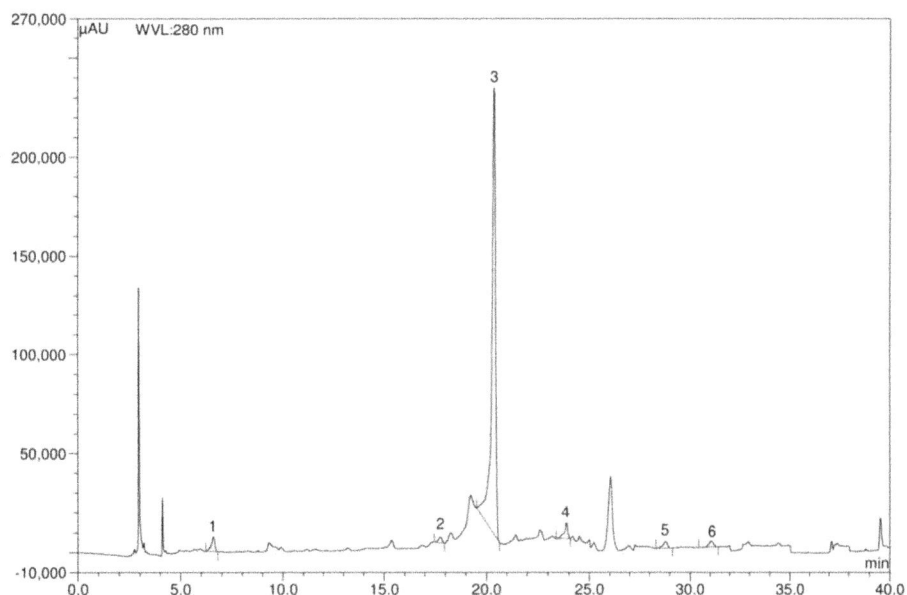

**Fig. 3** HPLC chromatogram of stem extract. (Peaks:1: gallic acid; 2: (+)-catechin; 3: vanillic acid; 4: vanillin; 5: ellagic acid; 6: benzoic acid)

**Table 1** Contents of polyphenolic compounds in the ethanol extract of leaf

| Polyphenolic compound | Ethanol extract of leaf | |
|---|---|---|
| | Content (mg/100 g of dry extract) | % RSD |
| GA | 7.25 | 0.07 |
| VA | 68.47 | 1.19 |
| VL | 10.09 | 0.11 |
| EA | 36.22 | 0.25 |

*RSD* Relative Standard Deviation

### Reducing power assay

At the concentrations of 10, 20, 40, 60, 80 and 100 µg/mL leaf and stem extract showed absorbance of 0.094, 0.108, 0.137, 0.186, 0.196, 0.217 and 0.127, 0.147, 0.194, 0.237, 0.295, 0.327 respectively while standard ascorbic acid showed absorbance of 0.493, 0.509, 0.518, 0.601, 0.648, and 0.684 respectively.

### Analgesic activity

The leaves extract used orally at different doses (250 mg/kg and 500 mg/kg) showed significant ($p < 0.01$) and dose dependent inhibition of pain responses (32.55 and 59.09% respectively) as compared to control group. On the other hand the stem extract at the dose of 250 and 500 mg/kg showed significant ($p < 0.01$) inhibition of pain responses (40.19 and 65.91% respectively) whereas standard diclofenac sodium (25 mg/kg) showed 80.27% writhing inhibition (Table 3). The stem extract showed more significant writhing inhibition in comparison to leaves extract.

### Antidiarrhoeal activity

In the castor oil induced diarrhoeal method, the leaves and stem extracts of *B. gymnorrhiza* produced a marked antidiarrhoeal effect in mice, as shown in Table 4. Thirty minutes after castor oil administration, all of the mice in the control group produced copious diarrhea. Pretreatment of mice with both the leaves and stem extract (250, 500 mg/kg, p.o.) dose dependently and significantly ($p < 0.01$) delayed the onset of diarrhea and reduced the frequency of

**Table 2** Contents of polyphenolic compounds in the ethanol extract of stem

| Polyphenolic compound | Ethanol extract of stem | |
|---|---|---|
| | Content (mg/100 g of dry extract) | % RSD |
| GA | 8.91 | 0.08 |
| CH | 6.05 | 0.05 |
| VA | 132.51 | 2.41 |
| VL | 11.64 | 0.13 |
| EA | 39.22 | 0.29 |
| BA | 19.83 | 0.16 |

*RSD* Relative Standard Deviation

**Table 3** Effect of extracts in acetic acid induced writhing in mice

| Treatment | Dose (mg/kg) | % Writhing | % Inhibition of writhing |
|---|---|---|---|
| Control | – | 100 | – |
| Standard | 25 | 19.73 | 80.27 ± 0.52* |
| Leaf extract | 250 | 67.45 | 32.55 ± 0.58* |
| Leaf extract | 500 | 40.91 | 59.09 ± 0.45* |
| Stem extract | 250 | 59.81 | 40.19 ± 0.58* |
| Stem extract | 500 | 34.09 | 65.91 ± 0.52 * |

*SD* standard deviation; *$p < 0.01$

defecation (Table 4). But the stem extract was more potent than leaves extract regarding the latent period and frequency of stool. Loperamide (3 mg/kg), a standard anti diarrhoeal drug markedly ($p < 0.01$) inhibited the diarrhoea.

### Acute toxicity test

The oral acute toxicity assessment of the extract at 100, 200, 400, 800 and 1000 mg/kg body weight resulted in no mortality and no observable signs of acute toxicity throughout 14 days. These results pointed out that the $LC_{50}$ (lethal concentration in 50%) value of the extract was greater than 1000 mg/kg body weight.

### Brine shrimp lethality bioassay

The cytotoxic activity of stem and leaves extracts of *B. gymnorrhiza* assayed by the brine shrimp lethality bioassay test. The effect of the extract was dose dependent. In this assay the leaves and stem extracts showed $LC_{50}$ value of 201.31 µg/ml and 232.09 µg/ml respectively whereas standard vincristine sulphate showed $LC_{50}$ value of 0.7158 µg/ml. No mortality was found in control group.

### Discussion

*Bruguiera gymnorrhiza* is ethnopharmacologically used for the treatment of various complaints. The therapeutic benefit of medicinal plants is usually attributed to their antioxidant properties. Phenolic compounds are known as high level antioxidants because of their ability to

**Table 4** Effect of leaf and stem extract on the latent period and of mean stool count of castor oil induced diarrhoeal episode in mice

| Treatment | Dose (mg/kg) | Mean Latent period (hr) | Mean no. of stools |
|---|---|---|---|
| 1% Tween 80 in water | – | 0.47 ± 0.03 | 5.66 ± 0.82 |
| Standard | 3 | 2.85 ± 0.07* | 2.17 ± 0.75* |
| Leaf extract | 250 | 0.58 ± 0.06* | 4.67 ± 0.52** |
| Leaf extract | 500 | 0.97 ± 0.14* | 4 ± 0.89* |
| Stem extract | 250 | 1.00 ± 0.14* | 3.83 ± 0.75* |
| Stem extract | 500 | 2.48 ± 0.18* | 3 ± 0.89* |

*SD* Standard Deviation; *$P < 0.01$; **$P < 0.05$

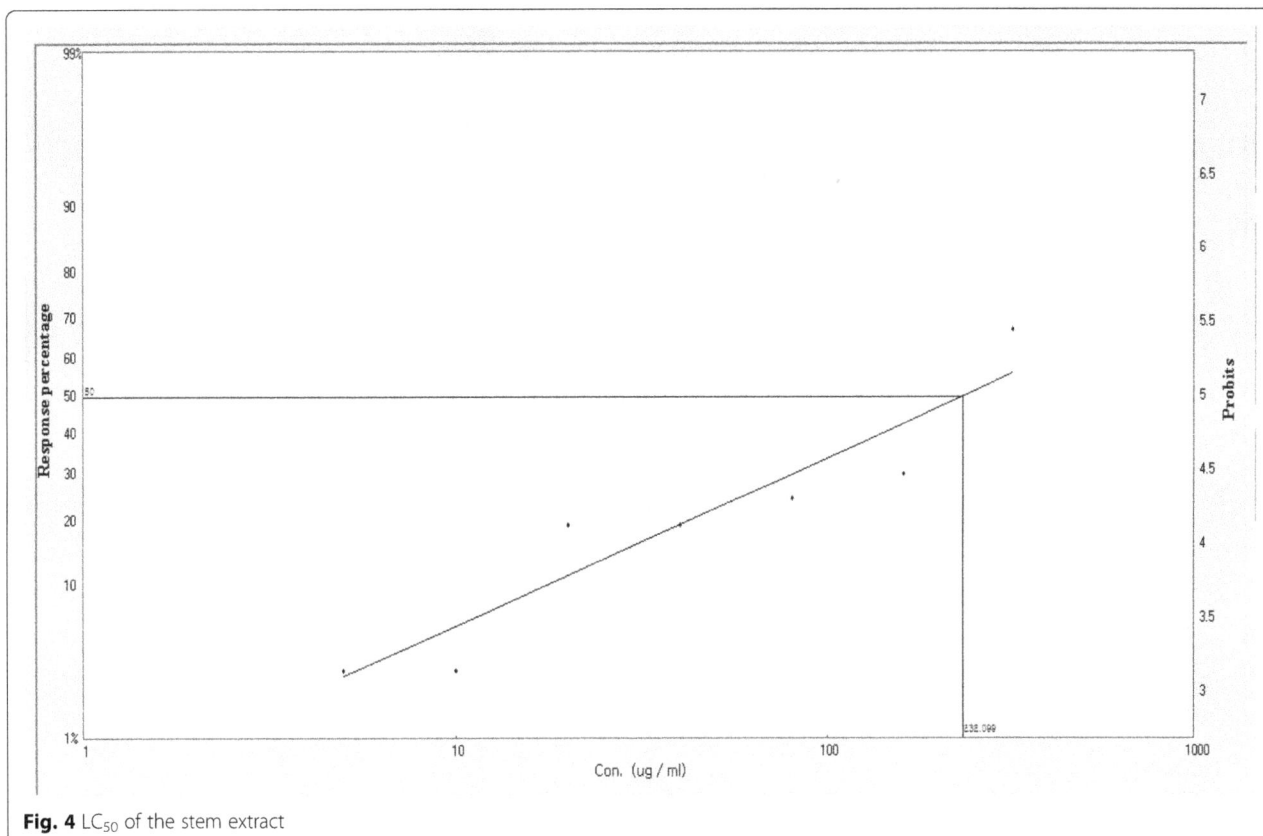

**Fig. 4** LC$_{50}$ of the stem extract

scavenge free radicals and active oxygen species such as singlet oxygen, superoxide anion radical and hydroxyl radicals [24, 25]. The structure as well as number and position of hydroxyl groups in polyphenols are essential for antioxidant activity [26–28]. The total polyphenol concentration of extract includes in addition to the principal phenolic antioxidants all the compounds that function as hydrogen donors in the plant material. Both extracts of B. gymnorrhiza contain significant amount of polyphenols and consequently significant antioxidant capacity found. Moreover, HPLC analyses of the both extracts indicate the presence of natural polyphenolic antioxidant compounds and it is supposed that these polyphenolic compounds may be responsible for antioxidant activity of the leaf and stem extract.

Analgesic activity of the both extracts was evaluated by acetic acid-induced writhing method that is the most sensitive and established method to assess analgesia. A few numbers of analgesics have been isolated from plants and thus require extensive studies to explore more analgesic agents from natural sources. Increased levels of local endogenous substances; PGE2, PGF2α as well as lipoxygenase derived eicosanoids in the peritoneal fluid have been reported to be responsible for pain sensation caused by intraperitoneal administration of acetic acid [29–31]. The writhing inhibition in mice

increased as concentration of the extracts was increased. From the present study it can be stated that stem extracts both at 250 and 500 mg per kg body weight were more potent than that of leaf (Table 3) as former produced remarkable writhing inhibition which was comparable to the standard diclofenac sodium. It is well established that various favonoids, alkaloids, steroids are involved in analgesic activity [32, 33]. In the phytochemical group tests of leaf extract, some major phytochemicals namely; alkaloids, steroids, glycosides, tannins, and flavonoids were identified whereas glycosides, flavonoids, alkaloids, tannin, saponins and gum were present in the stem extract. Besides, polyphenolic constituents namely (+)-catechin, ellagic acid and vannilin identified in the HPLC analysis, which showed analgesic activity in previous studies [34, 35]. Presence of slight increased amount of polyphenols as well as their synergistic action in stem extract may be responsible for more potent as an analgesic agent than other extracts.

Diarrhea can be described as the abnormally frequent defecation of feces of low consistency which may be due to a disturbance in the transport of water and electrolytes in the intestines. Although it is evidenced that ricinoleic acid produces diarrhea, recent study claims that nitric oxide in castor oil is responsible for the diarrheal effect [36, 37]. After oral ingestion of castor oil,

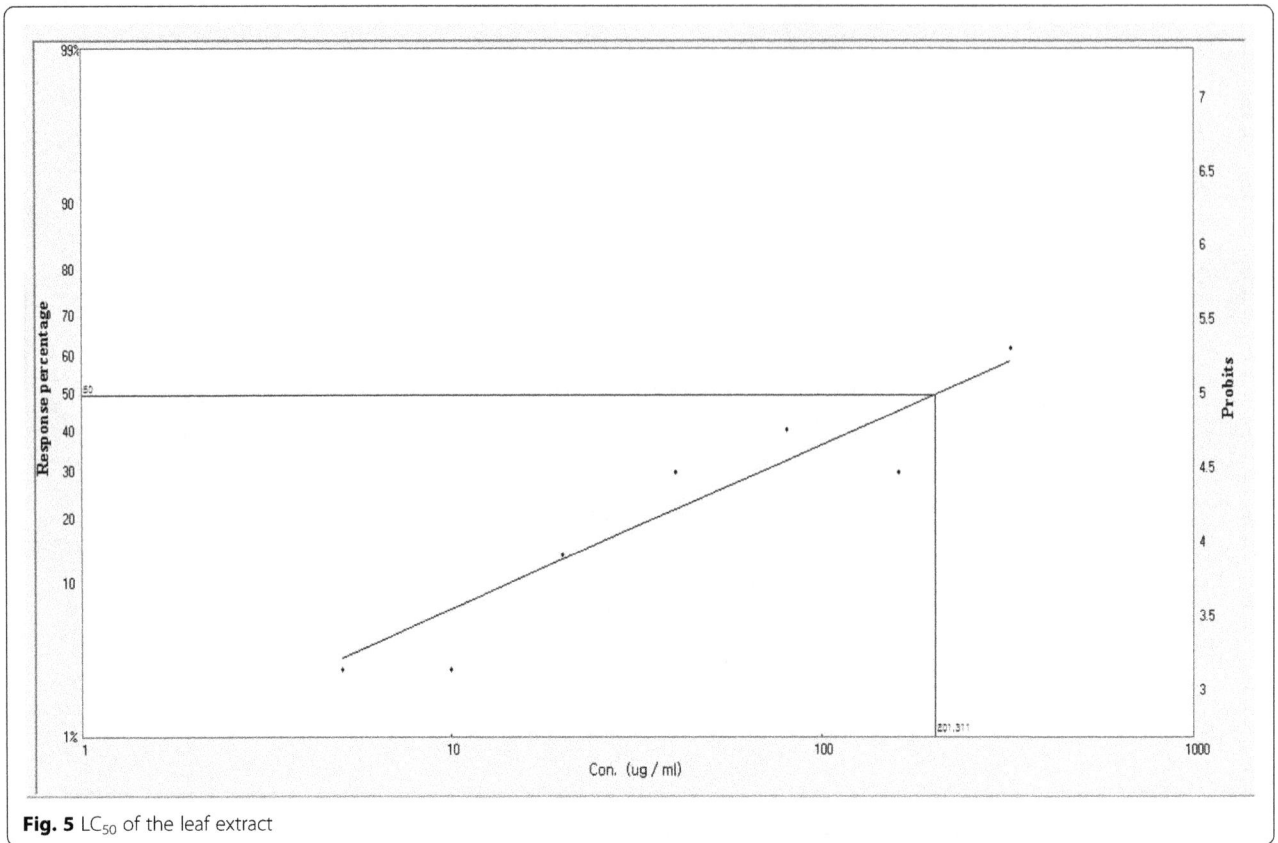

**Fig. 5** LC$_{50}$ of the leaf extract

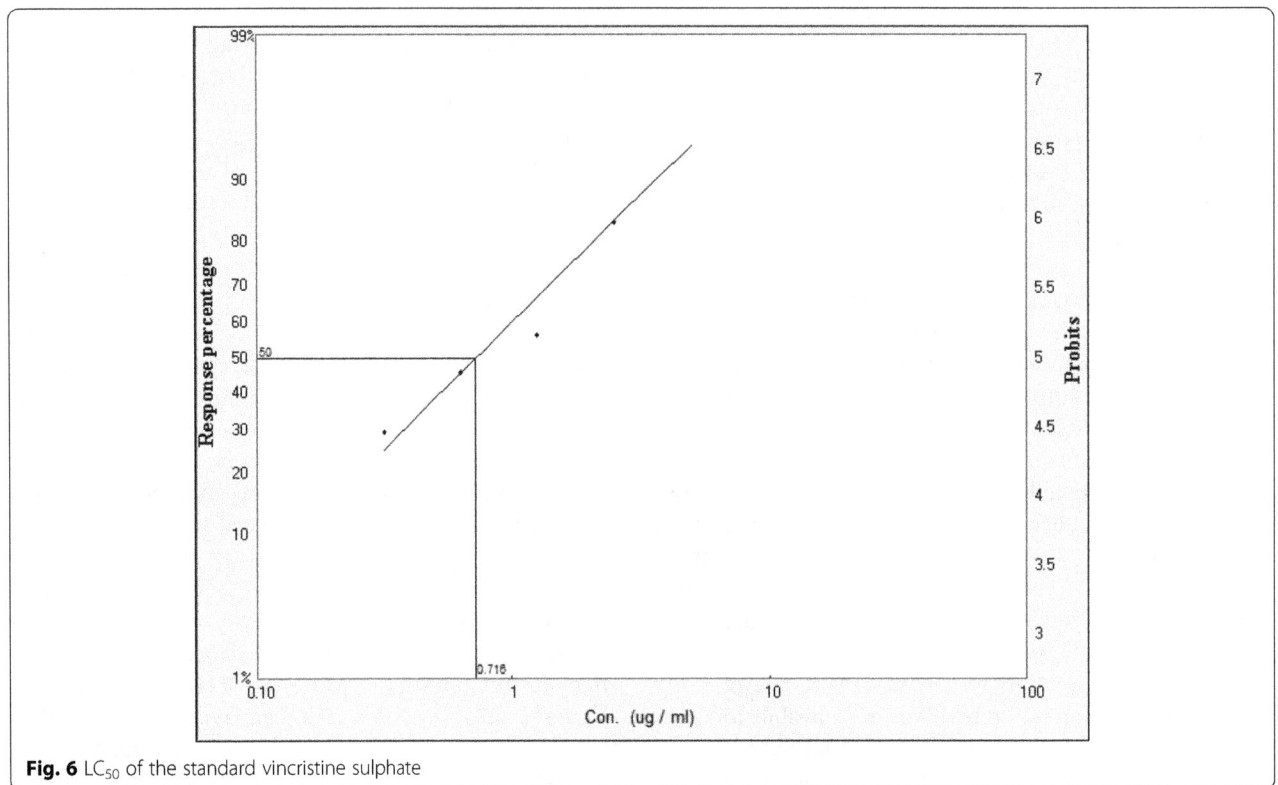

**Fig. 6** LC$_{50}$ of the standard vincristine sulphate

ricinoleic acid is released by lipases in the intestinal lumen, which causes irritation and inflammation in the intestinal mucosa, resulting in the release of inflammatory mediators (e.g., prostaglandins especially PGE series and histamine) [38, 39]. These mediators initiate vasodilatation, smooth muscle contraction, and mucus secretion in the small intestines. Also inhibition of intestinal Na + K+ ATPase activity, activation of adenylate cyclase and mucosal cAMP-mediated active secretion are the proposed mechanisms of diarrheal effect of castor oil [36]. Both the leaf and stem extracts of *B. gymnorrhiza* were found to inhibit the severity of diarrhoea induced by castor oil. The onset of diarrhea and frequency of defecation was reduced in dose dependent manner. Between the extracts, the stem extract was more potent than leaves extract regarding the latent period and frequency of stool. Antidiarrhoeal activity of tannins, flavonoids, polyphenols, saponins, alkaloids, sterols, reducing sugars and triterpenes was reported previously [40–42]. In the phytochemical group tests alkaloids, glycosides, tannins, and flavonoids were identified in both extracts. In addition to, (+)-catechin, ellagic acid, gallic acid and vannilin identified in the HPLC analysis, inhibited prostaglandins and consequently showed antidiarrhoel activity reported in previous studies [43, 44].

Most studies of polyphenols aimed to determine the protective effects of polyphenols against diseases and relatively few investigators have examined their possible toxicity. No acute toxicity was observed after oral administration of a grape seed proanthocyanidin extract at a dose of 2 g/kg and punicalagin (an ellagitannin present in pomegranate juice) at a dose of 60 g/kg body weight to rats or mice [45, 46]. Controversial results also have been reported in previous studies [45, 47, 48]. The risk of consuming high doses of polyphenols from naturally polyphenol rich foods is low. From our result of acute toxicity it can be supposed that both extracts were safe at high dose (1 g/kg body weight).

The brine shrimp lethality assay was considered as a convenient method for preliminary assessment of toxicity. It can also be used to extrapolate cell line toxicity and antitumor activity [36]. *B. gymnorrhiza* extracts were assessed for their cytotoxicity using the sensitive *in vitro* brine shrimp lethality bioassay (Figs. 4, 5 and 6). The leaves and stem extracts showed $LD_{50}$ value of 201.31 µg/ml and 232.09 µg/ml respectively. From the present study, it can be well predicted that the extracts do not have considerable cytotoxic activity.

## Conclusion

The crude ethanol extracts of the leaf and stem of *Bruguiera gymnorrhiza* revealed significant antioxidant, analgesic and antidiarrhoeal activities. The observed pharmacological activities may be due to the presence of

significant concentration of vanillic acid in the plant extracts. In addition, individual or synergistic activity of other phenolic constituents present in the extracts might be responsible for these pharmacological activities. Further pharmacological investigation and bioactivity guided studies are required to isolate the active principle (s) responsible for these activities.

**Abbreviations**
DAD: Diode array detector; DPPH; 2: 2-diphenyl-1-picryldydrazyl; GAE: Gallic acid equivalent; HPLC: High performance liquid chromatography; $IC_{50}$: 50% Inhibitory concentration; $LC_{50}$: Lethal concentration in 50% test animal; OD: Optical density; QE: Quercetin equivalent; $R^2$: Coefficient of determination; RSD: Relative standard deviation

**Acknowledgements**
The authors are grateful to the authority of International Centre for Diarrhoeal Disease and Research, Bangladesh (ICDDR, B) for providing experimental mice.

**Funding**
Not applicable.

**Authors' contributions**
This work has been carried out in collaboration among authors. IM and MNHZ have performed the extraction, antioxidant and other pharmacological activities. NNB and BB managed the literature searches, performed phytochemical screening, HPLC analysis and carried out the statistical analysis. BB designed the study. BB and MNHZ drafted the manuscript. All authors read and approved the final manuscript.

**Competing interests**
The authors declare that they have no competing interests.

**References**
1.  Phang CW, Malek SN, Ibrahim H. Antioxidant potential, cytotoxic activity and total phenolic content of *Alpinia pahangensis* rhizomes. BMC Complement Altern Med. 2013;13:243. doi:10.1186/1472-6882-13-243.
2.  Doss A. Preliminary phytochemical screening of some Indian medicinal plants. Ancient Sci Life. 2009;29(2):12–6.
3.  Balaji G, Chalamaiah M, Ramesh B, Amarnath YR. Antidiarrhoeal activity of ethanol and aqueous extracts of *Carum copticum* seeds in experimental rats. Asian Pac J Trop Biomed. 2012. doi:10.1016/S2221-1691(12)60376–1.
4.  Coe FG, Anderson GJ. Screening of medicinal plants used by the Garífuna of eastern Nicaragua for bioactive compounds. J Ethnopharmacol. 1996;53:29–50.
5.  Hassan MM, Khan SA, Shaikat AH, Hossain ME, Hoque MA, Ullah MH, et al. Analgesic and anti-inflammatory effects of ethanol extracted leaves of selected medicinal plants in animal model. Vet World. 2013;6(2):68–71. doi:10.5455/vetworld.2013.68-71.
6.  Azam MNK, Rahman MM, Biswas S, Ahmed MN. Appraisals of Bangladeshi medicinal plants used by folk medicine practitioners in the prevention and management of malignant neoplastic diseases. Int Scholarly Res Not. 2016. doi:10.1155/2016/7832120.
7.  Tumpa SI, Hossain MI, Ishika T. Ethnomedicinal uses of herbs by indigenous medicine practitioners of Jhenaidah district, Bangladesh. J Pharmacogn Phytochem. 2014;3(2):23–33.

8. Shaikh JU, Grice ID, Tiralongo E. Cytotoxic effects of Bangladeshi medicinal plant extracts. Evid Based Complement Alternat Med. 2011. doi:10.1093/ecam/nep111.

9. Li H, Xueshi H, Sattler I, Dahse HM, Hongzheng F, Grabley S, Wenhan L. Three new pimaren diterpenoids from marine mangrove plant, *Bruguiera gymnorrhiza*. Pharmazie. 2005;60:705–7. doi:10.1002/chin.200601187.

10. Li H, Xueshi H, Isabel S, Moellmann U, Hongzheng F, Wenhan L, et al. New aromatic compounds from the marine mangrove *Bruguiera gymnorrhiza*. Planta Med. 2005;71:160–4. doi:10.1055/s-2005-837784.

11. Xiang-Xi Y, Jia-Gang D, Cheng-Hai G, Xiao-Tao H, Fei L, Zhi-Ping W, Er-Wei H, Yan X, Zheng-Cai D, Hui-Xue H, Ri-Ming H. Four new cyclohexylideneacetonitrile derivatives from the hypocotyl of mangrove (*Bruguiera gymnorrhiza*). Molecules. 2015;20:14565–75.

12. Ghani A. Practical phytochemistry. Dhaka: Parash Publishers; 2005.

13. Zilani MNH, Amirul MI, Sharmin SK, Jamil AS, Mustafizur MR, Golam MH. Analgesic and antioxidant activities of *Colocasia fallax*. Orient Pharm Exp Med. 2016;16:131–7. doi:10.1007/s13596-016-0222-1.

14. Anisuzzman M, Nazmul MHZ, Sharmin SK, Asaduzzman M, Golam MH. Antioxidant, antibacterial potential and HPLC analysis of *Dioscorea alata* bulb. Indonesian J Pharm. 2016;27(1):9–14.

15. Salma AS, Siraj MA, Hossain A, Mia MS, Afrin S, Rahman MM. Investigation of the key pharmacological activities of *Ficu sracemosa* and analysis of its major bioactive polyphenols by HPLC-DAD. Evid Based Complement Altern Med. 2016. doi:10.1155/2016/3874516.

16. Sanjib S, Jamil AS, Himangsu M, Royhan G, Morsaline B, Lutfun N, et al. Bioactivity studies on *Musa seminifera* Lour. Pharmacogn Mag. 2013;9:315–22. doi:10.4103/0973-1296.117827.

17. Rahmat AK, Muhammad RK, Sumaira S, Mushtaq A. Evaluation of phenolic contents and antioxidant activity of various solvent extracts of *Sonchus asper* (L.) Hill. Chem Cent J. 2012;6:12.

18. Usha V, Suriyavathana M. Free radical scavenging activity of ethanolic extract of *Desmodium gangeticum*. J Acute Med. 2012;2:36–42.

19. Khirul MI, Nripendra NB, Sanjib S, Hemayet H, Ismet AJ, Tanzir AK, et al. Antinociceptive and antioxidant activity of *Zanthoxylum budrunga* Wall (Rutaceae) Seeds. Sci World J. 2014. doi:10.1155/2014/869537.

20. Islam MA, Ahmed F, Das AK, Bachar SC. Analgesic and anti-inflammatory activity of *Leonurus sibiricus*. Fitoterapia. 2005;76:359–62.

21. Bishwajit B, Nazmul MHZ, Aparajita M, Debendra NR, Jamil AS, Samir KS. Study of analgesic and antidiarrhoeal activities of *sonneratia caseolaris* (linn.) Leaf and stem using different solvent system. Indonesian J Pharm. 2013;24:255–60.

22. Abdulwali A, Jamaludin M, Khalijah A, Jamil AS, Aditya A. Evaluation of antidiabetic and antioxidant properties of *Brucea javanica* seed. Sci World J. 2014. doi:10.1155/2014/786130.

23. Meyer BN, Ferrigni NR, Putnum JE, Jacobson LB, Nicholos DE, McLaugline JL. Brine shrimp: a convenient general bioassay for active plant constituents. Planta Med. 1982;45:31–4.

24. Kanti BP, Syed IR. Plant polyphenols as dietary antioxidants in human health and disease. Oxid Med Cell Longev. 2009;2:270–8. doi:10.4161/oxim.2.5.9498.

25. Dejan ZO, Neda MM, Marina MF, Slobodan SP, Emilija ĐJ. Antioxidant activity relationship of phenolic compounds in *Hypericum perforatum* L. Chem Cent J. 2011;5:34. doi:10.1186/1752-153X-5-34.

26. Bendary E, Francis RR, Ali HMG, Sarwat MI, Hady SE. Antioxidant and structure–activity relationships (SARs) of some phenolic and anilines compounds. Ann Agric Sci. 2013;58(2):173–81.

27. Rong T. Chemistry and biochemistry of dietary polyphenols. Nutrients. 2010;2:1231–46. doi:10.3390/nu2121231.

28. Małgorzata M, Irena P. Antioxidant activity of the main phenolic compounds isolated from hot pepper fruit (*Capsicum annuum* L.). J Agric Food Chem. 2005;53:1750–6.

29. Himangsu M, Sanjib S, Khalijah A, Hemayet H, Abdulwali A, Khirul MI, et al. Central-stimulating and analgesic activity of the ethanolic extract of *Alternanthera sessilis* in mice. BMC Complement Altern Med. 2014;14:398. doi:10.1186/1472-6882-14-398.

30. Dhara AK, Suba V, Sen T, Pal S, Chaudhuri AK. Preliminary studies on the anti-inflammatory and analgesic activity of methanolic fraction of the root of *Tragia involucrate*. J Ethnopharmacol. 2000;72:265–8.

31. Shafiur R. Antioxida nt, analgesic, cytotoxic and antidiarrh eal activities of ethanolic *Zizyphus mauritiana* bark extract. Orient Pharm Exp Med. 2012;12: 67–73. doi:10.1007/s13596-011-0042-2.

32. Kumar S, Pandey AK. Chemistry and biological activities of flavonoids: an overview. Sci World J. 2013. doi:10.1155/2013/162750.

33. Bhaskar VH, Balakrishnan N. Analgesic, anti-infammatory and antipyretic activities of *Pergularia daemia* and *Carissa carandas*. DARU J Pharm Sci. 2009;17:168–74.

34. Cássia C, Thacyana TC, Miriam SNH, Felipe AP, Victor F, Marília FM, et al. Vanillic acid inhibits inflammatory pain by inhibiting neutrophil recruitment, oxidative stress, cytokine production, and NFκB activation in mice. J Nat Prod. 2015;78:1799–08. doi:10.1021/acs.jnatprod.5b00246.

35. Yrbas ML, Morucci F, Alonso R, Gorzalczany S. Pharmacological mechanism underlying the antinociceptive activity of vanillic acid. Pharmacol Biochem Behav. 2015;132:88–95. doi:10.1016/j.pbb.2015.02.016.

36. Khalilur MR, Soumitra B, Fokhrul MI, Rafikul MI, Sayeed MA, Shahnaj P, et al. Studies on the anti-diarrheal properties of leaf extract of *Desmodium puchellum*. Asian Pac J Trop Biomed. 2013;3:639–43.

37. Khalilur MR, Ashraf MUC, Taufiqual MI, Anisuzzaman MC, Erfan MU, Chandra DS. Evaluation of antidiarrheal activity of methanolic extract of *Maranta arundinacea* linn. Leaves. Adv Pharmacol Sci. 2015. doi:10.1155/2015/257057.

38. Qnais EY, Elokda AS, Abu Ghalyun YY, Abdulla FA. Antidiarrheal activity of the aqueous extract of *Punica granatum* (Pomegranate) peels. Pharm Biol. 2007;45:715–20.

39. Balaji G, Chalamaiah M, Ramesh B, Amarnath RY. Antidiarrhoeal activity of ethanol and aqueous extracts of *Carum copticum* seeds in experimental rats. Asian Pac J Trop Biomed. 2012;2(2):S1151-55.

40. Ibrahim OMS, Shwaysh MM. Evaluation of Punica granatum peels extracts and its phenolic, alkaloid and terpenoid constituents against chemically induced diarrhoea in rats. Adv Anim Vet Sci. 2016;4:161–8. doi:10.14737/journal.aavs/2016/4.3.161.168.

41. Chanchal NR, Balasubramaniam A, Sayyed N. Antidiarrheal potential of *Tabernaemontana divaricata*. Phytopharmacology. 2013;4:61–8.

42. Ezeigbo II, Ezeja MI, Madubuike KG, Ifenkwe DC, Ukweni IA, Udeh NE, Akomas SC. Antidiarrhoeal activity of leaf methanolic extract of *Rauwolfia serpentine*. Asian Pac J Trop Biomed. 2012;2:430–2.

43. Ihekwereme CP, Erhirhie EO, Mbagwu IS, Ilodigwe EE, Ajaghaku DL, Okoye FB. Antidiarrheal property of *Napoleona imperialis* may be due to procyanidins and ellagic acid derivatives. J App Pharm Sci. 2016;6:101–6.

44. Hai-Tao X, Siu-Wai T, Hong-Yan Q, Franky FK, Choia ZY, Quan-Bin H, Hu-Biao C, Hong-Xi X, Hong S, Ai-Ping L, Zhao-Xiang B. A bioactivity-guided study on the anti-diarrhea activity of *Polygonum chinense* Linn. J Ethnopharmacol. 2013;149:499–505. doi:10.1016/j.jep.2013.07.007.

45. Louise IM, Walker R, Catherine BP, Augustin S. Risks and safety of polyphenol consumption. Am J Clin Nutr. 2005;81:326S–9.

46. Cerda B, Ceron JJ, Tomas-Barberan FA, Espin JC. Repeated oral administration of high doses of the pomegranate ellagitannin punicalagin to rats for 37 days is not toxic. J Agric Food Chem. 2003;51:3493–501.

47. Joshua DL, Mary JK, Shengmin S, Kenneth RR, Jihyeung J, Chung SY. Hepatotoxicity of high oral dose (−)-Epigallocatechin-3-Gallate in mice. Food Chem Toxicol. 2010;48(1):409–16. doi:10.1016/j.fct.2009.10.030.

48. Isomura T, Suzuki S, Origasa H, Hosono A, Suzuki M, Sawada T, Terao S, Muto Y, Koga T. Liver-related safety assessment of green tea extracts in humans: a systematic review of randomized controlled trials. Eur J Clin Nutr. 2016;70:1221–9.

# 7

# Evaluation of phytochemical composition and antioxidative, hypoglycaemic and hypolipidaemic properties of methanolic extract of *Hemidesmus indicus* roots in streptozotocin-induced diabetic mice

Ankita Joshi, Harsha Lad, Harsha Sharma and Deepak Bhatnagar[*]

## Abstract

**Background:** *Hemidesmus indicus* is an important medicinal plant and extensively used in Ayurvedic and Unani system of medicine. The aim of the study was to evaluate the antioxidant, hypoglycaemic and hypolipidemic potential of methanolic extract of roots of *Hemidesmus indicus* (HIE) in streptozotocin (STZ) induced diabetic mice.

**Methods:** HIE was analyzed by LC-MS to determine its phytochemical composition. The in-vitro antioxidant activity of HIE was analyzed through inhibition of free radical scavenging activity (FRSA), total antioxidant power (TAP) and reducing power. Diabetes in mice was induced by a single dose of STZ followed by HIE treatment. The antioxidative, hypoglycaemic and hypolipidemic activity were studied ex-vivo in tissues of diabetic mice.

**Results:** Phytochemical composition of *hemidesmus indicus* roots (HIE) revealed the presence of phenols, flavanoids, terpenoids and about 40 different phytoconstituents by LC-MS analysis. Inhibition of lipid peroxidation (LPO) and modulation in superoxide dismutase (SOD), catalase (CAT), glutathione-S- transferase (GST) activity and glutathione (GSH) content showed potent antioxidant activity of HIE in STZ induced diabetic mice, which was also substantiated by in-vitro antioxidant assays. The decrease in fasting blood glucose and serum lipid profile was also observed in mice administered HIE.

**Conclusion:** It is proposed that HIE modulates the oxidant/antioxidant in favor of reducing oxidative stress, hypoglycemia and improved the lipid profile in treated groups.

**Keywords:** Streptozotocin, Hypoglycaemic, Hypolipidaemic, Lipid peroxidation, Antioxidants, *Hemidesmus indicus*

## Background

Diabetes mellitus is a complex chronic metabolic disorder characterized by alterations in carbohydrate, protein and fat metabolism. The metabolic changes are caused by the insufficiency of secretion or action of endogenous insulin [1]. Oxidative stress is suggested to be one of the mechanism underlying diabetes and diabetic complications. It results from an oxidant/antioxidant imbalance in favour of oxidants leading to damage of various intracellular components such as proteins, lipids and nucleic acid as well as extracellular matrix components such as proteoglycans and collagens. Free radicals are formed by glucose oxidation, non enzymatic glycation of proteins, oxidative degradation of glycated proteins and increased lipid oxidation (LPO), which may promote oxidative stress and lead to the development of insulin resistance [2]. The harmful effects of oxidative stress are counteracted by the cellular defense mechanism, which consists of enzymes, nonenzymatic and metabolic antioxidants. To treat diabetes various oral antihyperglycaemic agents have been developed over the past years, which include sulphonylureas, biguanides, α-glucosidase inhibitors and thiazolidinediones [3]. Hypoglycaemia, lactic acidosis and gastrointestinal

* Correspondence: bhatnagarbio@gmail.com
School of Biochemistry, Devi Ahilya University, Khandwa Road, Indore, MP 452017, India

intolerance are some of the adverse effect of these drugs. These side-effects of synthetic drugs along with drug-resistance have led to the resurgence of phytomedicine and search for novel type of antioxidant and antidiabetic from medicinal plants.

*Hemidesmus indicus* belongs to the family Periplocaceae and is distributed throughout India. Roots and stems of *H. indicus* act as laxative, diaphoretic, diuretic and are useful in treatment of syphilis, cough, asthma and leucoderma. *H. indicus* roots (Fig. 1) contains steroids, terpenoids, flavonoids, saponins, phenolic compounds, tannins and lignins, inulins, cardiac glycosides, proteins and carbohydrates [4]. Pregnenolone glycosides such as hemidesmosides A–C and 2-hydroxy-4-methoxybenzoic acid, 2-hydroxy-4- methoxybenzaldehyde, and 3-hydroxy-4-methoxybenzaldehyde were reported in *H. indicus* roots [5, 6]. These phytoconstituents are accountable for its different biological actions. The phenolic and flavanoid content found in aqueous extract of *H. indicus* corresponds to its reported antioxidant activity [7, 8] The present study was undertaken to investigate the effects of methanolic extract of *H. indicus* roots on lipid peroxidation, antioxidant enzyme activity, lipid profile and fasting blood glucose of STZ induced diabetic mice.

## Methods
### Chemicals and reagents
Streptozotocin, 2,2-diphenyl-1-p-picryl- hydrazyl (DPPH), ursolic acid and quercitrin hydrate were procured from Sigma Chemical Co. St. Louis, Missouri, USA. HPLC grade acetonitrile were purchased from Merck Chemicals, Mumbai, India. Pyrogallol, ethylenediamine tetra acetic acid (EDTA) and other chemicals and solvents of AR grade were purchased from Hi Media Co. Mumbai, India.

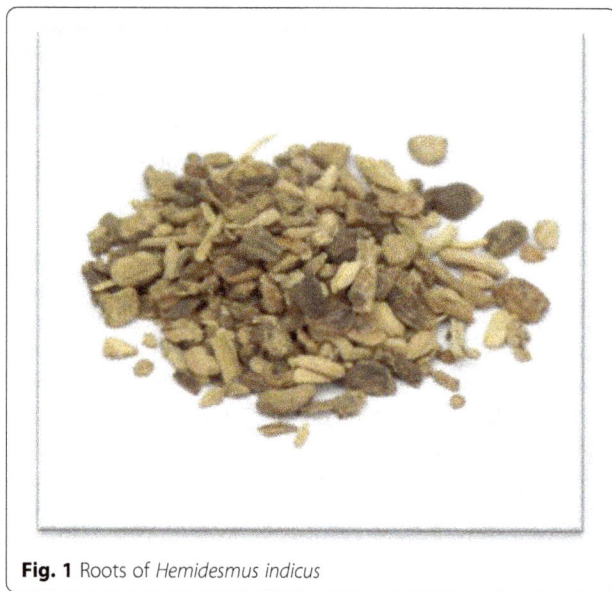

**Fig. 1** Roots of *Hemidesmus indicus*

### Plant material and preparation of the extract
*H. indicus* roots were procured from the local market. The plant roots were authenticated by Prof. A.B. Seerwani, Department of Botany, Holkar Science College, Indore. The dried powder of roots of *H. indicus* (HIE) (50 g) were extracted in methanol (300 ml) by the Soxhlet apparatus at 40 °C for 8 h. The extract was concentrated by evaporation at 35 °C in water bath. The yield of dried extract was 13.48% (w/w). The reconstitution of HIE was done in methanol to prepare stock solution of 100 mg/ml for photochemical and in vitro analysis and in 1% DMSO for in vivo dosage preparation. These extracts were stored at 4 °C for analysis.

### Animals
Healthy colony bred mice of Swiss albino strain of both sex weighing 20 ± 5 g were kept in polypropylene cages at an ambient temperature. Animals had free access to feed (M.P. Livestock and Poultry Development Corporation, Indore) and water. The experiments were performed according to the guidelines of the Institutional Animal Ethics Committee (IAEC) (CPCSEA/2015/01 dt. 4/7/2015). The standard necropsies procedures were carried out at the termination of study to collect the required tissues and blood sample for various analyses from mice of both sexes, as the study does not involve any gender specific parameters.

### Total phenol content
Total phenol content of HIE was determined using the Folin–Ciocalteu method by Singleton and Rossi [9]. Propyl gallate solution (1 mg/ml, 0–30 μg) was used as standard.

### Total flavonoid content
Total flavonoids were estimated according to the aluminum chloride method of Zhang et al., (2011) [10]. Quercitrin hydrate (1 mg/ml in ethanol, 0–250 μg) was used as a standard.

### Total triterpenoid content
Total triterpenoid content was estimated by the method of Chang and Lin [11]. Ursolic acid (1 mg/ml in methanol, 0–50 μg) was used as standard.

### Liquid chromatography-mass spectroscopy (LC-MS)
LC-MS analysis of the methanolic extract of *Hemidesmus indicus* roots was carried out using Agilant (6550 iFunnel Q-TOFs) system consisting of Hip sampler, binary pump, column component, Q-TOF having dual ion source and electrospray ion generation (ESI) with Agilent Jet Stream (AJS). Chromatographic separations were performed using 5 μl of methanolic sample injected with needle wash onto an Agilent 1290 infinity UHPLC system fitted with a Zorbax Eclipse C18 column (2.1 × 150 mm, 5 μ) and flow

rate was 200 μl/min. The column was held at 95% Solvent A (water) and 5% Solvent B (acetonitrile) for 2 min, followed by an 20 min step gradient from 5% B to 95% B, then 5 min with 5% A, 95% B. Then the elution was achieved with a linear gradient from 5% A to 95% A for 4 min. The following parameters were used throughout the MS experiment: for electro spray ionization with positive ion polarity, the capillary voltage was set to 3500 V, the capillary temperature to 250 °C, the nebulizer pressure to 35 psi and the drying gas flow rate to 13 L/ min. Data acquisition and mass spectrometric evaluation were carried out using software Agilent Mass Hunter Qualitative analysis B.06.

### Free radical scavenging activity using 1, 1, 2, 2-diphenyl-p-picryl hydrazyl

The method is based on the reduction of an ethanolic solution of DPPH by hydrogen donating groups of antioxidant substance [12]. The decrease in DPPH absorption at 517 nm was measured.

### Total antioxidant power using ferric reducing antioxidant power

The total antioxidant capacity (TAC) of HIE was determined using the ferric reducing antioxidant power (FRAP) [13].

### Reducing power

The reducing power of the test samples was determined according to the method of Oyaizu [14]. The reductive ability was measured by the reduction of $FeCl_3$ in presence of plant extracts. Ascorbic acid dissolved in distil water having concentration ranging from 0 to 17.6 μg was used as positive control.

### Induction of diabetes

A single dose of freshly prepared STZ (180 mg/kg body wt.) in cold 0.01 M citrate buffer (pH 4.5) was administered intraperitonially to overnight fasted mice to induce diabetes [15]. Streptozotocin causes β-cell toxicity via mechanism involving both free radical mediated damage and alkylation of DNA [16]. Mice were orally administered 10% ($w/v$) glucose for 24 h after STZ injection to overcome hypoglycaemic shock and after 72 h, fasting blood glucose (FBG) was measured. Mice having FBG levels above 250 mg/dl were considered diabetic and were selected for further experiments. The FBG of the animals were estimated by glucometer (Akkiscan, Nempro Care, India) at every 3rd day, after the induction of diabetes up to the end of treatment (day 12th). The variation in the body weight during the study period was recorded (provided in Additional file 1) and the food and water intake was monitored in the animals.

### Experimental design

The mice were divided into four groups of 6 animals each. The groups of animals were control mice without any treatment (Group 1), STZ induced diabetic mice (Group 2), mice treated with glibenclamide (10 mg/kg/day, orally) from 1st day of diabetes induction to 12th day (Group 3) and mice treated with HIE (35 mg/kg/day, orally) from 1st to 12th day after the induction of diabetes (Group 4). The animals were observed for the development of diabetes up to day 5 of STZ administration. Treatments in group 3 and 4 were administered to diabetic mice for 12 days after development of diabetes.

### Collection and processing of biological samples

The animals were sacrificed under mild ether anesthesia. Liver and kidney homogenate (10%) was prepared using Potter-Elvehjem Homogenizer (Remi, Mumbai, India) in ice cold phosphate buffer saline (PBS) (1: 9, $v/v$) followed by centrifugation at 16000 xg for 30 min at 4 °C. Blood was collected by cardiac puncture in citrated tubes. Erythrocytes lysate was prepared as described earlier [17]. The supernatant obtained after centrifugation of tissue homogenate and erythrocytes lysate were immediately used to determine antioxidant enzymes and protein content.

### Measurement of serum biochemical parameters

Blood was collected from diabetic and treated groups and the serum samples were analyzed using commercially available kits (Beacon Diagnostics, Navsari, India) for cholesterol, HDL, LDL, VLDL triglycerides by ELISA plate reader (LISA Plus, Rapid Diagnostics, China) and spectrophotometer (Shimadzu, UV-1800, Japan). The quantitative estimations were performed according to the manufacturer's protocol.

### Determination of malondialdehyde levels

Malondialdehyde (MDA) content in liver, kidney and erythrocytes was measured by HPLC method [18].

### Determination of antioxidant status

The activity of superoxide dismutase (SOD), catalase (CAT) and glutathione-S-transferase (GST) was measured in tissue homogenates and erythrocytes lysate. The reduced GSH content was measured in tissue homogenates and blood [19–22].

### Statistical analysis

The results obtained were analyzed by the SPSS software package version 20. The mean values obtained for the different groups were compared by one-way ANOVA, followed by post hoc -Tukeys (HSD) test.

**Table 1** Estimation of phytoconstituents and total antioxidant power of HIE

| Constituents | Content |
|---|---|
| Total phenolic[a] | $12.95 \pm 0.77$ |
| Total triterpenoid[b] | $79.42 \pm 2.35$ |
| Total flavanoid[c] | $57.68 \pm 1.65$ |
| Total antioxidant power[d] | $77.36 \pm 1.59$ |

Values are Mean $\pm$ SE of four experiments
[a] mg GAE/g of dry wt.
[b] mg UAE /g of dry wt.
[c] mg QHE/g of dry wt.
[d] $\mu$M/g of dry wt.

## Results

### Determination of phytoconstituents
Phytochemical analysis of HIE was evaluated and the results are represented in Table 1.

### Qualitative mass spectral analysis
HIE showed 73 unique mass signals, out of which putative empirical formulas of 62 compounds were obtained and identified by comparison with phytochemical database {developed by Sophisticated Analytical Instrument Facility - Indian Institute of Technology, Bombay (SAIF-IITB) and Pubchem} and details of the compounds are provided in Additional file 1. The MS spectrum of some of the compounds is represented in Fig. 2.

### Total antioxidant power using ferric reducing antioxidant power
The results of total antioxidant power (TAP) using FRAP are presented in Table 1.

### Free radical scavenging activity
HIE showed FRSA by donating the hydrogen atom or electron to stable free radical DPPH. A linear relationship was observed in the DPPH radical scavenging activity and HIE concentrations (Fig. 3a). The FRSA of butylated hydroxyl toluene (BHT, 0.18 mg/ml) was found to be $55.51 \pm 0.69\%$. The $IC_{50}$ value for BHT and HIE were $0.06 \pm 0.02$ mg/ml and $0.10 \pm 0.03$ mg/ml respectively.

### Reducing power
The reduction of $FeCl_3$ in the presence of methanolic extract of HIE was monitored at 700 nm (Fig. 3 b). The higher absorbance of the reaction mixture indicated

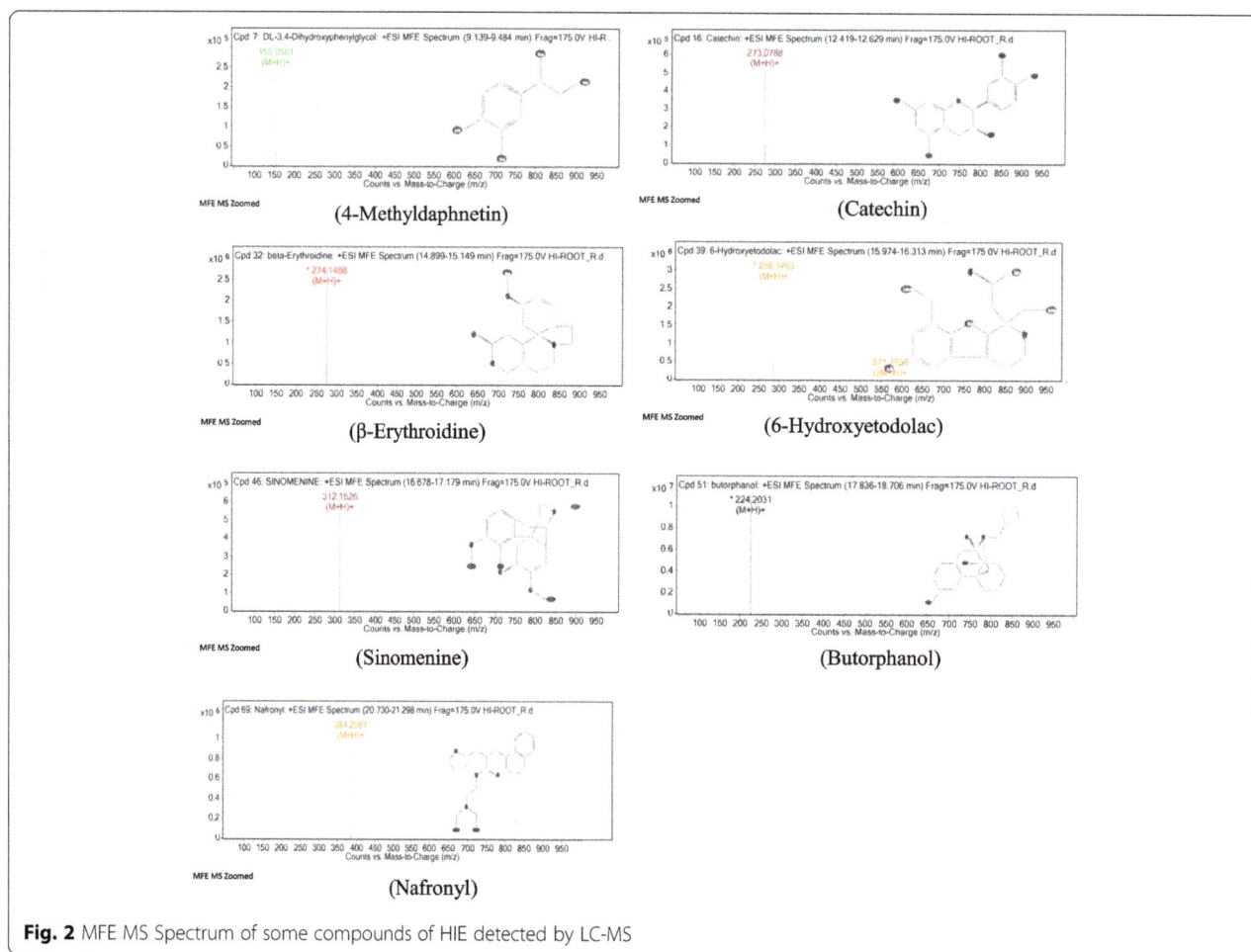

(4-Methyldaphnetin)

(Catechin)

(β-Erythroidine)

(6-Hydroxyetodolac)

(Sinomenine)

(Butorphanol)

(Nafronyl)

**Fig. 2** MFE MS Spectrum of some compounds of HIE detected by LC-MS

## a

## b

**Fig. 3** Effect of different concentration of HIE on (**a**) DPPH radical scavenging activity; (**b**) Reducing power. Values are Mean ± SE of four experiments

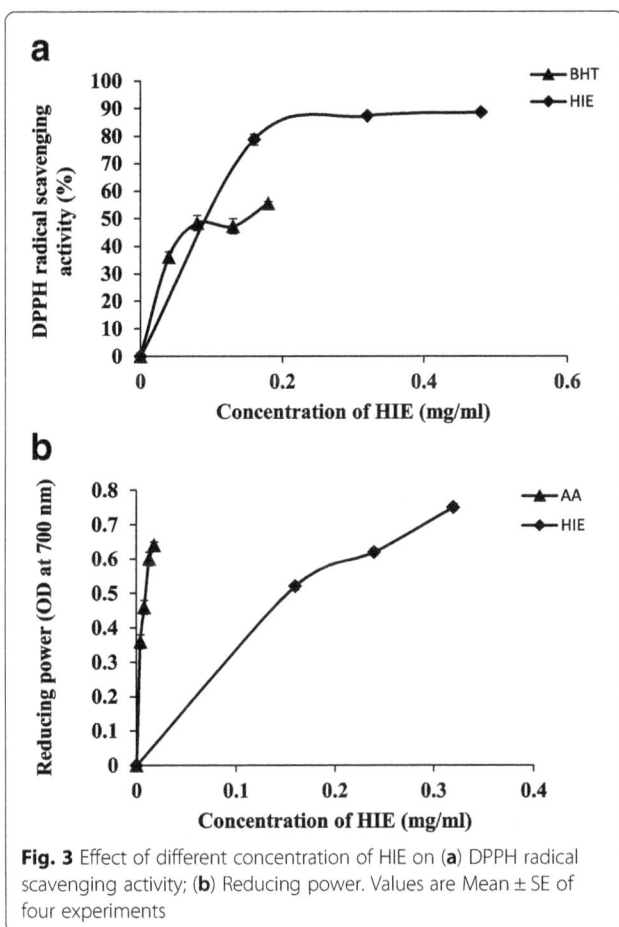

greater reducing power. Ascorbic acid showed the absorbance of $0.64 \pm 0.01$ at the concentration of 176 μg/ml.

The total phenolic content of HIE showed a strong and positive correlation with reducing power ($R2 = 0.997$, $p < 0.05$) and DPPH radical scavenging activity ($R2 = 0.851$) (Table 2). The total flavanoid content exhibited correlation of 0.997 ($p < 0.05$) with reducing power and 0.921 with DPPH radical scavenging activity. It is suggested that the radical scavenging activity and antioxidant activity of HIE is due to the presence of the phenolic and flavanoid compounds.

**Table 2** Correlation coefficient between phytoconstituents and antioxidant properties of HIE

| Antioxidant Properties | FRSA | RP |
|---|---|---|
| Phyto-Constituents | | |
| TPC | 0.851 | 0.997* |
| TFC | 0.921 | 0.997* |
| TTC | 0.921 | 0.997* |

FRSA Free radical scavenging activity
RP Reducing power
TPC Total phenolic content
TFC Total flavanoid content
TTC Total triterpenoid content
*Correlation coefficient is significant at $P < 0.05$

### Fasting blood glucose and lipid profile

The effect of HIE on fasting blood glucose is represented in Table 3. Glibenclamide and HIE (Group 3 and 4) produced significant decrease in blood glucose level when compared to the diabetic control (Group 2) after 6 days of treatment. Food intake and body weight showed mild decrease after development of diabetes and non-significant alterations in the body weight was observed in all groups throughout the study period (Additional file 2).

The results showed that there was significant decrease in serum cholesterol, triglycerides, LDL and VLDL in the glibenclamide and HIE treated mice (Table 4; Group 3 and 4) when compared to diabetic control (Group 2).

### Determination of MDA levels

MDA content was found significantly increased in the liver, kidney and erythrocytes of the diabetic group (Table 5; Group 2) as compared to control (Group 1). A significant inhibition in the liver and kidney LPO was observed with glibenclamide (Group 3) and HIE (Group 4) as compared to diabetic control (Group 2). The liver and kidney MDA content of HIE treated group of mice (Group 4) was comparable to that of control group (Group 1). Erythrocytes MDA content remained unaffected in glibenclamide and decreased in HIE treated mice as compare to diabetic control.

### Determination of antioxidant status

The decrease in SOD activity was significant in the liver, whereas it was increased in kidney and erythrocytes in diabetic mice, as compared to control (Table 6; Group 1). Glibenclamide and HIE (Group 3 and 4) significantly elevated the SOD activity in the liver, while in kidney it was comparable to control and in erythrocytes SOD activity was remarkably reduced as compared to diabetic control.

A significant increase in liver, kidney and erythrocyte catalase activity was observed in diabetic animals (Table 6; Group 2) when compared against the control (Group 1). The treatment with glibenclamide (Group 3) significantly decreased the catalase activity in liver, while in erythrocytes and kidney the change was non-significant as compared to diabetic control (Group 2). However, with HIE (Group 4) treatment, liver, kidney and erythrocytes catalase activity is normalized and significantly decreased as compared to diabetic control (Group 2).

GSH content increased in liver and decreased in kidney and erythrocytes of diabetic animal (Group 2) as compared to control (Table 7; Group 1). Glibenclamide treated animal showed low GSH content in liver, while with HIE treatment, the liver GSH content was near to normal. In kidney, both the treatment resulted in recovery of GSH content to normal, whereas for erythrocytes there was no reduction in GSH content in glibenclamide treatment as

**Table 3** Effects of HIE treatment on fasting blood glucose in streptozotocin induced diabetic mice

| Group | Day 1 | Day 3 | Day 6 | Day 9 | Day 12 |
|---|---|---|---|---|---|
| 1 | 91.75 ± 2.78 | 89.25 ± 2.72 | 96.25 ± 1.49 | 82.00 ± 2.27 | 92.00 ± 2.55 |
| 2 | 368.25 ± 12.29[**] | 294.25 ± 9.29[**] | 320.50 ± 16.06[**] | 312.25 ± 17.4[**] | 321.50 ± 22.77[**] |
| 3 | 470.00 ± 22.39[**#] | 276.75 ± 24[**] | 167.75 ± 5.71[*##] | 141.50 ± 6.96[*##] | 112.25 ± 5.76[##] |
| 4 | 541.75 ± 11.96[**##] | 374.57 ± 23.39[**] | 243.75 ± 13.29[**#] | 178.25 ± 8.12[**##] | 121.25 ± 5.22[##] |

Values are mean ± SE of 6 animals
[*]$P < 0.01$, [**]$P < 0.001$ = significant as compared to control (Group 1)
[#]$P < 0.01$, [##]$P < 0.001$ = significant as compared to diabetic control (Group 2)
Values of FBG are in mg %

compared to diabetic mice. Increase in GSH content of erythrocytes was observed in HIE as compared to diabetic group (Group 2).

GST activity in tissues and erythrocytes was significantly increased in diabetic animals (Table 7; Group 2) when compared against a control (Group 1), GST activity was not improved by the treatment with glibenclamide (Group 3) as compared to diabetic mice. HIE (Group 4) significantly reduced the liver and erythrocytes GST activity when compared to diabetic control (Group 2) whereas it is restored to normal in kidney.

## Discussion

ROS produced in various tissues leads to tissue injury as well as early events related to the development of diabetes mellitus and its complications [23]. HIE may have beneficial effects on type 1 and 2 diabetes, as the mechanism of development of both the diabetes involve oxidative stress. However, the animal model used represents only type 1 diabetes. Traditional plant remedies have been used in the treatment of diabetes but only a few have been scientifically evaluated [24]. Methanolic extract of *H. indicus* roots contained high quantity of flavanoid and triterpenoid than phenolic content and contributes to the observed antioxidant potential of the extract. The LC-MS analysis coupled with putative identification of compounds indicated the presence of phenolic and flavanoids such as DL-3,4-dihydroxyphenyl glycol, catechin, amiloxate (cinnamic acid derivative); 4-methyldaphnetin (coumarin), terpenoid such as punctaporin B and podocarpatriene derivative. Various

alkaloids such as ecgonine, homatropine, β-erythroidine, butorphanol, securinine along with other phytoconstituents such as phytosterols, lactones, prostaglandins, amino acids, lipids and fatty acids were also identified. Cholesterol lowering triparanol and nafronyl, which enhances cellular oxidative capacity and nudifloramide an end product of NAD degradation shown to potentially inhibit PARP-1 were found in HIE. Natural compounds having anti-inflammatory activity such as safroglycol, etodolac derivative, anisodamine, β santonin, nabumetone and securinine were identified by their molecular peak (base peak) [25–28].

The results of free radical scavenging activity showed that HIE reduced DPPH free radical to non-radical DPPH-H by compounds having hydroxyl groups (catechin) or compounds, which oxidise readily (sinomenine). The phenolics, flavanoids, diterpene and sesquiterpene compounds present in HIE can donate hydrogen to terminate the odd electrons of the DPPH radical. The scavenging ability of HIE can be attributed to these bioactive compounds. The higher FRAP value represents high total antioxidant power of HIE. The phenolic compounds reduce $Fe^{3+}$ to $Fe^{2+}$ and interrupt free radical chain reaction, either by hydrogen atom or electron transfer process and form phenoxyl radical [29]. The reducing power of HIE was positively correlated with the total phenolic, flavanoid and triterpenoid content also evident from mass spectral analysis. *H. indicus* is an edible plant and contains significant amount of total phenolics and reported to have antioxidant activity [30]. An earlier report by Rajan et al., [31] also showed the antioxidant activity of roots of *H. indicus* having

**Table 4** Effects of HIE treatment on serum lipid profile in streptozotocin induced diabetic mice

| Group | Cholesterol[a] | Triglycerides[a] | HDL[a] | LDL[a] | VLDL[a] |
|---|---|---|---|---|---|
| 1 | 125.03 ± 6.28 | 35.90 ± 7.68 | 101.82 ± 2.50 | 83.88 ± 3.76 | 7.18 ± 1.53 |
| 2 | 274.32 ± 15.82[**] | 63.90 ± 2.05[*] | 73.11 ± 3.17[*] | 160.84 ± 5.26[**] | 12.78 ± 0.41[*] |
| 3 | 122.74 ± 7.09[##] | 32.25 ± 6.24[##] | 113.31 ± 5.59[##] | 117.36 ± 7.59[*##] | 6.45 ± 1.25[##] |
| 4 | 122.77 ± 9.89[##] | 32.99 ± 0.18[##] | 122.74 ± 2.10[##] | 117.84 ± 5.87[*##] | 6.6 ± 0.04[##] |

Values are mean ± SE of 6 animals
[*]$P < 0.01$, [**]$P < 0.001$ = significant as compared to control (Group 1)
[#]$P < 0.01$, [##]$P < 0.001$ = significant as compared to diabetic control (Group 2)
[a]mg %

**Table 5** Effect of HIE on liver, kidney and erythrocytes LPO in STZ induced diabetic mice

| LPO$^a$ | | | |
|---|---|---|---|
| Group | Liver | Kidney | Erythrocytes |
| 1 | $31.72 \pm 1.43$ | $70.50 \pm 6.16$ | ND |
| 2 | $308.04 \pm 18.10^*$ | $340.53 \pm 10.71^*$ | $37.08 \pm 2.51^*$ |
| 3 | $133.75 \pm 8.78^{*\#}$ | $64.52 \pm 6.17^\#$ | $40.66 \pm 1.23^*$ |
| 4 | $33.77 \pm 1.99^\#$ | $58.82 \pm 9.17^\#$ | $21.89 \pm 0.86^{*\#}$ |

Values are mean $\pm$ SE of 6 animals
$^*P < 0.001$ = significant as compared to control (Group 1)
$^\#P < 0.001$ = significant as compared to diabetic control (Group 2).
ND = Not Detected
$^a$picomoles of MDA formed/mg protein for liver and kidney and nanomoles of MDA formed/gm Hb for erythrocytes

quantifiable amounts of phenolic compounds, tannins and flavonoids, as observed in the present study.

Free radicals are formed in diabetes by glucose autoxidation, polyol pathway and non-enzymatic glycation of proteins [32]. Streptozotocin selectively acts on pancreatic β-cells and cause enhanced ROS in pancreas, liver and other tissues. Increased ROS results in tissue damage and enhanced LPO i.e., oxidation of membrane lipid. Increased MDA in liver, kidney and erythrocytes of diabetic animals than those of control was due to ROS mediated propagation of chain reaction. The increase in MDA content may be due to diminished activity of an antioxidant defense system to sufficiently scavenge free radicals generated in STZ induced diabetes. It has been reported that the increase in MDA associated with diabetes may be reversed by treatment with combined vitamins C, E, and β-carotene [33]. HIE treatment showed a marked inhibition in LPO and thereby reduction in MDA content probably due to inhibition of propagation of LPO. Cellular defense mechanisms, which act against free radicals, include GSH and antioxidant enzymes such as SOD, CAT and GST respectively whose activities contribute to eliminate superoxide, hydrogen peroxide and hydroxyl radicals [34]. The activity of these antioxidant enzymes critically influences the susceptibility of various tissues to oxidative stress and is associated with the development of complications in diabetes. The superoxide

radicals are dismutated by SOD to form hydrogen peroxide followed by its decomposition into water and oxygen by catalase. Liver SOD activity was decreased in diabetic animals as compared to control. This may be due to excessive production of superoxide radical that inhibit the activity of SOD, which consequently improved after HIE treatment. The increased activity of kidney and erythrocytes SOD in diabetic mice may be a response to combat minor generation of ROS upon STZ administration, which was normalized in HIE treated diabetic mice. The increased activity of the liver, kidney and erythrocytes catalase was observed in STZ induced diabetes that was significantly restored by HIE. The elevation of CAT activity may be endogenous compensatory mechanism for prolonged over production of free radicals and oxidative stress [35].

Glutathione (GSH) efficient antioxidant present in almost all living cells and is considered as one of the biomarker of redox imbalance at cellular level. The present study showed decreased kidney and erythrocytes GSH content in diabetic control, which may be considered to be an indicator of increased free radical scavenger in the repair of radical caused biological damage. HIE treatment restores the GSH content, whereas glibenclamide treatment does not affect GSH content of STZ induced diabetic mice. Both liver GSH content and GST activity were increased in diabetic control suggesting that cellular antioxidant defense mechanism was triggered by STZ induced generation of ROS. There was a significant decrease in both liver GSH content and GST activity upon HIE treatment probably due to the up regulation of GSH redox system in liver to counteract oxidative stress, as GSH also act as cofactor for GST in this system.

The reduction in FBG upon HIE treatment in STZ induced diabetic mice, indicates that HIE has high antidiabetic potential probably due to the insulin secretagogue and antioxidative action of the *H indicus* root extract. Hyperglycaemia stimulates ROS formation and resulting oxidative stress triggers hyperglycaemia induced diabetic complications [36]. The hypoglycaemic and antioxidative effect of HIE may prevent development and progression of diabetic complications.

**Table 6** Effect of HIE on SOD and CAT in STZ induced diabetic mice

| SOD$^a$ | | | | CAT$^b$ | | | |
|---|---|---|---|---|---|---|---|
| Group | Liver | Kidney | Erythrocytes | Liver | Kidney | Erythrocytes |
| 1 | $19.19 \pm 0.50$ | $6.34 \pm 0.10$ | $120.83 \pm 4.64$ | $199.96 \pm 7.94$ | $187.28 \pm 5.13$ | $693.76 \pm 89.77$ |
| 2 | $2.97 \pm 0.05^{***}$ | $13.92 \pm 0.21^{***}$ | $263.95 \pm 9.96^{***\#}$ | $312.66 \pm 1.44^{***}$ | $243.86 \pm 10.68^*$ | $1652.21 \pm 85.34^{***}$ |
| 3 | $8.25 \pm 0.37^{***\#}$ | $5.32 \pm 0.12^{**\#}$ | $128.97 \pm 5.98^\#$ | $219.78 \pm 6.54^\#$ | $204.07 \pm 11.69^{NS}$ | $1444.72 \pm 27.18^{***}$ |
| 4 | $7.95 \pm 0.69^{***\#}$ | $6.96 \pm 0.17^\#$ | $27.34 \pm 2.28^{***\#}$ | $209.79 \pm 5.44^\#$ | $168.99 \pm 5.63^\#$ | $523.57 \pm 76.07^\#$ |

Values are mean $\pm$ SE of 6 animals
$^*P < 0.05$, $^{**}P < 0.01$, $^{***}P < 0.001$ = significant as compared to control (Group 1)
$^\#P < 0.001$ = significant as compared to diabetic control (Group 2). $^{NS}$Not significant
$^a$units/mg protein
$^b$μmoles $H_2O_2$ decomposed/min/mg protein

**Table 7** Effect of HIE on GSH and GST and in STZ induced diabetic mice

| GSH[a] | | | | GST[b] | | |
|---|---|---|---|---|---|---|
| Group | Liver | Kidney | Erythrocytes | Liver | Kidney | Erythrocytes |
| 1 | $19.27 \pm 0.62$ | $25.33 \pm 0.45$ | $25.05 \pm 0.91$ | $0.33 \pm 0.06$ | $0.36 \pm 0.07$ | $10.22 \pm 0.40$ |
| 2 | $31.60 \pm 1.98^*$ | $15.78 \pm 0.39^*$ | $7.31 \pm 1.11^*$ | $4.24 \pm 0.42^*$ | $1.37 \pm 0.13^*$ | $18.10 \pm 1.45^*$ |
| 3 | $13.93 \pm 1.78^{\#\#}$ | $25.66 \pm 1.61^{\#\#}$ | $7.94 \pm 0.21^*$ | $1.76 \pm 0.23^{*\#\#}$ | $1.11 \pm 0.08^*$ | $19.94 \pm 1.61^*$ |
| 4 | $22.04 \pm 0.67^{\#}$ | $38.26 \pm 0.61^{*\#\#}$ | $13.82 \pm 0.56^{*\#\#}$ | $0.16 \pm 0.02^{\#\#}$ | $0.30 \pm 0.05^{\#\#}$ | $6.97 \pm 0.30^{\#\#}$ |

Values are mean $\pm$ SE of 6 animals
$^*P < 0.001$ = significant as compared to control (Group 1)
$^{\#}P < 0.01, ^{\#\#}P < 0.001$ = significant as compared to diabetic control (Group 2)
[a]nanomoles of DTNB conjugated/mg protein for liver and kidney and $\mu$moles of DTNB conjugated/gm Hb for erythrocytes
[b]$\mu$moles of GSH conjugated/min/mg protein

Certain oxidative stress related defects in oxidative phosphorylation machinery and mitochondrial $\beta$-oxidation lead to excess accumulation of intracellular triglyceride in muscle and liver and subsequent insulin resistance [37]. As compared to diabetic control, glibenclamide and HIE treated mice, the total cholesterol, triglyceride, LDL and VLDL were significantly lowered with increased HDL indicating recovery of normal lipid metabolism in STZ induced diabetes. The results showed that HIE was found to be effective against diabetic dyslipidaemia.

## Conclusion

The methanolic extract of *H. indicus* roots contains various phytoconstituents having potent antioxidant, hypoglycaemic and hypolipidaemic activity. Oral administration of HIE, lowers the FBG of STZ induced diabetic mice as well as it modulates the intracellular antioxidant defense to overcome the oxidative damage and improves the serum lipid profile. It is suggested that the roots of *H. indicus* may serve as an important hypoglycaemic and hypolipidaemic agent to protect the cells by mitigating oxidative stress induced toxicity in STZ induced diabetes.

## Abbreviations

AJS: Agilent Jet Stream; CAT: Catalase; DPPH: 2,2-diphenyl-1-p-picryl-hydrazyl; ESI: Electrospray ion generation; FBG: Fasting Blood Glucose; FRAP: Ferric Reducing Antioxidant Power; FRSA: Free Radical Scavenging Activity; GSH: Glutathione; GST: Glutathione-S- Transferase; HDL: High Density Lipoprotein; HIE: Methanolic extract of *Hemidesmus indicus* roots; LC-MS: Liquid Chromatography-Mass Spectroscopy; LDL: Low Density Lipoprotein; LPO: Lipid Peroxidation; MDA: Malondialdehyde; NAD: Nicotinamide-adenine dinucleotide; PARP-1: Poly ADP ribose polymerase-1; PBS: Phosphate Buffer Saline; ROS: Reactive Oxygen Species; SOD: Superoxide Dismutase; STZ: Streptozotocin; TAP: Total Antioxidant Power; VLDL: Very Low Density Lipoprotein

## Acknowledgements

We acknowledge SAIF- IIT Bombay, India for providing LC-MS facility for analysis of samples. AJ is thankful to University Grant Commission, New Delhi for providing Golden Jubilee Fellowship under UGC XIIth Plan grant.

## Funding

The funding from Golden Jubilee Fellowship under University Grant Commission, New Delhi (UGC XII[th] Plan) was provided to Ankita Joshi for this research work.

## Authors' contributions

AJ: designed and performed the experiments, participated in data analysis and manuscript preparation. HL, HS and DB: participated in design of experiments and helped in manuscript preparation. All authors read and approved the final manuscript.

## Competing interests

The authors declare that they have no competing interests.

## References

1. Alberti KG, Zimmet PZ. New diagnostic criteria and classification of diabetes-again. Diabet Med. 1998;15:535–6.
2. Wolff SP, Jiang ZY, Hunt JV. Protein glycation and oxidative stress in diabetes mellitus and ageing. Free Radic Biol Med. 1991;10:339–52.
3. Scheen AJ, Lefèbvre PJ. Oral antidiabetic agents a guide to selection. Drugs. 1998;55:225–36.
4. Lakshmi T, Rajendran R. *Hemidesmus indicus* commonly known as Indian sarasaparilla- an update. Int J Pharm Bio Sci. 2013;4:397–404.
5. Zhao Z, Matsunami K, Otsuka H, Negi N, Kumar A, Negi DS. A condensed phenylpropanoid glucoside and pregnane saponins from the roots of *Hemidesmus indicus*. J Nat Med. 2013;67:137–42.
6. Fiori J, Leoni A, Fimognari C, Turrini E, Hrelia P, Mandrone M, Iannello C, Antognoni F, Poli F, Gotti R. Determination of phytomarkers in pharmaceutical preparations of *Hemidesmus indicus* roots by micellar electrokinetic chromatography and high-performance liquid chromatography–mass spectrometry. Anal Lett. 2014;47:2629–42.
7. Ravikiran T, Shilpa S, Praveen Kumar N, Sowbhagya R, Anand S, Anupama SK, Bhagyalakshmi D. Antioxidant activity of *Hemidesmus indicus* (L.) r.Br. Encapsulated poly (lactide-co-glycolide) (PLGA) nanoparticles. J Pharm Biol Sci. 2016;11:9–17.
8. Kumar S, Pooja M, Harika K, Haswitha E, Nagabhushanamma G, Vidyavathi N. In-vitro antioxidant activities, total phenolics and flavonoid contents of whole plant of *Hemidesmus indicus* (Linn.). Asian J Pharm Clin Res. 2013;6:249–51.
9. Singleton VL, Rossi JA. Colorimetry of total phenolics with phosphomolybdic-phosphotungstic acid reagents. Am J Enol Vitic. 1965;16:144–58.
10. Zhang L, Ravipati AS, Koyyalamudi SR, Jeong SC, Reddy N, Smith PT, Münch G, Wu MJ, Satyanarayanan M, Vysetti B. Antioxidant and anti-inflammatory activities of selected medicinal plants containing phenolic and flavonoid compounds. J Agr Food Chem. 2011;59:12361–7.
11. Chang CL, Lin CS. Phytochemical composition, antioxidant activity, and neuroprotective effect of *Terminalia chebula* Retzius extracts. Evid Based Compliment Alternat Med. 2012; https://doi.org/10.1155/2012/125247.
12. Mellors A, Tappel AL. The inhibition of mitochondrial peroxidation by ubiquinone and ubiquinol. J Biol Chem. 1966;241:4353–6.

13. Benzie IF, Strain JJ. The ferric reducing ability of plasma as a measure of antioxidant power: the FRAP assay. Anal Biochem. 1996;239:70–6.

14. Oyaizu M. Studies on product of browning reaction prepared from glucosamine. Jpn J Nutr. 1986;44:307–15.

15. Arora S, Ojha SK, Vohora D. Characterisation of streptozotocin induced diabetes mellitus in swiss albino mice. Glob J Pharmacol. 2009;3:81–4.

16. Lenzen S. The mechanisms of alloxan- and streptozotocin-induced diabetes. Diabetologia. 2008;51:216–26.

17. Kale M, Rathore N, John S, Bhatnagar D. Lipid peroxidative damage on pyrethroid exposure and alteration in antioxidant status in rat erythrocytes: a possible involvement of reactive oxygen species. Toxicol Lett. 1999;105: 197–205.

18. Tukozkan N, Erdamar H, Seven I. Measurement of total malondialdehyde in plasma and tissue by high performance liquid chromatography and thiobarbituric acid assay. Firat Tip Dergisi. 2006;11:88–92.

19. Marklund S, Marklund G. Involvement of the superoxide anion radical in autoxidation of pyrogallol and convenient assay for superoxide dismutase. Eur J Biochem. 1974;47:469–74.

20. Aebi H. Catalase. In: Bergmeyer HU, editor. Methods in enzymatic assay. 3rd ed. New York: Academic press; 1983. p. 276–86.

21. Habig WH, Pabst MJ, Jakoby WB. Glutathione-S-transferase, the first enzymatic step in mercapturic acid formation. J Biol Chem. 1974;249:7130–9.

22. Beutler E, Duran O, Kelly BM. Improved method for determination of blood glutathione. J Lab Clin Med. 1963;61:882–8.

23. Maritim AC, Sanders RA, Watkins JB 3rd. Diabetes, oxidative stress, and antioxidants: a review. J Biochem Mol Toxicol. 2003;17:24–38.

24. Gupta RK, Kesari AN, Diwakarc S, Tyagia A, Tandona V, Chandra R, Watal G. In vivo evaluation of anti-oxidant and anti-lipidimic potential of *Annona squamosa* aqueous extract in type 2 diabetic models. J Ethnopharmacol. 2008;118:21–5.

25. Steinberg D, Avigan J, Feigelson EB. Effects of triparanol (mer-29) on cholesterol biosynthesis and on blood sterol levels in man. J Clin Invest. 1961;40:884–93.

26. Martindale - the Extra Pharmacopoeia' (30th ed), edited by J. E. F. Reynolds. Pp 1310. London: The Pharmaceutical Press. 1993. ISBN 0 85369300 5.

27. Shibata K, Mushiage M, Kondo T, Hayakawa T, Tsuge H. Effects of vitamin B$_6$ deficiency on the conversion ratio of tryptophan to niacin. Biosci Biotechnol Biochem. 1995;59:2060–3.

28. Galvez-Llompart M, Zanni R, Domenech RG. Modeling natural anti-inflammatory compounds by molecular topology. Int J Mol Sci. 2011;12: 9481–503.

29. Steenken S, Neta P. One-electron redox potentials of phenols. Compounds of biological interest. J Phys Chem. 1982;86:3661–7.

30. Jayawardena N, Watawana MI, Waisundara VY. Evaluation of the total antioxidant capacity, polyphenol contents and starch hydrolase inhibitory activity of ten edible plants in an in vitro model of digestion. Plant Foods Hum Nutr. 2015;70:71–6.

31. Rajan S, Shalini R, Bharathi C, Aruna V, Thirunalasundari T, Brindha P. *In vitro* antioxidant screening of *Hemidesmus indicus* root from South India. Asian J Pharm Biol Res. 2011;1:222–31.

32. Obrosova IG, Fathallah L, Greene DA. Early changes in lipid peroxidation and antioxidative defense in diabetic rat retina: effect of DL-α-lipoic acid. Eur J Pharmacol. 2000;398:139–46.

33. Mekinova D, Chorvathova V, Volkovova K, Staruchova M, Grancicova E, Klvanova J, Ondreic R. Effect of intake of exogenous vitamins C, E and β-carotene on the antioxidative status in kidneys of rats with streptozotocin-induced diabetes. Nahrung. 1995;39:257–61.

34. Soto C, Recoba R, Barron C, Alverez C, Favari L. Silymarin increases antioxidant enzymes in alloxan-induced diabetes in rat pancreas. Comp Biochem Physiol. 2003;136:205–12.

35. Aksoy N, Vural H, Sabuncu T, Aksoy S. Effect of melatonin on oxidative-antioxidative status of tissues in streptozotocin induced diabetic rats. Cell Biochem Funct. 2003;21:121–5.

36. Valko M, Leibfritz D, Moncola J, Cronin MT, Mazura M, Telser J. Free radicals and antioxidants in normal physiological functions and human disease. Int J Biochem Cell Biol. 2007;39:44–84.

37. Rosca MG, Mustata TG, Kinter MT, Ozdemir AM, Kern TS, Szweda LI, Brownlee M, Monnier VM, Weiss MF. Glycation of mitochondrial proteins from diabetic rat kidney is associated with excess superoxide formation. Am J Physiol-Renal Physiol. 2005;289:F420–30.

# 8

# A herbal composition of *Scutellaria baicalensis* and *Eleutherococcus senticosus* shows vasocontrictive effects in an ex-vivo mucosal tissue model and in allergic rhinitis patients

Michael Katotomichelakis[1*], K. Van Crombruggen[2], G. Holtappels[2], F. A. Kuhn[3], C. E. Fichandler[3], C. A. Kuhn-Glendye[3], J. B. Anon[4], C. T. Melroy[3], B. Karanfilov[5], T. W. Haegen[6], I. Kastanioudakis[7], C. Bachert[2] and N. Zhang[2]

## Abstract

**Background:** This study aimed to investigate the nasal decongestive efficacy of an alternative to pharmacotherapy, a herbal nasal spray composed of *Scutellaria baicalensis* and *Eleutherococcus senticosus*.

**Methods:** *Scutellaria baicalensis* and *Eleuthrococcus senticosus* and control solutions were applied separately to isolated mucosal tissue from inferior turbinates. Vasoconstriction was measured as a change in isometric tension. Moreover, twenty allergic rhinitis patients with nasal stuffiness participated in a randomized, placebo-controlled clinical study with cross-over design; the same patients served as their placebo control group. Pre-and post-treatment nasal congestion and smell test scores were evaluated for the test and placebo spray using two validated questionnaires, the 5 question nasal congestion questionnaire and the 12 question Brief Smell Identification Test-Version B.

**Results:** In the ex-vivo mucosal tissue, the herbal compounds were demonstrated to induce vasoconstriction when applied at 10 mg/ml concentration. The combination of *S. baicalensis* and *E. senticosus* proved effective in relieving patients' nasal congestion and was statistically superior to placebo. No side effects were noted, and there was no difference between the pre-and post-study smell test results.

**Conclusions:** The combined *S. baicalensis* and *E. senticosus* herbal nasal spray relieved nasal congestion significantly better than placebo without any side effects.

**Keywords:** Herbal treatment, Scutellaria Baicalensis, Eleuthrococcus senticosus, Nasal congestion, Smell

## Background

The nose is the predominant contact point between the respiratory system and the external environment. Its primary function is to prepare the inspired air for the lungs. It acts not only as the primary low resistance conduit for air to reach the lungs, but to humidify, cleanse and warm the inspired air to protect the more delicate tissues of the

lower airways [1, 2]. As such, it is constantly exposed to aeroallergens, chemicals, pollutants and viral or bacterial organisms, which can induce inflammation that commonly manifests as nasal congestion or stuffiness [3, 4].

If the nose cannot perform its function, particularly as a low resistance air conduit due to obstruction, it adversely affects the entire organism. When the nose is obstructed, the individual's sleep is impaired, resulting in a deficit in daytime wakefulness and physical functions [5]. Chronic upper airway obstruction is frequently the presenting complaint in diseases such as allergic rhinitis (AR) and

* Correspondence: katotomihelakism@yahoo.gr
[1]Department of Otorhinolaryngology, Medical School, Democritus University of Thrace, Alexandroupolis, Greece
Full list of author information is available at the end of the article

chronic rhinosinusitis (CRS). These are among the most common disabling diseases, and respectively account for 20% and 11% of the European adult population [6, 7].

The most common remedy most patients resort to for nasal obstruction is nasal decongestant sprays or drops which work via alpha-adrenergic effects; unfortunately, these are associated with rebound congestion phenomena, which lead to repeated use and subsequent "rhinitis medicamentosa" [8, 9]. Consequently, it would be beneficial if a nasal spray could be developed based on other mechanisms, which did not have the associated rebound effects. As a result, an increasing number of patients have begun to look for an efficacious alternative, including herbal treatment options [10]. Over the last two decades interest has mounted regarding the mechanism of action of herbal therapies [10, 11]. Many attempts to identify the active components of herbal remedies have concluded that in general no single component may be responsible for the therapeutic capacity, but rather it is a complex and intricate interaction of various herbs, which may result in therapeutic efficacy. This therapeutic efficacy needs to be thoroughly documented and confirmed in randomized, blinded placebo-controlled trials. Moreover although the majority of herbal medications are delivered orally, topical applications have also been practiced. In 2007 Jung et al. [12] found that this combination of the herbals, *Scutellaria Baicalensis* (Baikal skullcap) and *Eleuthrococcus Senticosus* (Siberian ginseng) demonstrated significant suppression of inflammatory mediators, including IL-6, TNF-a, neutrophil density and prostaglandin E2 in the mouse model [12].

These two multipurpose herbs have been used in China traditionally for treatment of inflammation, hypertension, cardiovascular diseases, bacterial and viral infections with low toxicity [13–16]. Furthermore we have demonstrated before that the combination of both herbs has a strong anti-inflammatory activity equivalent to topical steroids, and reduce the release of mediators from mast cells upon stimulation, without any impairment of nasal ciliary beat frequency in human tissue [17].

Consequently, the purposes of this study was to explore the vasoconstrictive effects of *Scutellaria baicalensis* and *Eleutherococcus senticosus* in a human nasal mucosa ex-vivo organ bath model and to investigate the nasal decongestant effect of a combined commercial powder solution of the two herbs compared to placebo. Furthermore, we intended to monitor side effects on the sense of smell and rebound mucosal swelling as perceived by patients.

## Methods
### Ex-vivo nasal tissue organ bath model
Inferior turbinates (IT) from a total of five patients (mean age 34 years, range 22 to 65 years) suffering either from allergic rhinitis, deviated septum with turbinate hypertrophy or chronic rhinosinusitis were included in the study. Mucosal tissues from IT were obtained at the Department of Otorhinolaryngology, Ghent University Hospital, during routine surgery for nasal congestion complaints. Inferior turbinate hypertrophy was diagnosed by nasal endoscopy. None of the subjects received intranasal corticosteroids, anti-histamines, anti-leukotrienes, oral or intranasal decongestants, or intranasal anticholinergics within the 2 weeks prior to surgery. None of the subjects received oral and/or intramuscular corticosteroids within the 4 weeks prior to surgery. The ethical committee of the Ghent University Hospital approved the study, and all patients completed an IRB approved informed consent.

### IT tissue preparation
The inferior turbinates collected during surgery were immediately transported to the laboratory and placed in cold physiological salt solution (PSS in mM; NaCl: 118.5, KCl: 4.8, CaCl$_2$: 1.9, MgSO$_4$: 1.2, NaHCO$_3$: 25, KH$_2$PO$_4$: 1.2 and glucose: 10.1). The bony structures were carefully removed and 8 full-thickness strips ($3 \times 15$ mm) were cut along the transverse axis.

### Isometric tension recording
The strips -prepared as describe above- were mounted in 10 ml organ baths containing aerated (5% CO$_2$ in O$_2$) PSS, maintained at 37 °C.

Vasodilatation (responsible for nasal congestion) and vasoconstriction (relief of nasal congestion) were measured as a change in isometric tension by means of a MLT0201 force transducer (Panlab, Spain) attached to a Power lab/8sp data recording system (AD Instruments, U.K.). The signals were captured and analysed with Lab Chart 6 Pro software.

Because nasal mucosa contains no contractile elements other than the smooth muscles of the blood vessels, the changes in isometric tension in this tissue are exclusively mediated by the vascular smooth muscle cells. Relaxations consequently equal vasodilatation and contractions are vasoconstrictions.

### Patients study group
This study was conducted in 2011 as a double-blind placebo-controlled randomized cross-over trial (DBPCR). Twenty allergic rhinitis (AR) patients (mean age 55 years, range 24 to 67 years) whose presenting complaint was nasal stuffiness participated in the study. The inclusion criteria were age ≥ 18 years, male or female, current complaint of nasal congestion for > 4 weeks. Exclusion criteria were nasal polyps, an acute viral URI or bacterial infection. The same patients were used as the placebo-control (CO) group. Diagnosis of AR was based on history of nasal stuffiness, nasal endoscopy and skin prick test (SPT) with a battery of common aeroallergens. Only subjects who fulfilled the criteria of AR according to the

ARIA guidelines [18] and were sensitized exclusively to *HDM, grass* and *tree* pollens were included. The Memorial Health University Hospital Research Committee of 2011 approved the study and all patients completed an IRB approved informed consent before participating in the prospective, randomized, double blind, placebo-controlled crossover study.

The Test Spray (provided by BreatheZen, Znova LLC, Pikesville, MD, USA) contained the two herbs Scutellaria baicalensis and Eleuthrococcus senticosus, in solution with potassium sorbate and ascorbic acid in Ringer's lactate solution; the placebo spray included all elements aside from the two herbs, including Ringer's lactate solution, potassium sorbate, and ascorbic acid. The test and placebo sprays were randomly assigned to bottles A&B in order to vary the starting order of drug or placebo. The contents of bottles A&B were blinded to both patient and clinical examiner. The patients sprayed each nostril twice, 3 x per day with bottle A for 7 days, did not spray for 3 days as a "wash out" period and then sprayed each nostril twice, 3 x per day with bottle B for 7 days. Three days were chosen to have no remaining effect from the ingredients of bottle A (> 5 times the half-life of the anti-obstructive effect).

At the start and the end of the study periods A and B, patients were asked to fill in two validated widely used questionnaires for nasal congestion evaluation, the 5 question nasal congestion questionnaire [19] and the 12 question Brief Smell Identification Test-Version B [20]. Both questionnaires were administered before the study, after bottle A and after bottle B. Pre-and post-treatment nasal congestion scores as well as smell test scores were evaluated for verum (test spray) and placebo sprays, and side effects were monitored. The 5 question nasal congestion questionnaire (CQ5) is derived from the CQ7, which is reliable, valid, and responsive to differences in severity of nasal congestion. However, a MCID has not been elaborated.

## Statistical analysis

A Wilcoxon test for paired samples was used to reveal improvement from baseline with both the herbal spray and placebo. The Mann-Whitney $U$ test was used for between-group (unpaired) comparisons. $P$ values of less than 0.05 were considered statistically significant.

## Results

### Nasal mucosal tissue organ bath model

*10 mg/ml Eleutherococcus senticosus*, equivalent to the formulation of the spray, induced a vasoconstrictive response in nasal mucosal strips similar in magnitude to vasoconstrictive stimuli such as electrical field stimulation (EFS; 8 Hz) and $10^{-6}$ M phenylephrine. Given the fact that in patients allergic to *HDM* the response to

exogenous applied allergen still clearly induced a relaxation indicates that the action by *Eleutherococcus senticosus* is exclusively vasoconstrictive and not inhibitory against allergen-induced responses (Fig. 1). The contractions by *Eleutherococcus senticosus* are not mediated via a similar mechanism of action as traditional nasal decongestions as interference with adrenoceptor-related mechanisms by means of guanethidine and phentolamine have no effect on the magnitude of the contraction. The exact mechanism of action remains unknown but the involvement of prostaglandins or neuronal components that indirectly release other contractile substances could be excluded as indomethacin and tetrodotoxin was ineffective, respectively.

The nasal mucosal tissue showed normal responses to know stimuli such as EFS, 15 V, 8 Hz, 20 s, and phenylephrine $10^{-6}$ M, and HDM-induced relaxation (Fig. 2).

*Scutellaria baicalensis* could not be tested in the organ bath model due to foam formation.

## Patients DBPCR trial

All patients completed the study schedule, receiving two treatments (randomized selection of test sprays first or placebo spray first) and a 3 day wash-out period in between the treatment phases in a cross-over study design. There was a significant improvement from baseline nasal stuffiness with both the herbal spray ($p = 0.0002$) and placebo spray ($p = 0.002$) (Fig. 3). Furthermore, the change from baseline was significantly superior for the Herbal spray compared to placebo, and the two groups were significantly different at end of treatment in relieving nasal congestion ($p = 0.026$) (Wilcoxon Test for paired samples).

17/20 patients completed all 3 smell tests. The pre-test score total for all patients was 172 (improvement of 0.33/patient). Most patients had the same score before and after the study, a few patients had an improved score, none had a decreased score. There was consecutively no change in the smell test results with either spray, nor any significant differences between the pre-study and post-study smell test results. There were no adverse events reported from either treatment. No patient developed rhinitis medicamentosa-like symptoms (rebound congestion) from continued use of either spray, nor after cessation of use.

## Discussion

Nasal congestion is a quality of life concern that variably affects every individual [6]. When this becomes chronic, several systemic or topical decongestants are available, but all have undesired side effects. Topical nasal decongestants commonly produce rhinitis medicamentosa [8, 9]. Oral decongestants may be also a problem for patients with hypertension, pulmonary disease or prostate hypertrophy.

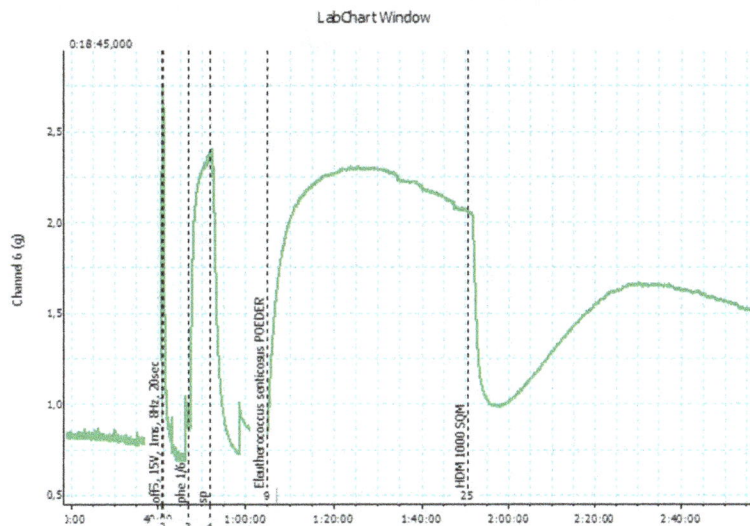

**Fig. 1** Responses to electricfield stimulation (EFS, 8 Hz) and the know vasoconstrictor phenylephrine ($10^{-6}$ M), followed by response to *Eleutherococcus senticosus* (10 mg/ml) and HDM (1000 SQM)

Nasal saline irrigations, which have become very popular may in fact interfere with ciliary beat frequency. Unal et al. [3] found that patients who used post operative Ringer's lactate irrigation, had significantly better mucocillary transport times than patents using isotonic saline. They concluded that Ringer's lactate is a better solution for nasal irrigation than 0.9% saline.

*Scutellaria baicalensis* and *Eleuthrococcus senticosus* are two herbs, which have been used for many years in Eastern medicine and have recently been shown to have strong anti-inflammatory effects [13–16]. Specifically, in our previous study in a human nasal mucosal model we found that the combination of these two herbs suppresses PGD-2, histamine, IL-5 and pro-inflammatory cytokines equal to or better than fluticasone nasal spray [17]. Our conclusion was that the combination of *S. baicalensis* and *E. senticosus* may be able to significantly block allergic early-and late-phase mediators and substantially suppress the release of proinflammatory and Th1-, Th2-, and Th17- derived cytokines [17]. This suggests that the combination of *Scutellaria baicalensis* and *Eleutherococcus senticosus* may be as good

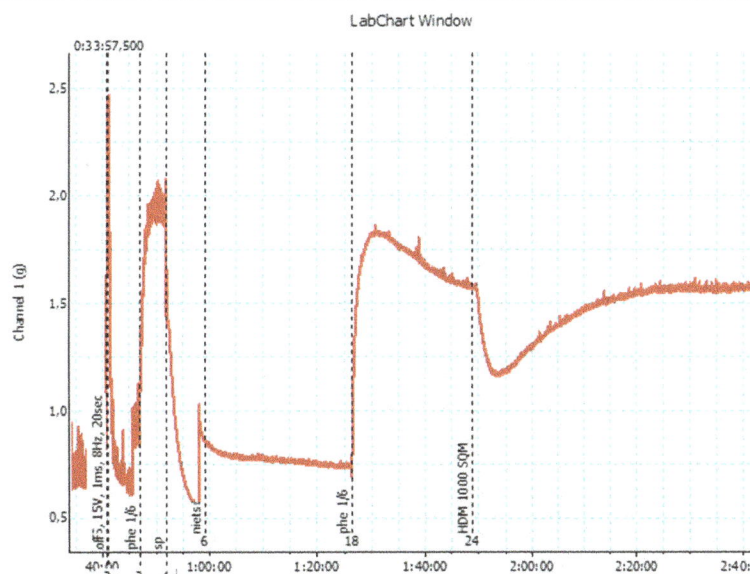

**Fig. 2** Positive controls: normal responses to EFS (8 Hz) and phenylephrine ($10^{-6}$ M) followed by response to HDM (1000 SQM) on a phenylephrine-precontracted tissue

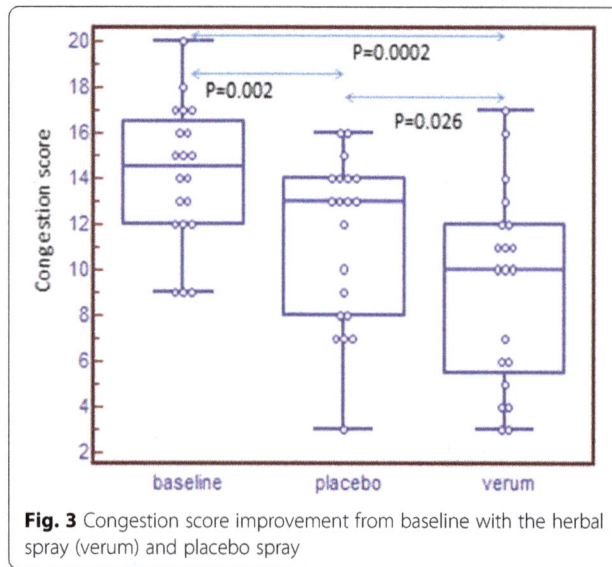

**Fig. 3** Congestion score improvement from baseline with the herbal spray (verum) and placebo spray

as nasal corticosteroid sprays in controlling allergic rhinitis, without the concern for HPA axis suppression. Further studies will be required to establish this.

The purpose of this study was to demonstrate that these herbal compounds reduce nasal congestion. Indeed, we found significant improvement of the 5 question nasal congestion questionnaire scores [19]- in patients who used the herbal nasal spray, compared to the placebo control group ($p = 0.026$) and to the baseline score ($p = 0.0002$). The Smell Test demonstrated no difference between the pre and post study smell test results (Brief Smell Identification Test-Version B [20].

Furthermore, experiments in ex vivo human mucosal tissue from inferior turbinates showed *Eleutherococcus senticosus* to induce a vasoconstrictive response when given to an organ bath setup. This vasoconstrictive effect at 10 mg/ml was similar in magnitude to vasoconstrictive stimuli such as electrical field stimulation (EFS; 8 Hz) and $10^{-6}$ M phenylephrine.

The given data in this study reveal that the herbal spray is safe for nasal use and effectively reduces nasal congestion more significantly than the base solution of Ringer's lactate, vitamin C and potassium sorbate. It does not affect the patients' sense of smell and does not cause any rebound nasal congestion. The clinical application of this herbal spray has the potential to benefit a wide array of patients who suffer from nasal congestion, but do not want the rebound phenomena associated with other nose sprays or cannot use oral decongestants secondary to comorbidities or paradoxical side effects. The potential antibacterial and possible antiviral properties and its anti-inflammatory effect, make this an attractive alternative to current nasal decongestant sprays. Further studies are needed to more completely

evaluate this herbal medication's efficacy and range of application.

## Conclusion

We found that the *Scutellaria baicalensis* and *Eleuthrococcus senticosus* herbal nasal spray relieved nasal congestion in a mucosal model and in clinic significantly better than placebo without any reported rebound effect and no effect on the sense of smell. The potential uses for this spray include use in acute and chronic sinusitis, allergic rhinitis, viral upper respiratory infections and even peri-operative application. Further evaluation of the safety and efficacy of this herbal spray in rhinitis patients is pending.

**Abbreviations**
AR: Allergic rhinitis; CO: Control; CQ5: 5 question nasal congestion questionnaire; CRS: Chronic rhinosinusitis; DBPCR: Double-blind placebo-controlled randomized cross-over trial; EFS: Electrical field stimulation; IT: Inferior turbinates; SPT: Skin prick test; URI: Upper respiratory infection

**Acknowledgements**
Not applicable.

**Funding**
No funding

**Authors' contributions**
KM and KI analyzed the data and drafted manuscript; VCK and HG carried out the human nasal mucosa ex-vivo organ bath model and drafted manuscript; KA, FCE, KGCA and MCT participated in the design of the study, carried out the double-blind placebo-controlled randomized cross-over trial in patients, and analyzed the data; AJB, KB and HTW participated in the design of the study and coordination and drafted manuscript; BC and ZN designed, conceived the study and coordination, analyzed the data and drafted manuscript. All authors read and approved the final manuscript.

**Competing interests**
The authors declare that they have no competing interests.

**Author details**
[1]Department of Otorhinolaryngology, Medical School, Democritus University of Thrace, Alexandroupolis, Greece. [2]Upper Airways Research Laboratory (URL), Ghent University Hospital, Ghent, Belgium. [3]Georgia Nasal & Sinus Institute, Savannah, GA, USA. [4]ENT Specialists of Northwest Pennsylvania, Erie, PA, USA. [5]Ohio Sinus Institute, Dublin, OH, USA. [6]Arizona Sinus Center, Phoenix, AZ, USA. [7]Department of Otorhinolaryngology, Medical School, University of Ioannina, Ioannina, Greece.

## References

1. Geurkink N. Nasal anatomy, physiology, and function. J Allergy Clin Immunol. 1983;72:123–8.
2. Bachert C. Clinical aspects of environmental illnesses of the nose and paranasal sinuses–science and clinical practice. Eur Arch Otorhinolaryngol Suppl. 1996;1:73–153.
3. Unal M, Görür K, Ozcan C. Ringer-lactate solution versus isotonic saline solution on mucociliary function after nasal septal surgery. J Laryngol Otol. 2001;115:796–7.
4. Naclerio RM, Bachert C, Baraniuk JN. Pathophysiology of nasal congestion. Int J Gen Med. 2010;3:47–57.
5. Osborn JL, Sacks R. Chapter 2: nasal obstruction. Am J Rhinol Allergy. 2013; 27(Suppl 1):S7–8.
6. Bachert C, Van Cauwenberge P, Olbrecht J, Van Schoor J. Prevalence, classification and perception of allergic and nonallergic rhinitis in Belgium. Allergy. 2006;61:693–8.
7. Hastan D, Fokkens WJ, Bachert C, et al. Chronic rhinosinusitis in Europe-an underestimated disease. A GA2LEN in study. Allergy. 2011;66:1216–23.
8. Ramey JT, Bailen E, Lockey RF. Rhinitis medicamentosa. J Investig Allergol Clin Immunol. 2006;16:148–55.
9. Scadding GK. Rhinitis medicamentosa. Clin Exp Allergy. 1995;25:391–4.
10. Li XM, Brown L. Efficacy and mechanisms of action of traditional Chinese medicines for treating asthma and allergy. J Allergy Clin Immunol. 2009;123: 297–306.
11. Eisenberg DM, Kessler RC, Foster C, Norlock FE, Calkins DR, Delbanco TL. Unconventional medicine in the United States. Prevalence, costs, and patterns of use. NEJM. 1993;328:246–52.
12. Jung SM, Schumacher HR, Kim H, Kim M, Lee SH, Pessler F. Reduction of urate crystal-induced inflammation by root extracts from traditional oriental medicinal plants: elevation of prostaglandin D2 levels. Arthritis Res Ther. 2007;9:R64.
13. Huang CH, Kimura R, Bawarshi-Nassar R, Hussain A. Mechanism of nasal absorption of drugs. II: absorption of L-tyrosine and the effect of structuralmodification on its absorption. J Pharm Sci. 1985;74:1298–301.
14. Gulla J, Singer AJ, Gaspari R. Herbal use in ED patients. Acad Emerg Med. 2001;8:450.
15. Eisenberg DM, Kessler RC, Foster C, Norlock FE, Calkins DR, Delbanco TL. Unconventional medicine in the United States. Prevalence, costs, and patterns of use. N Engl J Med. 1993;328:246–52.
16. Ueda S, Nakamura H, Masutani H, Sasada T, Takabayashi A, Yamaoka Y, Yodoi J. Baicalin induces apoptosis via mitochondrial pathway as prooxidant. Mol Immunol. 2002;38:781–91.
17. Zhang N, Van Crombruggen K, Holtappels G, Bachert C. A herbal composition of Scutellariabaicalensis and Eleutherococcussenticosus shows potent anti-inflammatory effects in an ex vivo human mucosal tissue model. Evid Based Complement Alternat Med. 2012;2012:673145.
18. Bousquet J, Khaltaev N, Cruz AA, et al. Allergy. 2008;63(Suppl 86):8–160.
19. Stull DE, Meltzer EO, Krouse JH, Roberts L, Kim S, Frank L, Naclerio R, Lund V, Long A. The congestion quantifier five-item test for nasal congestion: refinement of the congestion quantifier seven-item test. Am J Rhinol Allergy. 2010;24:34–8.
20. Doty RL, Marcus A, Lee WW. Development of the 12-item Cross-Cultural Smell Identification Test (CC-SIT). Laryngoscope. 1996;106:353–6.

# 9

# Evaluation of wound healing effect of herbal lotion in albino rats and its antibacterial activities

T. Dons[*] and S. Soosairaj

## Abstract

**Background:** This particular study emphasis on the in vivo wound healing and in vitro antibacterial activity of herbal lotions preparated from Ethanolic extract of Justicia tranquebariensis, *Aloe vera* and *Curcuma longa*.

**Methods:** Each plant powder (10 g) was soaked in 30 ml of ethanol in a sterile bottle for 48 h at 4 °C. Herbal lotion formulation I (10%) and II (20%) was prepared. Antibacterial activity by Agar Well diffusion method for three medicinal plant lotions was tested against skin and wound pathogens, like *Staphylococcus aureus*, Bacillus subtilis, *Escherichia coli* and *Klebsiella pneumoniae*. The excision wound model was employed for wound healing activity in albino rats. Healthy albino rats (150-200 g) of either sex were taken for excision wound model. Animals were divided into four groups of six animals in each. The Group 1 is control. The Groups 2 and 3 animals were treated with 10% and 20% ointment of herbal lotion and Group 4 animals were treated with Soframycin that served as standard. All animals had free access to pelleted food and water. Temperature was maintained at 23 ± 1 °C. The results were expressed as mean ± SEM. Further sample tissues were fixed in 10% buffered formalin, processed and blocked with paraffin at 40–60 °C, and then sectioned into 5 µm thick sections. The significance of differences between the means was analyzed by student's t- test followed by Turkey's test.

**Results:** Complete wound healing was observed with lotion formulation I and II treated rats in 15 days as that of Soframycin ointment. These findings were further confirmed by histological examination of granulation tissue with a lesser amount of collagination and absence of inflammatory cells.

**Conclusion:** The findings from this research indicates that the ethanol extract of Justicia tranquebariensis, *Aloe vera* and *Curcuma longa* are effective in inhibiting the growth of wound associated pathogen and faster the process of wound healing.

**Keywords:** Justicia tranquebariensis, *Curcuma longa*, *Aloe vera*, Lotion, Wound healing and histochemical studies

## Background

Wound is the disruption of cellular and anatomic continuity of living tissue produced by physical, chemical, electrical or microbial insults to the tissue. Wound healing is the dynamic process of regeneration or repair of broken tissue [1]. Normal wound-healing response begins with injury and is a concentrated sequence of events. The healing cascade is activated when platelets aggregate and the release of clotting factors resulting in the deposition of fibrin clot at the site of injury [2]. The fibrin clot serves as a provisional matrix and sets the stage for the subsequent events of healing.

Inflammatory cells also arrive along with the platelets at the site of injury providing key signals known as cytokines or growth factors. The fibroblast is the connective tissue responsible for collagen deposition that is needed to repair the tissue injury. In normal tissues, collagen provides strength, integrity, and structure. When tissues are disrupted following injury, collagen is needed to repair the defect and restore anatomic structure and function [3].

Hence, there is a need for herbal based wound healing agents. *Curcuma longa* has anti-inflammatory, antimicrobial and wound healing property [4]. *Aloe* has anti-inflammatory activity, increase degree of cross-linking [5] and also used as moisturizing agent.

* Correspondence: dona.thiraviadoss@gmail.com
Department of Botany, St. Joseph's College, Trichy, India

The rationale behind the selection of above microbial stains is based on the literature survey as referred below. *Staphylococcus aureus* and *Escherichia coli* were the most common causative agent of wound infections [6, 7]. *Klebsiella pneumoniae* was associated with nosocomial infections burn wound infection and sepsis in surgical wounds [8]. *Bacillus subtilis* was associated with nosocomial infection and could cause secondary diseases and infections such as bacteremia, septicemia, and wound infection in hospitalized patients, especially patients who had the impaired immune system [9].

In present study herbal lotion was prepared and its feasibility was checked by wound healing activity in albino rats as compared to Soframycin ointment.

## Methods
### Plant collection and processing
Stem of *Justicia tranquebariensis*, succulent leaves of *Aloe vera* and rhizome of *Curcuma longa* were collected from Semmalai hills. Their taxonomic identify was confirmed using local flora [10]. The plants were washed three times in running tap water to remove the soil particles and other unwanted waste materials. Cleaned plants were chopped into small pieces and shade dried at room temperature. The dried plant samples were pulverized using a blender and the powder were collected in a clean glass bottles and stored until further use.

### Preparation of NA broth
*Staphylococcus aureus, Bacillus subtilis, Escherichia coli,* and *Klebsiella pneumoniae* were procured from Doctors Diagnostic Centre, Tiruchirappalli and subculture in nutrient broth with the help of sterile inoculation loop. The pure cultured nutrient broth was kept overnight at 37 °C. After that, the culture was maintained in freezer for further use [11].

### Preparation of plant extract
Each plant powder (10 g) was soaked in 30 ml of ethanol in a sterile bottle for 48 h at 4 °C. There after the extract was filtered and allowed to evaporate and the residue was weighed. The solvent free dried extract residues were resuspended in ethanol and stored in refrigerator for herbal lotion preparation [12].

### Herbal lotion
Herbal lotion formulation I (10%) and II (20%) was prepared by dissolving *Justicia tranquebariensis, Aloe vera* and *Curcuma longa* extracts as given in (Table 1). To this Petroleum Jelly and White soft paraffin was added and the mixture was stirred. Petroleum jelly and white soft paraffin, (British Pharmacopoeia, 1988) was used as a hydrocarbon (oleaginous) base.

**Table 1** Constituents of herbal lotion

| Ingredients | Formulation I (10%) (in g) | Formulation II (20%) (in g) |
|---|---|---|
| *Justicia tranquebariensis* | 1 | 2 |
| *Aloe vera* | 0.75 | 1.5 |
| *Curcuma longa* | 0.5 | 1 |
| Petroleum Jelly | 6.75 | 13.5 |
| White soft paraffin | 1 | 2 |

### Antibacterial activity by agar well diffusion method
The prepared lotion was studied for its activity against gram positive bacteria (*Staphylococcus aureus, Bacillus subtilis*) and gram negative bacteria (*Escherichia coli, Klebsiella pneumoniae*).

The antibacterial activity of the extracts was determined by agar well diffusion technique. 20 ml of nutrient agar media was transferred into petriplates and they were left undisturbed for 1-2 h. Bacterial culture (0.5 µl) was transferred into petriplates using cotton stick and evenly spread with the help of sterile bent glass rod. Cups was made in Petri plates using sterile cork borer having diameter of 6 mm and each formulation was added into well. Then bacterial plates were incubated at 37 °C 24 h [13]. Antibacterial activity was determined by measuring the zone of inhibition around each well using zone reader [14]. Measured inhibition zones were recorded as mean diameter in mm.

### Evaluation of in vivo wound healing activity
#### Study setting
Ethical approval to the study was obtained from the Srimad Andavan Arts and Science College institutional animal ethics committee (Vide No. SAC/IAEC/BC/2016/Ph.D-001) (Appendix - I). Albino rats (150-200 g) were housed in standard plastic rat cages with stainless steel coverlids and wheat straw was used as bedding material. The animals were kept at the animal house of Department of Biochemistry, Srimad Andavan Arts and Science College, Tiruchirappalli. All animals had free access to pelleted food and water. Temperature was maintained at 23 ± 1 °C.

The animals were divided in to four groups as given below. Each group consisted of six animals each.

- Group I – Normal Excision wounded animals without treatment
- Group II – Normal Excision wounded animals with Low dose (10%) treated for 15 days.
- Group III – Normal Excision wounded animals with High dose (20%) treated for 15 days.
- Group IV - Normal Excision wounded animals with Standard Drug Soframycin treated for 15 days.

**Excision wound model** The rats weighing (150 to 200 g) were selected and their hairs from dorsal thoracic central region were shaved after anaesthetized to a diameter of 30 mm with the aid of rizor blades. The anticipated area of the wound was marked on the shaved skin. Skin wound were created with aid of toothed forceps, surgical blades and pointed scissors. The wound was cleaned with cotton swab soaked in alcohol.

The two herbal formulations and Soframycin ointment were applied on wound once daily for 15 days starting from the first day of wounding. Wound contraction was measured for 15 days at interval of 2 days [15]. Contraction which mainly contributes for wound closure was studied by tracing the raw wound area on transparent paper every alternate day till wounds were completely covered with epithelium. These wound tracings were retraced on a millimeter scale graph paper, to determine the wound area. Wound contraction (WC) was calculated as a percentage change in the initial wound size i.e.

$$Percentage\ Wound\ Closure = \frac{(Initial\ wound\ size - specific\ day\ wound\ size)}{Initial\ Wound\ size} \times 100$$

Epithalization period was monitored by noting the number of days required for Escher to fall away, leaving no raw wound behind.

**Histopathology study of wounds** The healing tissues from all groups of animals were obtained on 15th day and processed for histological study. Sample tissues were fixed in 10% buffered formalin, processed and blocked with paraffin at 40–60 °C, and then sectioned into 5 μm thick sections with the help of microtome section and stained with hematoxylin-eosin and observed under microscope for any histological changes [16]. The different animal groups were assessed and the results were compared with control groups.

**Statistical analysis** The results were expressed as mean ± SEM. The significance of differences between the means was analyzed by student's t- test followed by Turkey's test. A $P$-value< 0.05 was considered significant.

## Results and discussion
### Antibacterial activity of plant lotion
The lotions I & II exhibited excellent antibacterial activity against all the selected bacteria. Among the four test organisms E. coli, and Klebsiella pneumoniae were inhibited by formulation I and II. Moderate inhibition was noticed against Staphylococcus aureus and Bacillus subtilis. It was observed that, inhibitory action was highest for gram negative bacteria, followed by gram positive bacteria Table 2.

J. tranquebariensis; A. vera and C. longa were part of the traditional system of medicine for treating skin conditions by topical applications onto the affected area [17–19]. All

**Table 2** Results of antibacterial activity of herbal lotion by agar well diffusion method

| Test organism | Zone of Inhibition in mm** | |
|---|---|---|
| | 10% | 20% |
| Staphylococcus aureus | 10,11,13 | 12,13,15 |
| Bacillus subtilis | 10,12,13 | 11,13,15 |
| E. coli | 10,11,12 | 12,14,15 |
| Klebsiella pneumoniae | 11,12,13 | 12,13,14 |

**Zone measurement

chronic wounds were colonized by bacteria, with low levels of bacteria being beneficial to the wound healing process. Wound infection was detrimental to wound healing, but the diagnosis and management of wound infection was controversial, and varies between clinicians. There was increasing recognition of the concept of critical colonization or local infection, when wound healing may be delayed in the absence of the typical clinical features of infection. The progression from wound colonization to infection depends not only on the bacterial count or the species present, but also on the host immune response, the number of different species present, the virulence of the organisms and synergistic interactions between the different species [20]. There was increasing evidence that bacteria within chronic wounds lived within communities, in which the bacteria were protected from host defences and develop resistance to antibiotic treatment.

An appreciation of the factors affecting the progression from colonization to infection could help clinicians with the interpretation of clinical findings and microbiological investigations in patients with chronic wounds. An understanding of the physiology and interactions within multi-species wound may aid the development of more effective methods of treating infected and poorly healing wounds. The emergence of consensus guidelines has helped to optimize clinical management [21].

### Wound healing activity
In excision wound study, wound contraction rate was identical to the ointment and the herbal formulations (I and II). Complete healing was observed in 14th day in all treated groups Table 3 while untreated group

**Table 3** Rate of Wound Contraction and Epithelialization in experimental animals

| Groups | Wound Contraction (cm) | | Rate of Epithelialization (Days) |
|---|---|---|---|
| | 0th Day | 15th Day | |
| Group I | 2.08 ± 0.06 | 1.62 ± 0.05 | 15.50 ± 0.56 |
| Group II | 2.15 ± 0.02 | 1.23 ± 0.02 | 10.33 ± 0.42 |
| Group III | 2.13 ± 0.05 | 0.62 ± 0.04 | 6.83 ± 0.31 |
| Group IV | 2.17 ± 0.03 | 0.37 ± 0.04 | 4.50 ± 0.34 |

(control) and group IV (cream base) animals took more than 15 days for healing of wounds Fig. 1.

There was a significant increase in percentage of contractibility from day five onwards in herbal lotion treated rats when compared with control rats. The wound contracting ability of animals treated with ointment containing (20% $w$/w) herbal lotion was found to be significantly higher ($P < 0.001$) on 15th day when compared to the control group. A better healing pattern and reduction in period of epithalization was observed in herbal lotion 20% w/w treated group.

Results obtained in the present study suggested that treatment of excision wounds with herbal lotion of *J.tranquebariensis*, *A. vera* and *C. longa* has accelerated the wound healing process. The results showed that Soframycin increased the collagen content of the skin and contributed to wound strength. The wound healing potential of the herbal lotion may be attributed to the presence of a mixture of phytoconstituents including flavonoids and tannins [22].

Therapeutic use of medicinal plants was an alternative health care option for those living in rural areas. Dependence on medicinal plants by the rural people was governed by economic factors, ease of availability and the strong belief in the plant remedies. The use of medicinal plants for treating various ailments ranging from acute to chronic conditions has become a way of life for many indigenous people in rural communities. Based on regular usage, many indigenous people were familiar with the different uses, preparations and identification of medicinal plants. Traditional herbalists and herb-sellers were the main sources of distributing information and prescriptions on medicinal plant remedies in rural communities [23].

The histopathological studies revealed Fig. 2 that the wounds treated with herbal lotion (20%) showed a discontinuous epidermis, with mild vacuolization and less amount of collagination and absence of in inflammatory cells. The rats treated with (10%) herbal lotion showed extensive necrosis and collagination with disturbed epidermis. The Soframycin treated animals showed hyper granulation and evidences of inflammatory cells. Restoration of adnexa, and extensive fibrosis and collagen tissue within the dermis observed. The control group of rats showed normal histopathological architecture.

The maturation and remodeling phase of wound healing has cell population decreased and collagen deposition will be increased in granulation tissues which form

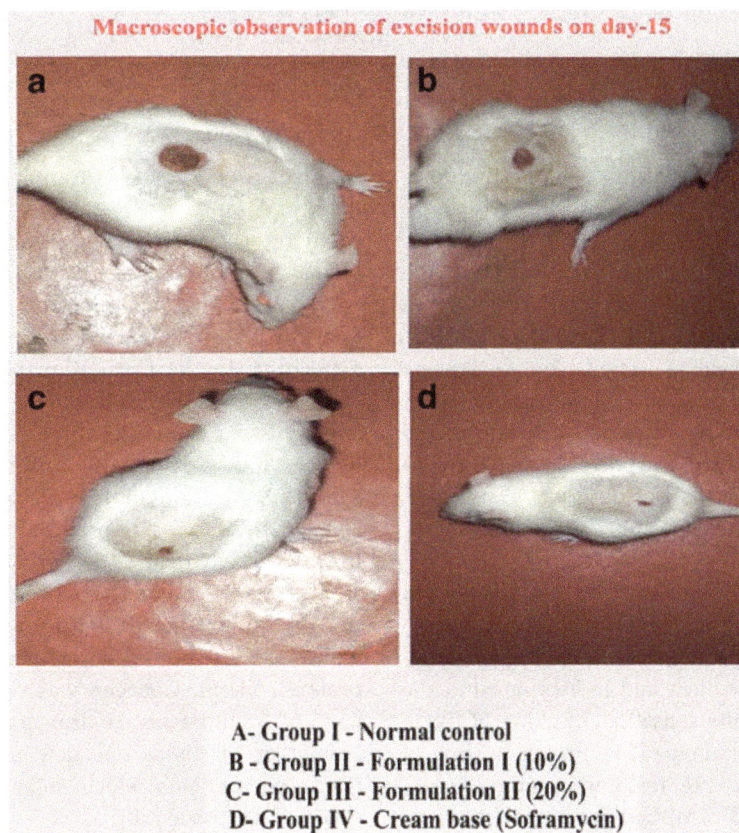

Macroscopic observation of excision wounds on day-15

A- Group I - Normal control
B - Group II - Formulation I (10%)
C- Group III - Formulation II (20%)
D- Group IV - Cream base (Soframycin)

**Fig. 1** Photographical representation of wound treatment

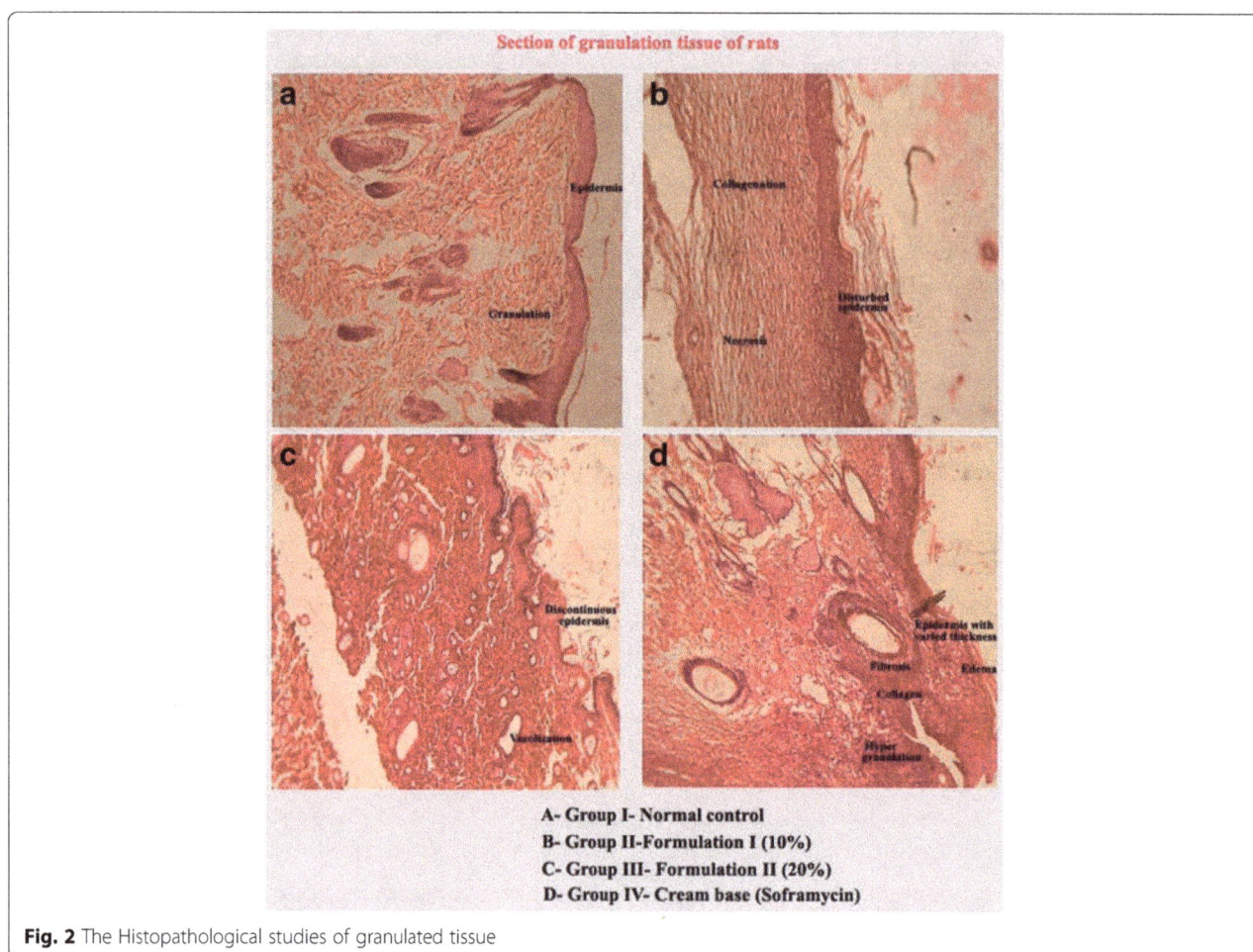

**Fig. 2** The Histopathological studies of granulated tissue

the scar. The Fig. 2 shows the histopathological studies of granulated tissue from control to treated group (GROUP-I, GROUP-II GROUP-III GROUP-IV). The hematoxylin and eosin staining were used for the complete loss of collagen and the same was observed in group-1 and group-3. The Group-3 (20%) dose resulted with significant wound-healing activity by decreasing period of vacuolization formation of granulation tissue. The synthesis of collagen by increased rate of wound contraction was compared to the control animals. Accumulation of inflammatory cells was observed in group-4, compared to treated groups of 2 and 3where the inflammatory cells were absent.

Wounds were physical injuries that resulted in an opening or break of the skin. The most common symptoms of wounds were bleeding, loss of feeling or function below the wound site, heat and redness around the wound, painful or throbbing sensation, swelling of tissue in the area and pus like drainage [24]. Proper healing of wounds was essential for the restoration of disrupted anatomical continuity and disturbed functional status of the skin. It was a product of the integrated response of several cell types to injury.

This process was a complex phenomenon and it mainly comprises of 3 phases: inflammatory phase, proliferative phase and maturational or remodeling phase. The inflammatory phase was characterized by haemostasis and inflammation. Proliferative phase was followed by epithelialization, angiogenesis and collagen deposition. In the maturation phase, the wound underwent contraction resulting in a smaller amount of apparent scar tissue [25–27]. Granulation tissue formed in the final part of the proliferative phase after the topical application of herbal lotion at both low (10%) and high (20%) was composed of collagen and epidermis. The high dose 20% herbal lotion treated animals showed better results than the reference drug Soframycin treated group though both the dose of herbal lotion treated group showed a significant increase in hydroxyproline content. Collagen was composed of hydroxyproline and amino acids. Hydroxyproline has been used as a biomarker for tissue collagen and the collagen was the major components which supports and strengthen the extracellular tissue [28].

The enhanced capacity of wound healing with the plant was on the basis of anti-inflammatory effects of the plant that were well documented in the literature [29]. Study on animal models showed enhanced rate of wound contraction and drastic reduction in healing time than control, which might be due to enhanced epitheliasation. Many studies indicated that plant products were potential agents for wound healing and were largely preferred because of the absence of unwanted side effects and their effectiveness [30]. Any agent who accelerates the above processes was a promoter of wound healing. The application of medicinal concoctions from plants to treat skin lesions, in particular wounds had a long tradition. Plants with wound healing activity have been reported and experimentally studied on various animal models to reveal the most active promising compounds [31].

## Conclusion

All the above results indicate the effectiveness of herbal lotions in enhancing wound healing activities. The herbal lotion prepared from extract of *Justicia tranquebariensis*, *Curcuma longa*, and *Aloe vera* showed marked reduction in wound area in comparison to control group when examined for wound healing activity by topical application in albino rat.

## Abbreviations

%: *Percentage*; $^0$C: Degree *Celsius*; C: Celsius; g: Gram; hrs: Hours; i.e.: id est.; ml: Millilitre; mm: Millimolar; NA: Nutrient agar; w/w: Weight per Weight; wc: Wound Contraction; μl: Microlitre

## Acknowledgements
The authors are thankful to the management Professors Agnel Arul John, and Ramesh Kannan, Department of Biochemistry of Srimad Andavan Arts and Science College and for providing facilities to carry out this work. We are also thankful to Dr. Karthik Mohan, and Dr. Benno Susai, Department of Biochemistry, St. Joseph's College, for their help in histopathology.

1. Dr. N. Agnel Arul John
   Assistant Professor.
   Department of Biochemistry.
   Srimad Andavan Arts and Science College.
   Trichy-2, India.
2. Dr. N. Ramesh Kannan
   Assistant Professor.
   Department of Biochemistry.
   Srimad Andavan Arts and Science College.
   Trichy, India.
3. Dr. Karthik Mohan
   Assistant Professor.
   Department of Biochemistry.
   St. Joseph's College.
   Trichy-2, India.
4. Dr. Benno Susai
   Assistant Professor.
   Department of Biochemistry.
   St. Joseph's College.
   Trichy-2, India.

## Funding
This study was not funded by any funding agency.

## Authors' contributions
TD - Major part of the research work was done. SS - Monitored the progress and edited the full text manuscript. Both authors read and approved the final manuscript.

## Competing interests
The authors declare that they have no competing interests.

## References
1. Farahpour MR, Habibi M. Evaluation of the wound healing activity of an ethanolic extract of *Ceylon cinnamon* in mice. Vet Med. 2012;57:53.
2. Eppley BL, Woodall JE, Higgins J. Platelet quantification and growth factor analysis from platelet-rich plasma: implications for wound healing. Plast Reconstr Surg. 2004;114:1502–8.
3. Madhava Chetty K, Sivaji K, Tulasirao K. Flowering plants of Chittor District, Andhra Pradesh. Tirupati, India: Students offset printers; 2008. p. 277.
4. Ukil A, Maity S, Karmakar S, Datta N, Vedasiromoni JR, Das PK. Curcumin, the major component of food flavour turmeric, reduces mucosal injury in trinitrobenzene sulphonic acid-induced colitis. Br J Pharmacol. 2003;139: 209–18.
5. Chithra P, Sajithal GB, Chandrakasan G. Influence of *aloe vera* on collagen characteristics in healing dermal wound in rats. Mol Cell Biochem. 1998;181: 71–6.
6. Bagdonas R, Tamelis A, Rimdeika R. *Staphylococcus aureus* in the surgery of burns. Medicina. 2003;39:1078–81.
7. Roesch M, Perreten V, Doher MG, Schaeren W, Schallibaum M, Blum JW. Comparison of antibiotic resistance of udder pathogens in dairy cows kept on organic and on conventional farms. J Dairy Sci. 2006;89:989–97.
8. Schwarz S, Chaslus-Dancla E. Use of anticrobials in veterinary medicine and mechanisms of resistance. Vet Res. 2001;32:201–25.
9. Azizi H, Saleh F, Khelrandish F, Azizi M. Molecular diagnosis and characterization of *Bacillus subtilis* isolated from burn wound in Iran. Res. Mol Med. 2014;2:40–4.
10. Matthew KM. The Flora of Tamil Nadu Carnatic. The Rapinet HerbariuM, St. Joseph's College. 1983; 1–3, Tiruchirapalli, India.
11. Kamal A, Swapna P, Shetti RV, Shaik AB, Narasimha Rao MP, Gupta S. Synthesis, biological evaluation of new oxazolidino-sulfonamides as potential antimicrobial agents. EurJMedChem. 2013;62:661–9.
12. Sebastian S, Thiraviadoss D. Spectral and antibacterial studies on some ethnobotanically important medicinal plants used by Thottianaickans of Semmalai. Indo Am J Pharm Res. 2015;5:2617–25.
13. Pesaramelli K, Vellanki J, Keerthi DV, Chaitanya SK. Evaluation of antibacterial activity of herbs. Int Res J Pharm. 2012;3:230–2.
14. Killedar SG, Harinath N. Antimicrobial and phytochemical screening of different leaf extracts of memecylon umbellatum burm. Int Res J Pharmacy. 2012;3:188–92.
15. Biswas TK, Maity LN, Mukherjee B. Wound healing potential of *Pterocarpus Santalinus* Linn: a pharmacological evaluation. International journal of low extreme. Wounds. 2004;3:143–50.
16. Sadaf F, Saleem R, Ahmed M, Ahmad SI, Navaid-ul-Zafar N. Healing potential of cream containing extract of *Sphaeranthus indicus* on dermal wounds in Guinea pigs. J Ethnopharmacol. 2006;107:161–3.
17. Agarry OO, Olaleye MT, Bello-Michael CO. Comparative antimicrobial activities of *Aloe vera* gel and leaf. Afr J Biotechnol. 2005;4:1413–4.
18. Jagtap NS, Khadabadi SS, Ghorpade DS, Banarase NB, Naphade SS. Antimicrobial and antifungal activity of Centella Asiatica (L.) urban, Umbiliferaceae. Research J Pharm Tech. 2009;2:328–30.
19. Santosh T, Patro MK, Bal AK, Choudhury A. Langerhans cell Histiocytosis on fine NeedleAspiration cytology: a report of 2 cases and review of literature. Orthop Muscul Syst. 2015;4:1–3.
20. Geraint Rogers B, Mary Carroll P, Kenneth BD. Studying bacterial infections through culture-independent approaches. J Medi Micro. 2009;58:1401–18.
21. Edwards R, Harding K. Bacteria and wound healing. Curr Opin Infect Dis. 2004;12(2):91–6.
22. Nayak BS, Sandiford S, Maxwell A. Evaluation of the wound-healing activity of ethanolic of Morinda Citrifolia L. leaf. Evid Based Complement Alternat Med. 2009;6:351–6.

23.  Matsiliza B, Barker NPA. Preliminary survey of plants used in traditional medicine in the Grahamstown area. S Afr J Bot. 2001;67:177–82.

24.  Gerald C, Walker MW, Criscione L, Gustafson EL, Batzl-Hartmann C, Smith KE, Vaysse P, Durki MM, Laz TM, Linemeyer DL, Schaffhauser AO, Whitebread S, Hofbauer KG, Taber RI, Branchek TA, Weinshank RLA. Receptor subtype involved in neuropeptide-Y-induced food intake. Nature. 1996;382:168–71.

25.  Phillips GD, Whitehe RA, Kinghton DR. Initiation and pattern of angiogenesis in wound healing in the rats. Am J Anat. 1991;192:257–62.

26.  Baie SH, Sheikh K. The wound healing properties of *Channastriatus*-cetrimide cream - wound contraction and glycosaminoglycan measurement. J Ethnopharmacol. 2000;73:15–30.

27.  Bonner J. Scar wars. Chem Ind (Lond). 2000;23:770–3.

28.  Pattanayak SP, Sunita P. Wound healing, anti-microbial and antioxidant potential of *Dendrophthoe falcata* (L.f) Ettingsh. J Ethnopharmacol. 2008;120: 241–7.

29.  Sarada DVL, Geethalakshmi R, Sakravarthi C, Kritika T, Arul Kirubakaran M. Evaluation of antioxidant and wound healing potentials of Sphaeranthus amaranthoides Burm, f. Biomed Res Int. 2013:1–7.

30.  Rashed H, Hesse R, DJW P. Origin of unusually thick ice-proximal Heinrich layers H1 to H3 in the northwest Labrador Sea. Earth Planet Sci Lett. 2003; 208:319–36.

31.  Abu-Al-Basal M. The Influence of Some Local Medicinal Plant Extracts on Skin Wound Healing Activity; Evaluated by Histological and Ultra-Structural Studies. Ph.D. Thesis, University of Jordan, Amman, Jordan. 2001.

# 10

# Toxicological implications of the therapeutic use of *Acalypha wilkesiana* leaves in traditional medicine

Kingsley Omage[1*], Marshall A. Azeke[2], Jerry N. E. Orhue[3] and Sylvia O. Iseghohi[3]

## Abstract

**Background:** In traditional medicine, *Acalypha wilkesiana* is frequently used solely or as a composite part of many herbal preparations for therapeutic purposes. This study was therefore conducted to evaluate the effects of oral administration of extracts of *Acalypha wilkesiana* leaves, on some serum diagnostic enzymes in normal experimental rabbits.

**Methods:** Eighteen adult male experimental rabbits were randomized into three groups (A, B and C), comprising of six animals each. Group A animals were given aqueous extracts of *Acalypha wilkesiana* leaves, while group B animals were given ethanol extracts of *Acalypha wilkesiana* leaves. The extracts were administered orally at a dose of 300 mg/kg body weight for a period of twenty-one (21) days. Group C animals were given water, thus they served as control. Data are represented as Mean ± S.E.M ($n = 6$). Significance of Difference was tested by ANOVA at $P < 0.05$.

**Results:** Administration of the aqueous or ethanol extracts, to the experimental animals resulted in a significantly ($P < 0.05$) higher alkaline phosphatase (ALP) and lactate dehydrogenase (LDH), non-significantly ($P > 0.05$) lower serum total bilirubin, direct bilirubin, Alanine aminotransferase (ALT), Aspartate aminotransferase (AST), gamma glutamyl transferase (GGT) and creatinine kinase (CK), as compared with the control animals.

**Conclusion:** In view of the effects of the plant extracts on ALP and LDH levels, the use of *Acalypha wilkesiana* leaf in traditional medicine should be with caution.

**Keywords:** *Acalypha wilkesiana*, Ethanol extract, Aqueous extract, Diagnostic enzymes, Bilirubin

## Background

The increase in demand for therapeutic drugs from natural products is traceable to the realization that plant products contain active constituents that are capable of curing majority of man's diseases. The use of plant, plant extract or plant-derived chemicals to treat diseases (whether topical, subcutaneous or systemic) has stood the test of time [1]. Medicinal herbs are plants which contain substances that can be used for therapeutic purposes, some of which are precursors for the synthesis of drugs [2]. Herbal medicines are the mainstay of about 75–80% of the world population (mainly in developing countries) for primary health care because of better cultural acceptability, regarding compatibility with the human body and less adverse effects [3–5]. In West Africa, new drugs are often beyond the reach of the poor and not less than 80% of the population use medicinal plants as remedy against infections and diseases [6, 7].

*Acalypha wilkesiana* is native to the south pacific islands and belongs to the Euphorbiaceae family. It is widely cultivated in the tropical and subtropical countries. The plant reportedly contains terpenoids; sesquiterpenes, monoterpenes, triterpenoids and polyphenols [8, 9]. The leaves are known to contain steroids, alkaloids, phytates, anthraquinones, oxalates, saponins, tannins, and glycosides [1, 9]. In view of the benefits of these compounds detected in *Acalypha wilkesiana* leaves, the plant can be seen as a potential source of useful drugs [10]. In traditional medicine, *Acalypha wilkesiana* is frequently used solely or as a composite part of many herbal preparations for therapeutic purposes. Although the leaves of this plant are eaten as vegetables in Southern Nigeria for therapeutic purposes,

* Correspondence: omagekingsley@yahoo.com
[1]Department of Biochemistry, College of Basic Medical Sciences, Igbinedion University, Okada, Edo State, Nigeria
Full list of author information is available at the end of the article

the scientific basis for its safety has not been fully established. Thus, the aim of this research is to evaluate the safety or otherwise of the use of *Acalypha wilkesiana* leaves in traditional medicine, by evaluating the effects of oral administration of extracts of *Acalypha wilkesiana* leaves on some serum diagnostic enzymes, in normal experimental rabbits.

## Methods
### Plant materials
Fresh *Acalypha wilkesiana* leaves, obtained from a local garden within Benin City were authenticated at the Department of Plant Biology and Biotechnology, of the University of Benin, Benin City. The leaves were properly washed, air-dried and ground into fine powder.

### Preparation of ethanol extract
One hundred gram of the powdered leaves was soaked in 400 ml of absolute ethanol (95%) for 72 h. The mixture was occasionally stirred using a magnetic stirrer, to ensure proper mixture of the vessel content. After 72 h, the mixture was filtered using a sintered funnel and the extract (filtrate) concentrated using a rotary evaporator. The concentrate of the extract was weighed and used for the study [10].

### Preparation of aqueous extract
One hundred gram of the powdered leaves was soaked in 400 ml of distilled water for 72 h, and treated as described above for ethanol extract [10].

### Experimental animals
Eighteen adult male experimental rabbits of the New Zealand strain, weighing between 0.9–1.5 kg were used for the study. The rabbits were housed in clean disinfected cages in the animal house of the Department of Biochemistry, University of Benin and maintained on a 12-h light and dark cycle. They were allowed to acclimatize to the new environment for a period of three weeks, with free access to feed (standard pelletized growers feed from UAC-Vital Feed, Jos, Plateau State) and water. The experimental procedures performed on the animals were approved by the Animal Ethics Committee of the Faculty of Life Sciences, University of Benin, Nigeria. The use of rabbits for the study was also according to the Ethical Guidelines Involving Whole Animal Testing of the Animal Ethics Committee, Faculty of Life Sciences, University of Benin. The experimental animals were then randomized into three groups (groups A, B and C) of six rabbits each [11].

### Experimental design
Groups A, B and C animals were treated as follows;

Group A Rabbits: Given Aqueous Extract of *Acalypha wilkesiana* leaves
Group B Rabbits: Given Ethanol Extract of *Acalypha wilkesiana* leaves
Group C Rabbits: Given distilled water (Control) [11]

### Administration of extracts
Five grams of the concentrated extracts were suspended in distilled water and measured amounts (dose) administered to the experimental animals with respect to their body weight. The extracts (aqueous or ethanol) were administered orally at a dose of 300 mg/kg body weight to the experimental rabbits for a period of twenty-one (21) days [11].

The dose "300 mg/kg body weight" was selected after a preliminary study (though unpublished) was done with graded doses (i.e. 200, 250, 300, 350 and 400 mg/kg body weight) of the plant extracts administered to salt loaded rabbits. The 300 mg/kg body weight dose was found to be more effective.

### Collection of blood
Prior to administration (Basal/day 0) with the extract, blood samples were collected from the veins located on the dorsal side of the ear lobes of the experimental rabbits, using sterilized hypodermic needles. At days 7, 14 and 21 after administration of the extracts, blood samples were also collected. Blood samples were collected in plane (universal) bottles immersed in ice. Immediately after collection of blood, the tubes were centrifuged at 3500 rpm for 10 min and clear serum obtained which were used for further analysis [11].

### Assay methods
Alanine aminotransferase (ALT) assay was done by the method of Reitman and Frankel (1957) [12]. ALT was measured by monitoring the concentration of pyruvate hydrazone formed with 2, 4 – dinitrophenyl hydrazine at 546 nm. Aspartate aminotransferase (AST) assay was also done by the method of Reitman and Frankel (1957) [12]. AST was measured by monitoring the concentration of oxaloacetate formed with 2, 4- dimtrophenyl hydrazine at 546 nm. Gamma Glutamyl Transferase (GGT) was determined by the method of Szasz (1969) [13]. The substrate L-γ-glutamyl-3-carboxy-4-nitroanilide, in the presence of glycylglycine was converted by γ-GT in the sample to 5-amino-2-nitrobenzoate which was measured at 405 nm, to determine the increase in absorbance. Alkaline Phosphatase (ALP) was determined by the method of Rec. GSCC (1972) [14], which measured the intensity of the yellow colour PNP formed from PNPP by ALP action at 405 nm. Lactate Dehydrogenase (LDH) was done by the method of Weissharr et al., (1975) [15]. The reduction of pyruvate to lactate involved the concomitant oxidation of NADH to

NAD$^+$ which was monitored at 340 nm. Creatinine Kinase was by the method of Bauer (1976) [16]. The creatine that was liberated reacted with diacetyl and α-naphtol to form a colored product which was read at 520 nm. Bilirubin was determined by the method of Jendrassik and Grof, (1938) [17]. The principle involves the reaction of direct (conjugated) bilirubin with diazotized sulphanilic acid in alkaline medium to form a blue colored complex. Total bilirubin was determined in the presence of caffeine, which released albumin bound bilirubin, by the reaction with diazotized sulphanilic acid and absorbance was read at 578 nm.

### Statistical analysis
Data are represented as Mean ± S.E.M ($n = 6$). Significance of Difference was tested by Student T-Test, ANOVA and Turkey-Kramer test, using the GraphPad Instat Version 3 (GraphPad Software Inc. San Diego, California U.S.A.). Statistical Significance was set at $P < 0.05$.

### Results
The effects of oral administration of extracts (aqueous or ethanol) of Acalypha wilkesiana leaves on some serum parameters in normal experimental rabbits, are as described below.

In Table 1, the treated groups (A & B) showed fluctuations in their mean serum alanine aminotransferase (ALT) levels, after extract administrations, with the changes significant ($p < 0.05$) at day 14 of extract administration. When compared with the control (group C), group A (given aqueous extract) showed ALT levels significantly ($p < 0.05$) lower at day 7.

At day 7 of treatment, the aqueous extract (group A) resulted in significantly ($P < 0.05$) lower AST levels as compared with the control, while the ethanol extract (group B) resulted in non-significantly ($P > 0.05$) lower AST levels as compared with the control. At day 14 of treatment, group A showed a non-significantly ($P > 0.05$) higher AST levels while group B showed a non-significantly ($P > 0.05$) lower AST levels, as compared with the control. At day 21 of treatment, group A showed a significantly ($P < 0.05$) lower AST levels, while group B showed a non-significantly ($P > 0.05$) lower AST levels as compared with the control.

Alkaline phosphatase (ALP) levels were also affected by treatment with Acalypha wilkesiana leaf extracts (aqueous or ethanol) as indicated in Table 2. At day 7 of extract administration, group A (given aqueous extract) showed a significantly ($P < 0.05$) higher ALP levels, while group B (given ethanol extract) showed a non-significantly ($P > 0.05$) higher ALP levels, as compared with group C (control). At day 14 of extract administration, there was no significant ($P > 0.05$) difference in the values of ALP (A & B compared with C). But at day 21 of extract administration, both test groups (A & B) showed significantly ($P < 0.05$) higher ALP levels, as compared with the control group (C).

At day 7 of extract administration, group A showed a non-significantly ($P > 0.05$) higher LDH levels, while group B showed a significantly ($P < 0.05$) higher LDH levels, as compared with group C. At day 14 of treatment, both test groups (A & B) showed significantly ($P < 0.05$) higher LDH levels, as compared with the control group (C). But, at day 21 of treatment, group A showed a non-significantly ($P > 0.05$) higher LDH levels, while group B showed a significantly ($P < 0.05$) higher LDH levels, as compared with group C. Thus, administration of the extracts (aqueous and ethanol) resulted in

**Table 1** Serum ALT and AST of normal rabbits treated with extracts of Acalypha wilkesiana leaves

| Treatment or group | | | |
|---|---|---|---|
| | A (Aq. Ext) | B (Et. Ext) | C (Control) |
| Serum ALT (U/L) | | | |
| DAY 0 | 30.83 ± 5.05$^{xa}$ | 32.50 ± 3.50$^{xa}$ | 37.83 ± 4.00$^{xa}$ |
| DAY 7 | 25.00 ± 0.87$^{xa}$ | 34.00 ± 1.53$^{ya}$ | 38.00 ± 3.88$^{ya}$ |
| DAY 14 | 48.83 ± 2.35$^{xb}$ | 51.83 ± 3.09$^{xb}$ | 45.33 ± 5.86$^{xa}$ |
| DAY 21 | 33.83 ± 0.67$^{xa}$ | 43.50 ± 2.18$^{xa}$ | 45.67 ± 4.76$^{xa}$ |
| Serum AST (U/L) | | | |
| DAY 0 | 45.67 ± 2.03$^{xa}$ | 36.00 ± 8.54$^{xa}$ | 60.67 ± 5.36$^{xa}$ |
| DAY 7 | 24.00 ± 3.62$^{xa}$ | 28.00 ± 1.80$^{ya}$ | 52.83 ± 18.70$^{ya}$ |
| DAY 14 | 89.67 ± 0.33$^{xb}$ | 41.83 ± 4.97$^{ya}$ | 60.17 ± 15.48$^{ya}$ |
| DAY 21 | 32.33 ± 1.96$^{xa}$ | 54.00 ± 7.51$^{yb}$ | 62.83 ± 8.73$^{ya}$ |

Data represent Means ± S.E.M ($n = 6$). Means with different letter [a, b] superscripts, along column, are significantly different ($p < 0.05$). Means with different letter [x, y] superscripts, along row, are significantly different ($p < 0.05$)

**Table 2** Serum ALP and LDH of normal rabbits treated with extracts of Acalypha wilkesiana leaves

| Treatment or group | | | |
|---|---|---|---|
| | A (Aq. Ext) | B (Et. Ext) | C (Control) |
| Serum ALP (IU/L) | | | |
| DAY 0 | 10.55 ± 0.36$^{xa}$ | 11.52 ± 1.44$^{xa}$ | 11.37 ± 1.68$^{xa}$ |
| DAY 7 | 17.69 ± 0.77$^{xb}$ | 14.50 ± 1.67$^{ya}$ | 13.93 ± 0.53$^{ya}$ |
| DAY 14 | 11.95 ± 0.66$^{xa}$ | 11.22 ± 0.12$^{xa}$ | 11.53 ± 1.52$^{xa}$ |
| DAY 21 | 24.31 ± 1.19$^{xb}$ | 20.61 ± 0.34$^{xb}$ | 15.93 ± 1.03$^{ya}$ |
| Serum LDH (U/L) | | | |
| DAY 0 | 12.91 ± 3.23$^{xa}$ | 16.14 ± 6.46$^{xa}$ | 29.05 ± 14.79$^{xa}$ |
| DAY 7 | 48.42 ± 11.18$^{xb}$ | 87.15 ± 29.58$^{yb}$ | 41.96 ± 17.08$^{xa}$ |
| DAY 14 | 96.83 ± 5.59$^{xc}$ | 119.42 ± 46.89$^{xc}$ | 58.10 ± 14.79$^{ya}$ |
| DAY 21 | 167.84 ± 26.42$^{xd}$ | 203.34 ± 39.13$^{yd}$ | 151.70 ± 44.84$^{xa}$ |

Data represent Means ± S.E.M ($n = 6$). Means with different letter [a, b, c, d] superscripts, along column, are significantly different ($p < 0.05$). Means with different letter [x, y] superscripts, along row, are significantly different ($p < 0.05$)

a steady and significant ($p < 0.05$) increases in serum LDH levels all through the period of administration.

In Table 3, the test groups, given the aqueous or ethanol extract showed non-significantly ($P > 0.05$) higher gamma glutamyl transferase (GGT) levels, as compared to the control group, at day 7 of treatment. But at day 14 of treatment, the test groups showed non-significantly ($P > 0.05$) lower GGT values, as compared with the control. However, at day 21 of treatment, there was no significant difference in the values of GGT in all the groups (A & B compared with C).

After 7 days of extract administration, group A (given aqueous extract) showed a significantly ($P < 0.05$) lower CK levels, while group B (given ethanol extract) showed a non-significantly ($P > 0.05$) lower CK levels, as compared with group C (control). After 14 days of treatment, both test groups (A or B) showed non-significantly ($P > 0.05$) lower CK levels, as compared with the control group (C). However, at day 21 of treatment, group A showed a significantly ($P < 0.05$), lower CK levels while group B showed a non-significant ($P > 0.05$) lower CK levels, as compared with group C. Thus, treatment with the extracts resulted in decreases in serum CK levels.

Serum total bilirubin (mg/dl) levels (Table 4) were shown to be non-significantly ($P > 0.05$) lower in groups A & B as compared to group C, at day 7 of extracts administration. But at day 14, group A (given aqueous extract) showed a significantly ($P < 0.05$) lower total bilirubin levels as compared with group C (control), while group B (given ethanol extract) showed a non-significantly ($P > 0.05$) lower values as compared with group C. However, at day 21 of extract administration, there was no significant difference ($P > 0.05$) in serum total bilirubin levels of all the groups (tests compared with control).

**Table 3** Serum GGT and CK of normal rabbits treated with extracts of *Acalypha wilkesiana* leaves

| | Treatment or group | | |
|---|---|---|---|
| | A (Aq. Ext) | B (Et. Ext) | C (Control) |
| Serum GGT (U/L) | | | |
| DAY 0 | 3.86 ± 0.39[xa] | 3.86 ± 0.39[xa] | 4.63 ± 0.67[xa] |
| DAY 7 | 5.02 ± 0.39[xa] | 4.63 ± 0.67[xa] | 4.24 ± 0.39[xa] |
| DAY 14 | 3.09 ± 0.38[xa] | 3.48 ± 1.16[xa] | 4.24 ± 0.77[xa] |
| DAY 21 | 4.24 ± 0.39[xa] | 4.63 ± 0.67[xa] | 4.63 ± 0.67[xa] |
| Serum CK (U/L) | | | |
| DAY 0 | 53.65 ± 2.38[xa] | 53.65 ± 4.13[xa] | 48.15 ± 3.64[xa] |
| DAY 7 | 31.64 ± 3.64[xb] | 39.89 ± 1.38[yb] | 44.02 ± 4.96[ya] |
| DAY 14 | 42.65 ± 1.38[xb] | 33.01 ± 4.13[xb] | 45.40 ± 4.77[xa] |
| DAY 21 | 15.13 ± 1.38[xc] | 23.39 ± 3.64[yc] | 31.64 ± 1.38[ya] |

Data represent Means ± S.E.M ($n = 6$). Means with different letter [a, b, c,] superscripts, along column, are significantly different ($p < 0.05$). Means with different letter [x, y] superscripts, along row, are significantly different ($p < 0.05$)

**Table 4** Serum total bilirubin and direct bilirubin of normal rabbits treated with extracts of *Acalypha wilkesiana* leaves

| | Treatment or group | | |
|---|---|---|---|
| | A (Aq. Ext) | B (Et. Ext) | C (Control) |
| Serum total bilirubin (mg/dl) | | | |
| DAY 0 | 2.34 ± 0.83[xa] | 2.53 ± 0.22[xa] | 2.20 ± 0.45[xa] |
| DAY 7 | 1.52 ± 0.20[xa] | 1.24 ± 0.10[xa] | 1.83 ± 0.33[xa] |
| DAY 14 | 1.04 ± 0.78[xa] | 2.65 ± 0.45[ya] | 3.67 ± 0.45[yb] |
| DAY 21 | 0.87 ± 0.30[xa] | 0.66 ± 0.11[xb] | 0.82 ± 0.08[xa] |
| Serum direct bilirubin (mg/dl) | | | |
| DAY 0 | 4.31 ± 0.38[xa] | 4.66 ± 1.57[xa] | 4.69 ± 0.56[xa] |
| DAY 7 | 5.20 ± 1.69[xa] | 3.36 ± 0.29[xa] | 4.56 ± 1.86[xa] |
| DAY 14 | 5.03 ± 0.25[xa] | 3.59 ± 0.29[xa] | 5.28 ± 1.22[xa] |
| DAY 21 | 2.21 ± 0.29[xb] | 2.76 ± 0.41[xa] | 3.26 ± 0.57[xa] |

Data represent Means ± S.E.M ($n = 6$). Means with different letter [a, b] superscripts, along column, are significantly different ($p < 0.05$). Means with different letter [x, y] superscripts, along row, are significantly different ($p < 0.05$)

Serum direct bilirubin levels (Table 4) were shown to be non-significantly ($P > 0.05$) higher in group A and non-significantly ($P > 0.05$) lower in group B as compared with group C, at day 7. But at day 14, only group B showed a non-significantly ($P > 0.05$) lower values as compared with group C. While at day 21 of treatment, both groups (A & B) showed non-significantly ($P > 0.05$) lower serum direct bilirubin levels as compared with the control group (C).

## Discussion

The rationale for assaying enzyme activities is based on the premise that changes in activities reflect changes that have occurred in a specific tissue or organ. ALT is found mainly in the liver, but also in smaller amounts in the kidneys, heart, muscles, and pancreas. Low levels of ALT are normally found in the blood. But when the liver is damaged or diseased, it releases ALT into the bloodstream, which makes ALT levels increase. Most increases in ALT levels are caused by liver damage. The treated groups showed fluctuations in their mean serum alanine aminotransferase (ALT) levels, with the changes significant at day 14 of extract administration. Fluctuation of ALT levels is normal over the course of the day, and ALT levels can also increase in response to strenuous physical exercise. Significantly elevated levels of ALT (SGPT) often suggest the existence of other medical problems such as viral hepatitis, diabetes, congestive heart failure, liver damage, bile duct problems, infectious mononucleosis, or myopathy. For this reason, ALT is commonly used as a way of screening for liver problems.

Mean serum aspartate aminotransferase (AST) levels, showed a different trend from that of ALT. As observed, treatment with the plant extracts resulted in lower levels of serum AST of the test groups as compared with the control. Here, the effect of the aqueous extract is shown to be more significant. This possibly suggests a protective role or a non toxic effect of the plant on the various organs or tissues where this enzyme is found. AST is found in many tissues throughout the body, including the liver, heart, muscles, kidney, and brain. If any of these organs or tissues is affected by disease or injury, AST is released into the bloodstream. This means that AST is not as specific an indicator of liver damage as ALT. Damage to these tissues normally causes the enzymes to leak out into the blood, thus increasing the levels in the blood above normal. The decreases in the activities of AST as occasioned by the administration of the extract, tends to portend a protective role of the plant on this tissues. Aspartate aminotransferase (AST) exists in human tissues as two distinct isoenzymes, one located in the cytoplasm (c-AST), and the other in mitochondria (m-AST). Striated muscle, myocardium, and liver tissues are the main sources of AST. A growing body of information suggests that determination of AST isoenzymes in human serum is useful in evaluating damage to some of these organs [18].

Alkaline phosphatase (ALP) levels were also affected by treatment with *Acalypha wilkesiana* leaf extracts (aqueous or ethanol). Administration of the extracts resulted in significantly higher serum ALP levels of the test groups, with the aqueous extract more implicated. This may portend possible toxicity of the plant. The majority of sustained elevated ALP levels are associated with disorders of the liver or bone, or both. Therefore, these organ systems are of prime consideration in the differential diagnosis. Diseases of bone associated with increased serum ALP are restricted to the presence of osteoblastic activity. High ALP levels can show that the bile ducts are blocked. Levels are significantly higher in children and pregnant women. Also, elevated ALP indicates that there could be active bone formation occurring as ALP is a byproduct of osteoblast activity (such as the case in Paget's disease of bone). Levels are also elevated in people with untreated Celiac Disease [19]. Because of the cellular distribution of ALP, increased serum activity may be caused by a wide variety of disorders involving multiple organs. Attempts to define organ source by isoenzyme study may be met with limited success because of technical limitations; accurate measurement of different isoenzymes contributing to total serum ALP activity is not currently possible. However, the presence of the intestinal or placental isoenzyme may be revealed by selected methods.

Administration of the extracts (aqueous or ethanol) resulted in a steady and significant increases in serum LDH levels all through the period of administration. Increases in serum LDH levels of the test groups (as compared with the control), all through the period of treatment with the extract portends a negative implication. LDH is present in almost all body tissues, so the LDH test is used to detect tissue alterations and as an aid in the diagnosis of heart attack, anemia, and liver disease [20]. When disease or injury affects tissues containing LDH, the cells release LDH into the blood stream, where it is identified in higher than normal levels. The LDH is also elevated in disease of the liver, in certain types of anemia, and in cases of excessive destruction of cells, as in fractures, trauma, muscle damage and shock [20]. Even though an LDH test is useful in diagnosing tissue damage, other tests are usually necessary to pinpoint the location of the damage. One such test is the LDH isoenzymes test. LDH isoenzymes are five kinds of the LDH enzyme that are found in specific concentrations in different organs and tissues. By measuring the blood levels of these isoenzymes, the type, location, and severity of the cellular damage, can be understood. Thus, to ascertain the origin of the increased serum LDH as occasioned by treatment with extract, the differential diagnosis may need to be carried out. However, the plant may be selectively toxic with respect to the tissues. The ethanol extract was shown to be more potent in this respect.

Gamma-glutamyl transferase (GGT) is a metabolic enzyme expressed primarily in the liver, kidneys and other organs. Organ damage, especially damage to the liver, causes the release of this enzyme into the blood. Elevation of GGT levels is often an indication of liver damage and has been associated with liver injury as well as pancreatic and myocardial disorders. The results indicate that the plant (extracts) had no adverse effects on the serum GGT levels of the experimental animals. The slight increase and subsequent reduction in the serum GGT levels may be more of protective function than damage to the tissues of the test animals. GGT is also a very useful tool for preclinical investigation of experimental drug formulations and GGT levels are commonly used to monitor and attenuate the toxic effects of experimental drug formulations in rodents [21]. Although it is considered to be an index of hepatobiliary dysfunction and alcohol abuse [22], recent epidemiology and pathology studies have suggested its independent role in the pathogenesis and clinical evolution of cardiovascular diseases brought on by atherosclerosis [22, 23].

Serum creatinine kinase (CK) levels were affected after administration of extracts. Treatment with the extracts resulted in decreases in serum CK levels. The aqueous extract, as observed caused more significant decreases in the serum creatinine kinase levels than the ethanol extract, all through the treatment period. CK is an important enzyme involved in energy maintenance and energy transfer in muscle and brain cells. Four different isoforms of CK are expressed in a tissue-specific and developmentally regulated manner. Elevation of CK is an indication of damage to muscle. It is therefore indicative of injury, rhabdomyolysis, myocardial infarction, myocitis and myocarditis. For years, the gold standard for diagnosis of myocardial necrosis was the cardiac-specific isoenzyme of creatinine kinase (CK-MB). Previously, the myocardial fraction of lactate dehydrogenase and even aspartate aminotransferase were used to diagnose myocardial necrosis [24]. Isoenzyme determination has been used extensively as an indication for myocardial damage in heart attacks. The plant may therefore be protective against damages to muscles and possibly brain cells.

As observed, the ethanol extract tends to be more effective at reducing the levels of both serum total and direct bilirubin. Total bilirubin concentration reflects the levels of both the conjugated and unconjugated fractions of bilirubin. Total bilirubin levels are elevated in various forms of liver disease such as cirrhosis, hepatitis, and obstructions of the hepatobiliary system such as gallstones or tumors. Elevated total bilirubin levels are also observed in cases of intravascular hemolysis [25]. A high level of conjugated bilirubin in the blood can also be detected in the urine. In hepatitis, fibrosis, and cirrhosis, high amounts of unconjugated bilirubin means the liver cells are not conjugating bilirubin normally, causing it to build up in the blood. Bilirubin is not normally found in the urine but if it is, that is an indication of either liver cell damage or blockage of the flow of bile from the liver or gallbladder. These adverse effects of increased or elevated bilirubin in the system may possibly be countered by the plant, as it tends to help in the excretion of bilirubin, thus reducing its concentration in the blood.

## Conclusion

Treatment with both extracts resulted in fluctuations (no significant effect) in the levels of serum ALT and decreases in the levels of serum AST, total bilirubin and direct bilirubin of the test animals. Administration of the extracts resulted in significant increases in serum ALP and LDH levels of the test animals (which portends a negative implication). However, the serum GGT levels were not significantly affected, while the serum CK levels were reduced. In view of the effects of the plant extracts on ALP and LDH levels, the use of *Acalypha wilkesiana* leaf in traditional medicine should be with caution.

## Abbreviations

ALP: Alkaline Phosphatase; ALT: Alanine Aminotransferase; Aq.: Aqueous; AST: Aspartate Aminotransferase; CK: Creatinine Kinase; Et.: Ethanol; Ext.: Extract; GGT: Gamma Glutamyl Transferase; LDH: Lactate Dehydrogenase; S.E.M: Standard Error of Mean

## Acknowledgments

The Authors are grateful to the authorities of Department of Biochemistry, University of Benin (Edo State, Nigeria) for providing the necessary laboratory facilities.

## Declaration

We the authors declare that this manuscript is original, has not been published before and is not currently being considered for publication elsewhere. We confirm that the manuscript has been read and approved by all authors

## Authors' contributions

OK: Concepts, Design, Experimental Studies, Data acquisition and Analysis, Manuscript preparation, Statistical Analysis. AAM: Concepts, Design, Experimental Studies, Data acquisition and Analysis, Manuscript preparation, Statistical Analysis. ONEJ: Concepts, Design, Experimental Studies, Data acquisition and Analysis. IOS: Design, Experimental Studies, Data acquisition and Analysis. All authors read and approved the final manuscript.

## Competing interest

The authors wish to state that there are no competing interests associated with this publication and there has been no significant financial support for this work that could have influenced its outcome.

## Author details

[1]Department of Biochemistry, College of Basic Medical Sciences, Igbinedion University, Okada, Edo State, Nigeria. [2]Department of Biochemistry, Faculty of Natural Sciences, Ambrose Alli University, Ekpoma, Edo State, Nigeria. [3]Department of Biochemistry, Faculty of Life Sciences, University of Benin, Benin City, Edo State, Nigeria.

## References

1. Oladunmoye MK. Comparative Evaluation of Antimicrobial Activities and Phytochemical Screening of Two Varieties of *Acalypha Wilkesiana*. Trends in Appl Sci Res L. 2006;1(5):538–4.
2. Sofowora A. African Medicinal Plants. Ile Ife, Nigeria: University of Ife Press; 1984. p. 104.
3. Kamboj VP. Herbal Medicine. Curr Sci. 2000;78(1):35–9.
4. Cummingham JG, Klein BG. The systemic and pulmonary circulations. In: Textbook of Veterinary Physiology. 4th ed., USA: Saunders Elsevier. 2007. p 250.
5. Sapna S, Ravi TK. Approaches Towards Development and Promotion of Herbal Drugs. Pharmacogn Rev. 2007;1(1):180–4.
6. Kirby GC. Medicinal plants and the control of protozoal disease, with particular reference to malaria. Trans R Soc Trop Med Hyg. 1996;90:605–9.
7. Hostettmann K, Marston A. Twenty years of research into medicinal plants: Results and perspectives. Phytochem Rev. 2002;1:275–85.
8. Akinde BE. Phytochemicals and microbiological evaluation of the oils from the leaves of *Acalypha wilkesiana*. In: Sofowora A, editor. The state of medicinal plant research in Nigeria. Nigeria: University of Ibadan Press; 1986. p. 362–3.
9. Omage K, Azeke AM, Ihimire II, Idagan AM. Phytochemical, Proximate and Elemental Analysis of Acalypha wilkesiana leaves. Scientific Journal of Pure and Applied Sciences. 2013;2(9):323–31.
10. Omage K, Azeke AM. Medicinal Potential of *Acalypha wilkesiana* Leaves. Advances in Research. 2014;2(11):655–65.
11. Omage K, Azeke AM, Orhue NEJ. Implications of Oral Administration of Extracts of *Acalypha wilkesiana* leave on Serum Electrolytes, Urea and Creatinine in Normal Experimental Rabbits. Biokemistri. 2015;27(2):56–62.
12. Reitman S, Frankel S. A colorimetric method for the determination of serum glutamic oxalacetic and glutamic pyruvic transaminases. Amer J Clin Pathol. 1957;28:56–63.
13. Szasz G. A Kinetic Photometry Method for Serum γ-Glutamyl Transpeptidase. Clin Chem. 1969;15:124–36.
14. Rec. GSCC. Determination of Alkaline Phosphatase. Z Clin Chem Klin Biochemist. 1972;10:281–91.
15. Weissharr D, Gossrau E, Faderl B. Normal ranges of alpha-HBDH, LDH, AP and LAP as measured with substrate optimated test charges. Med Welt. 1975;26:387–92.

16. Bauer S. Dense growth of aerobic bacteria in a bench-scale fermentor. Biotechnol Bioeng. 1976;18:81–94.

17. Jendrassik L, Gróf P. Vereinfachte photometrische Methoden zur Bestimmung des Blutbilirubins. Biochem Z. 1938;297:82–9.

18. Panteghini M. Aspartate aminotransferase isoenzymes. Clin Biochem. 1990; 23(4):311–9.

19. Preussner HT. Detecting celiac disease in your patients. Am Fam Physician. 1998;57(5):1023–34.

20. David JS. Laboratory Test Handbook. 4th ed. New York: Lexi Comp. Inc; 1996.

21. Vázquez-Medina JP, et al. Prolonged fasting increases glutathione biosynthesis in post weaned northern elephant seals. J Exp Biol. 2011;214: 1294–9.

22. Whitfield JB. Gamma glutamyl transferase. Crit Rev Clin Lab Sci. 2001; 38(4):263–355.

23. Pompella A, Emdin M, Passino C, Paolicchi A. The significance of serum γ-glutamyltransferase in cardiovascular diseases. Clin Chem Lab Med. 2004;42:1085–91.

24. Sharif AH, Kristin LN, Magnus OE. Biomarkers in Cardiovascular Clinical Trials: Past, Present. Future Clinical Chemistry. 2012;58:145–53.

25. Burtis CA, Ashwood ER. Tietz Textbook of Clinical Chemistry and Laboratory Medicine. 3rd Ed. Philadelphia PA: W.B. Saunders Company. 1999. 1915.

# 11

# Sinupret® as add-on therapy to saline irrigation for children with acute Post-Viral Rhinosinusitis

Vasyl I. Popovich[1][*] and Ivanna V. Koshel[2]

## Abstract

**Background:** The present randomized controlled study investigated the efficacy of the complex herbal medicine Sinupret® syrup in the treatment of acute post-viral rhinosinusitis in children.

**Methods:** The patients were children aged from 6 to 11 years (mean 9.4 years old).
They were randomized into two groups. Both groups received a standard treatment including a symptomatic therapy and a saline therapy. Isotonic sea salt solution was given four times daily for a period of 14 days.
The treatment group received an additional treatment with Sinupret® syrup 3-times daily.
Using a 5-point scale (0–4 points), the physician evaluated the following symptomatic parameters at four successive visits (days 0, 5, 10 and 14): nasal congestion, nasal discharge, post-nasal drip and headache. Presence of cough in each group was recorded separately. Also using a 5-point scale (0–4 points), each patient gave a daily self-assessment of the following parameters from day 1 to day 10: rhinorrhea, headache, facial pain.

**Results:** Relative to symptomatic therapy + saline irrigation, significant improvements were found in seven of the eightsymptomatic parameters under complex treatment including Sinupret® syrup. The differences in facial pain and the incidence of cough in groups were not significant. The need for prescription of antibiotics in the treatment group was 28.5% less than in the control group. No adverse reactions to the herbal medicine occurred during the study period.

**Conclusion:** The complex herbal medicine Sinupret® syrup alleviates effectively the symptoms of acute post-viral rhinosinusitis in children. Furthermore, the prescription of antibiotics was also reduced.

**Keywords:** Rhinosinusitis, Herbal medicine, Sinupret syrup, Rhinorrhoea

## Background

Acute rhinosinusitis (ARS) is an inflammatory disease of the nose and paranasal sinuses. It is most commonly caused by viral infections, mainly rhino- or adenoviruses [1].

ARS is a self-limiting disease lasting 7–14 days. In Ukraine approximately 54% of patients with ARS show a self-healing within this period. 46% of ARS patients suffer from prolonged symptoms or complications.

ARS comprises of viral ARS (common cold) and post-viral ARS. In the EPOS 2007 the term non-viral ARS was chosen to indicate that most cases of ARS are not bacterial. However this term led to confusion and in the EPOS 2012 guidelines the term post-viral ARS expressedthe same phenomenon. A small percentage of the patients with post-viral ARS can have bacterial ARS [2]. Acute post-viral rhinosinusitis is defined as an increase of symptoms after 5 days or persistence of symptoms after 10 days with less than 12 weeks duration.

Post-viral ARS is a common condition in the community, usually following viral Upper Respiratory Tract Infections. Post-viral ARS should not be diagnosed in patients with symptoms for less than 10 days unless a marked worsening of symptoms occurs after 5 days, and features of severe pain and a pyrexia of >38 °C are present. Symptoms occurring for longer than 12 weeks indicate the presence of chronic rhinosinusitis.

* Correspondence: popovych_ent@ukr.net; popovychvasyl@gmail.com
[1]Department of Otorhinolaryngology, Ivano-Frankivsk University, Ivano-Frankivsk, Ukraine
Full list of author information is available at the end of the article

According to the "European position paper on rhinosinusitis and nasal polyps" (EPOS), drug treatments for alleviating symptoms in post-viral ARS include topical corticosteroids, herbal medicine and aspirin. Therapeutic irrigation with isotonic saline is also used to reduce intranasal pressure.

While diagnosis of viral ARS is very frequent, with about 6.3 million diagnoses per year only in Germany [3], the number of post-viral ARS patients is not exactly known. Nonetheless, the post-viral ARS is of great socio-economic importance. It leads to major direct therapy costs and important indirect costs caused by loss of productivity and more days of absence from work in comparison to viral ARS [2].

Only about 0.5% of cases of ARS can be characterized as acute bacterial rhinosinusitis (ABRS). Typical symptoms of ABRS include purulent nasal discharge, tooth pain, facial pain, and unilateral tenderness to palpation in the projection of the maxillary sinus, worsening of symptoms after initial improvement, hyperthermia and neutrocytosis.

However, acute rhinosinusitis is the fifth most frequent diagnosis for the prescription of antibiotics, even though there is no proof that this shortens the duration of the illness. The frequent and unnecessary treatment with antibiotics has led to the development of increased resistance and, for this reason, alternative evidence-based treatment strategies are urgently necessary. One possible approach is to use herbal medicines [4–6].

The potential role of herbal therapy is particularly great in the treatment of post- viral ARS. As there is no evidence that infectious factors play a role in the aetiology of post-viral ARS, it is appropriate to employ symptomatic or pathogenetic treatment, rather than to use antivirals and antibiotics.

It is commonly known that the pathogenesis of post-viral ARS lies in the development of inflammation and related mucosal oedema, primarily in the osteomeatal complex (OMC). The function of the mucociliary transport system (MTS) is impaired against the background of the growing frontal ostium and sinus dysfunction and increased production of pathologically altered mucus. These changes result in progressive deterioration in OMC function, particularly in the ventilation and drainage of the paranasal sinuses.

Unsuccessful attempts have been made to treat post-viral ARS with several conventional agents, including decongestants, antibiotics, antiseptics, antihistamines, homeopathic products and secretolytics. Thus, treatment of post-viral ARS remains a topical problem.

One promising approach is to use a preparation which is capable of inhibiting a variety of pathological processes. One of these preparations is the complex herbal medicine Sinupret which is based on gentian, evening primrose, elder, verbena and sorrel. This herbal medicine has been shown to enhance ciliary activity in vitro [7] and to have anti-inflammatory activity in animal experiments [8]. It has a wide spectrum of pharmacological properties, including secretolytic, secretomotoric, antiviral, anti-inflammatory, and immunomodulatory effects. Jund et al. [9] performed a double blind randomized placebo-controlled study on 386 adult patients with acute viral rhinosinusitis. The active treatment group was given a daily dose for 15 days of $3 \times 160$ mg herbal medicine. The active treatment group showed more significant improvements in the sino-nasal outcome test, including the total score, the nasal symptoms, the rhinogenic symptoms and general quality of life.

Until now, no GCP-compliant analysis of Sinupret syrup has been carried out in the treatment of post-viral ARS in children of school-age (6–11 years).

We now report a similar study to Jund et al. on children aged 6–11 years, employing a syrup formulation of the herbal medicine.

## Methods
### Study design
The study was a prospective multicentre non-interventional randomized study on the treatment of post-viral ARS in children aged 6 to 11 years. The study compared a treatment with a complex herbal medicine - Sinupret® syrup - and standard treatment, as summarized in Table 1.

Sinupret is a phytopharmaceutical widely utilized for a variety of respiratory ailments including rhinosinusitis and bronchitis. The compound is a mixture derived from parts of five plants: gentian root (Radic Gentianae); primrose flowers with calyx (Flores Primulae cum Calibus), European vervain herb (Nebra Verbenae), sorrel grass (Herba Rumicis); Flowers of elderberry (Flores

**Table 1** Study Treatments over 14 days

| Groups | Pharmaceutical drug | Dosage | Duration |
|---|---|---|---|
| Treatment | • Therapeutic irrigation (isotonic sea salt solution) | 4 times daily | 14 days |
| | • Phytopreparation, syrup (Sinupret) | (3.5 ml), 3 times daily | |
| | • Symptomatic medications (episodically): paracetamol, nasal decongestants | Age-specific dosage | |
| Control | • Therapeutic irrigation (isotonic sea salt solution) | 4 times daily | 14 days |
| | • Symptomatic medications (episodically): paracetamol, nasal decongestants | Age-specific dosage | |

Sambuci) (1: 3: 3: 3: 3). Table 1: Study Treatments over 14 days

Both groups were given symptomatic medication (paracetamol or nasal decongestants if necessary and both were treated with therapeutic irrigation with isotonic sodium chloride solution 4 times daily. The treatment group was given the herbal medicine – Sinupret syrup – 3 times daily at the age-specific dosage of 3.5 ml, additionally.

## Study population

The study population consisted of 120 children, 64 boys and 56 girls, aged 6 to 11 years (mean 9.4 years old) and with acute post-viral rhinosinusitis. The treatment group contained 65 children and the control group 55.

The number of patients with prolonged symptom > 10 days and those which had severe symptoms after 5 days is shown in Table 2.

### Inclusion criteria

The principle inclusion criteria was acute post-viral rhinosinusitis, with persistence of acute symptoms for 10 days or exacerbation of symptoms after day 5.

The following *five key symptoms* were rated by the physician with 0–4 points on the major sinusitis severity score (MSS score): nasal discharge, nasal congestion, postnasal drip, headache, facial pain, with a total score of up to 15 points (of the maximum possible sum 20 points). The scale of the scores is as follows: 0 absent, 1 slight, 2 moderate, 3 severe, 4 very severe.

### Exclusion criteria

- Administration of the herbal preparation within 30 days prior to the episode of rhinosinusitis
- Diagnosis of allergic rhinosinusitis
- Known intolerance to primrose drugs
- Severe acute disease requiring hospitalization or treatment with antibiotics
- Immune deficiency

**Table 2** Number of the patients with prolonged symptom > 10 days and those which had severe symptoms after 5 days

| Groups | Patients with prolonged symptoms > 10 days | | Patients with severe symptoms after 5 days | |
|---|---|---|---|---|
| | Number of patients | % | Number of patients | % |
| All patients n = 120 | 101 | 84.2% | 19 | 15.8% |
| Treatment group n = 65 | 54 | 83.2% | 11 | 16.8% |
| Control group n = 55 | 47 | 85.4% | 7 | 12.6% |

- Chronic pathology and anatomical anomalies of the osteomeatal complex, which may influence the outcome of the disease

### Withdrawal criteria

- Indications for antibiotic therapy
- Adverse reactions to the study drug
- Protocol violation

### Research methodology

During the study period four visits were conducted: visit 1 (day 0), visit 2 (day 5), visit 3 (day 10) and visit 4 (day 14). Symptoms were assessed by the physician and the patients. The five key symptoms were assessed by the physician at each visit. In addition, the key complaints of rhinorrhea, headache, facial pain, were assessed by the patients on a 0–4 point scale daily. Presence of cough was recorded separately.

### Efficacy criteria

The primary criteria were the improvements in symptoms. The secondary criteria was the frequency of transition to prescription of antibiotics to assess the transition from post-viral ARS to acute bacterial rhinosinusitis (ABRS).

### Data analysis

The data were presented descriptively. Differences between the two groups were tested with the paired test, using a two-sided 95% Confidence-Intervall (95% CI) with the significance $p \leq 0.05$.

## Results

### Study population

All the 120 patients completed the study period of 14 days.

Five (5) patients in the treatment group and nine patients in the control group were excluded from the study for reasons of protocol violation and data of these patients were excluded from analysis. These patients were offset by recruitment of additional patients.

### Antibiotics therapy

Five (5/65) of the patients (7.7%) in the treatment group had to be treated with antibiotics, in comparison to six (6/55) patients (10.9%) in the control group. This difference was not statistically significant ($p > 0.05$). In most cases (9 patients), treatment with antibiotics was started at visit 3 due to repeated increase in the temperature (39 °C and higher), re-worsening severity of sinusitis symptoms.

## Symptoms assessed by the physician

Figure 1 shows the physician's assessment of the nasal congestion symptom at visit 1 to 4. Both groups showed comparable symptoms at visit 1 (v1). At visit 2 (v2), nasal congestion was significantly less in the treatment group than in the control group ($p = 0.041$). From visit 3 (v3) to visit 4 (v4) nasal congestion of both groups showed further reduced symptoms to zero at visit 4.

Figure 2 shows the physician's assessment of the nasal discharge symptom at visits 1 to 4. The differences at v2 and v3 are statistically significant ($p < 0.038$).

The physician's assessment of post-nasal drip was also significantly lower in the treatment than in the control group at v2 (1.33 vs. 0.83, $p = 0.044$).

The physician's headache assessment also showed that this symptom was lower in the treatment group compared to the control one at v2. (0.45 vs. 0.32, $p = 0.048$).

There was a trend to less facial pain in the treatment group at v2, but the differences were not statistically significant (0.27 vs. 0.42, $p = 0.1$).

Furthermore, cough was observed in 60.8% of the patients of the treatment group and in 59.7% of the patients from the control. At the time of the visit 2 (Day 5) cough was recorded in 37.4% of the patients of the treatment group and in 43.2% of the patients from the control but these were not statistically significant.

## Symptoms assessed by the patients

Figure 3 shows the patient's self-assessment of rhinorrhea for the first 10 days of treatment. At the beginning of the study (day 1 and day 2) the rating of the patients in both groups was comparable. Significantly less rhinorrhea was found in the treatment group on days 3, 4, 5, 6 and 7 (all $p < 0.05$). Similar results were obtained for self-assessed headache and facial pain.

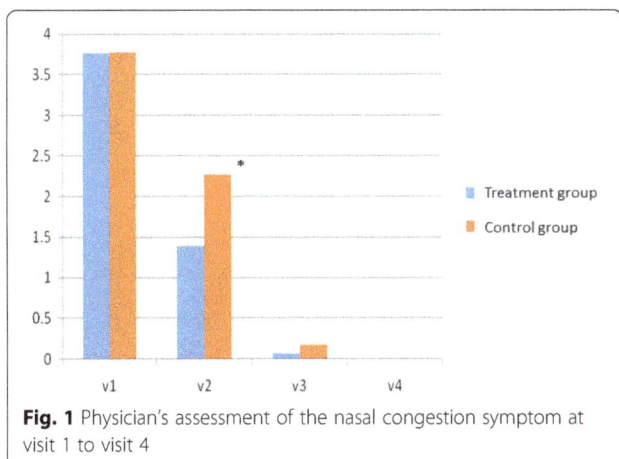

**Fig. 2** Physician's assessment of the nasal discharge symptom at visit 1 to visit 4. The differences at v2 and v3 are statistically significant ($p < 0.05$)

## Discussion

Acute post-viral rhinosinusitis is a very common and economically important condition, involving inflammation of the nasal mucous membranes and paranasal sinuses [2, 3]. The principle symptoms are inflammation and mucosal oedema, primarily in the osteomeatal complex. The function of the mucociliary transport system is impaired against the background of increased production of pathologically altered mucus. These symptoms develop after the acute viral infection and can be considered as the next stage of development of the disease after acute viral sinusitis when the symptoms persist for more than 10 days. Antiviral treatment is ineffective. Saline irrigation proved efficient for improving the symptoms in randomized, placebo-controlled studies [10]. International and Ukrainian guidelines consider irrigation therapy as a relevant treatment to enable a better secret mobilization for all the forms of ARS. Because of these benefits, we used irrigation therapy in both groups as a component of the basic therapy with local activity. If there would be an impact of irrigation therapy, the impact

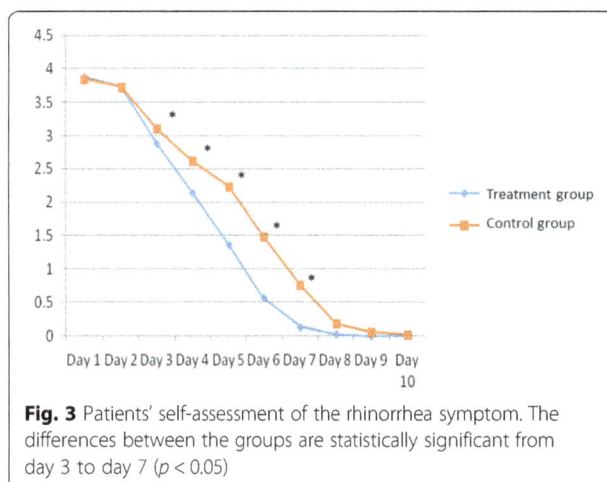

**Fig. 1** Physician's assessment of the nasal congestion symptom at visit 1 to visit 4

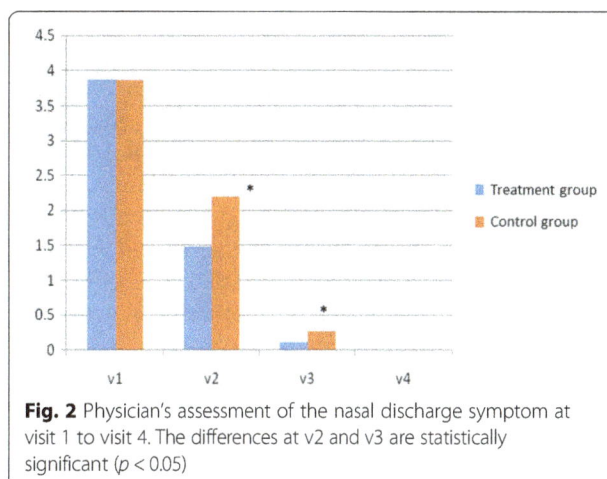

**Fig. 3** Patients' self-assessment of the rhinorrhea symptom. The differences between the groups are statistically significant from day 3 to day 7 ($p < 0.05$)

can be assumed as similar in both groups, since the group parameters are comparable. Evaluated differences in severity of symptoms between the treatment groups can therefore be assumed to be related to the herbal medicine. An additional herbal medicine with multiple systematic activities could be useful in alleviating the symptoms of acute post- viral rhinosinusitis and might inhibit the transition to a bacterial infection. There is an extensive evidence from in vitro and animal studies that the complex herbal medicine Sinupret possesses a variety of such relevant activities.

Rossi et al. [8] investigated the effects of Sinupret in an in vivo model of acute inflammation, carrageenan-induced pleurisy in rats. Sinupret significantly reduced exudate volume and leukocyte numbers in the pleural exudate. There were also parallel reductions in the expression of the enzyme cyclooxygenase-2, which forms pro-inflammatory prostaglandin $E_2$. Zhang et al. [7] showed that Sinupret promotes transepithelial chloride transport, and enhances ciliary beat frequency and airway surface liquid depth. Taken together, these activities would tend to enhance mucus clearance. In vitro studies suggest that one underlying mechanism may be the binding of antioxidant components of the herbal medicine to CFTR (cystic fibrosis transmembrane conductance regulator), resulting in direct activation and enhanced chloride transport [11].

The present randomized controlled study investigated the efficacy of Sinupret in alleviating the symptoms of acute post-viral rhinosinusitis in children aged 6 to 11 years. Relative to standard treatment, significant improvements were found in the treatment group in five key symptoms as assessed by the physician and in three key symptoms as assessed by the patient. There was also a reduction in the number of patients given antibiotic treatment. Similar findings have been made in a study with adult patients [9].

During the study period none of the patients showed any adverse reactions to Sinupret. That supports the safety of the treatment in children.

## Limitations

This was a randomized non-interventional study. Limitations include the lack of virological information and the lack of radiological measurements.

## Conclusion

Sinupret is an effective treatment for the symptoms of acute post-viral rhinosinusitis in children. Sinupret could also encourage reduction in the unnecessary prescription of antibiotics for this condition. This is important in the light of the development of bacterial resistance.

**Abbreviations**
ABRS: Acute bacterial rhinosinusitis; CFTR: Cystic fibrosis transmembrane conductance regulator; MSS score: Major sinusitis severity score; v1, 2, 3, 4: visits 1, 2, 3, 4

**Acknowledgements**
None.

**Authors' contributions**
VP: creation of the study design, protocol, data processing and interpretation. IK: work with patients, data collection. Both authors read and approved the final manuscript.

**Authors' information**
Prof. Popovich is the Head of the Department of Otolaryngology at Ivano-Frankivsk University, Ukraine.
Dr. Koshel is an associated professor of the ENT-department of Otolaryngology at Ivano-Frankivsk University, Ukraine.

**Competing interests**
The authors declare that they have no competing interests.

**Declarations**
The authors confirmed the absence of conflict of interests.

**Author details**
[1]Department of Otorhinolaryngology, Ivano-Frankivsk University, Ivano-Frankivsk, Ukraine. [2]Ivano-Frankivsk University, Galitskaya str. 2, 76000 Ivano-Frankivsk, Ukraine.

**References**
1. Chang CC, Incaudo GA, Gershwin ME. Diseases of the sinuses: a comprehensive textbook of diagnosis and treatment. 2nd Ed, New York: Springer-Verlag; 2014; p 99-107.
2. Fokkens W, Lund V, Mullol J, et al. EPOS 2012: European position paper on rhinosinusitis and nasal polyps. Rhinology. 2012;supplement 23:1–299.
3. Hellgren J, Cervin A, Nordling S, Bergman A, Cardell LO. Allergic rhinitis and the common cold – high cost to society. Allergy. 2010;65(6):776–83.
4. Bachert C, Schapowal A, Funk P, Kieser M. Treatment of acute rhinosinusitis with the preparation from Pelargonium sidoides EPs 7630: a randomized, double-blind, placebo-controlled trial. Rhinology. 2009;47(1):51–8.
5. Timmer A, Günther J, Rücker G, Motschall E, Antes G, Kern WV. Pelargonium sidoides's extract for acute respiratory tract infections. Cochrane Database Syst Rev. 2013;Issue 10. Art. No.: CD006323. doi:10.1002/14651858.CD006323.pub3.
6. Guo R, Canter PH, Ernst E. Herbal medicines for the treatment of rhinosinusitis: a systematic review. Otolaryngol Head Neck Surg. 2006;135:496–506.
7. Zhang S, Skinner D, Hicks SB, Bevensee MO, Sorscher EJ, Lazrak A, Matalon S, McNicholas CM, Woodworth BA. Sinupret activates CFTR and TMEM16A-dependent transepithelial chloride transport and improves indicators of mucociliary clearance. PLoS One. 2014;9(8):PMID 25117505. doi:10.1371/journal.pone.0104090.
8. Rossi A, Dehm F, Kiesselbach C, Haunschild J, Sautebin L, Werz O. The novel Sinupret® dry extract exhibits effectiveness in vivo. Fitoterapia. 2012;83:715–20.
9. Jund R, Mondigler M, Steindl H, Stammer H, Stierna P, Bachert C. Klinische Wirksamkeit eines pflanzlichen Kombinationspräparates in der Behandlung der akuten viralen Rhinosinusitis. MMW-Fortschritte der Medizin. 2015;157(S4):6–11.
10. Pynnonen MA, Mukerji SS, Kim HM, Adams ME, Terrell JE. Nasal saline for chronic sinonasal symptoms: a randomized controlled trial. Arch Otolaryngol Head Neck Surg. 2007;133(11):1115–20.
11. Zhang S, Smith N, Schuster D, Azbell C, Sorscher EJ, Rowe SM, Woodworth BA. Quercetin increases CFTR mediated chloride transport and ciliary beat frequency: therapeutic implications for chronic rhinosinusitis. Am J Rhinol Allergy. 2011;25(5):307–12.

# 12

# Neuroprotective effects of *Peltophorum pterocarpum* leaf extract against hydrogen peroxide induced oxidative stress and cytotoxicity

Theanmalar Masilamani[1*], Thavamanithevi Subramaniam[1], Norshariza Nordin[2] and Rozita Rosli[3]

## Abstract

**Background:** *Peltophorum pterocarpum* is a plant from the family of Leguminosae and a tropical tree found in South East Asia region. The leaves of the plant is rich in anti-oxidant polyphenols. Traditionally this plant was used to cure intestinal disorders and as a relief for sprain, bruise, muscular pain and sores and for pain during child birth. Since oxidative stress is a major contributing factor towards neurodegenerative diseases the leaves of this plant was explored for its neuroprotective properties.

**Method:** In this study, we report the neuroprotective properties of the ethanolic extract of *Peltophorum pterocarpum* leaf against oxidative stress induced cell death by $H_2O_2$, in an in vitro model of neuronally differentiated IMR32 neuroblastoma cells. Hydrogen peroxide was used as an inducer for oxidative stress. Cell viability was determined using MTT assay, apoptosis studies were carried out using Annexin V-FITC and Caspase 3 assays, mitochondrial membrane potential was examined using JC1 staining. The oxidative stress induced by $H_2O_2$ was determined by quantifying the intracellular reactive oxygen species production using DCF-DA staining. Mitogen activated protein kinase signaling pathway of the neuroprotective effect of PTE was also elucidated since oxidative stress activates this pathway signaling.

**Results:** *Peltophorum pterocarpum* leaf extract did not exhibit any cytotoxicity to differentiated IMR32 cells at the tested concentration of 7.8 μg/ml till 250 μg/ml. Pre-treatment of differentiated IMR32 with *Peltophorum pterocarpum* leaf extract prior to exposure to 300 μM hydrogen peroxide significantly ameliorated neuronal cell death and apoptosis in a dose-dependent manner. Hydrogen peroxide induced oxidative stress caused the reduction of mitochondrial membrane potential in differentiated IMR32 cells. *Peltophorum pterocarpum* leaf extract conferred neuroprotection to differentiated IMR32 by increasing the mitochondrial membrane potential in a dose-dependent manner which was significantly higher at 125 μg/ml and 250 μg/ml. PTE pre-treatment attenuated the increase of intracellular reactive oxygen species induced by hydrogen peroxide in a dose-dependent manner up till concentration of 125 μg/ml. Western blot analysis on mitogen activated protein kinases (MAPKs) revealed that neuroprotection of *Peltophorum pterocarpum* leaf extract against hydrogen peroxide induced cytotoxicity was achieved by complete inhibition of the activation of phospho-p-38 phosphorylation and attenuation of phospho-ERK1/2.

**Conclusion:** This study thus suggests that *Peltophorum pterocarpum* leaf extract has neuroprotective activity against oxidative-stress induced neuronal cell death.

**Keywords:** Antioxidant, Neuroprotective, Apoptosis, Oxidative stress, Reactive oxygen Species, *Peltophorum pterocarpum*

* Correspondence: thean@sirim.my; malarthean@gmail.com
[1]SIRIM Bhd, Industrial Biotechnology Research Centre (IBRC), No 1, Persiaran Dato Menteri Seksyen 2, 40700 Shah Alam, Selangor, Malaysia
Full list of author information is available at the end of the article

## Background

Oxidative stress due to the over production of reactive oxygen species (ROS) during normal aerobic respiration in the neurons play an important role in the pathophysiology of many neurodegeneration diseases. Alzheimer's disease (AD), Parkinson's disease (PD), Amyotropic Lateral Sclerosis (ALS), and Huntington's disease (HD) are irreparable and debilitating neurodegenerative diseases that causes gradual damage to the structure, function and finally death of neurons [1]. Neuronal cells are particularly sensitive to oxidative stress because they are deficient in their internal anti-oxidant defense mechanism against damage by free radicals or ROS [2]. Since neurons are post-mitotic cells, neuronal cell death is irreversible. Thus, in order to prevent neuronal damage, anti-oxidant based natural products are much sought after for use as a preventive measure to combat oxidative stress induced cell death in neurons. There have also been a continuous effort to use natural based anti-oxidant compounds as neuroprotective adjunct in the prevention of neuronal cell death. Natural compounds such as curcumin [3, 4], huperzine A [5] and a standardized extract from Gingko biloba leaf (EGb761) [6] are some of the plant based compounds that have neuroprotective effect.

*Peltophorum pterocarpum* is a plant from the family of Leguminosae and a tropical tree found in South Eastern Asia. The leaves of *Peltophorum pterocarpum* have been reported to be hepatoprotective against paracetamol induced liver toxicity in albino Wistar rats mainly due to its anti-oxidant effect [7]. The methanolic extract of the bark of this plant was found to be neuroprotective against scopolamine induced memory loss in rats [8]. However, studies on the neuroprotective effect of the leaves have not yet been done. In this study, the PTE extract was explored for its in vitro neuroprotective properties against $H_2O_2$ induced cell death and oxidative stress on the differentiated IMR32 neuroblastoma cells (dIMR32).

## Methods
### Plant material and extraction

Fresh leaves of the *Peltophorum pterocarpum* were obtained from Block 19 of SIRIM Bhd, Shah Alam, Malaysia. The plant was authenticated by an herbalist from the Forest Research Institute of Malaysia (FRIM), Kepong. The leaves of the plant were washed with distilled water and dried in an oven at 40 °C. The dried leaves were then powderized and extraction was carried out at room temperature for 24 h in an orbital shaker (at 200 rpm) using absolute ethanol (analytical grade, Merck) at concentration of 1:20 (*w/v*) where 10 g of the leaves were extracted in 200 ml of ethanol. After 24 h the suspension was filtered using a 114 Whatman filter paper and filtrate

collected. The solvent filtrate was concentrated using a rotary evaporator.

### HPLC profiling of PTE Extract

The HPLC profiling of ethanolic extract of *Peltophorum pterocarpum* leaves (PTE) was carried using Shimadzu HPLC instrument with UV visible PDA detector at 254 nm. Chromatographic separation was accomplished by injecting the sample onto a Novapak C18 column (250 × 4.6 mm, 5-μm). The mobile phase consisted of solvent A: 0.1% formic acid in water and solvent B: 0.1% formic acid in acetonitrile; gradient starting from 10% B and 90% A for 14mins, 100% B and 0% A for 11 min, 10% B and 90% A for another 5 min; then re-equilibrating prior to the next injection. The detection wavelength was 254 nm with a flow rate of 0.8 ml / min and an injection volume of 10 μl was used.

### IMR32 cell culture and differentiation

IMR32 (ATCC® CCL-127™) neuroblastoma cell line, was purchased from ATCC. IMR32 cells were routinely maintained in complete Eagle's Minimum Essential Medium (EMEM, GIBCO) supplemented with 1 mM sodium pyruvate, 1 mM non-essential amino acids (NEAA, GIBCO), 10% fetal bovine growth serum (FBS, HyClone) and 1X antibiotic/antimycotic (HyClone) containing 10,000 units of penicillin, 10,000 μg of streptomycin, and 25 μg of Amphotericin B per milliliter. The cells were maintained in humidified 5% $CO_2$ incubator and passaged according to the recommended dilutions and confluency by ATCC. Differentiation of the IMR32 cells were carried out using RPMI medium (Gibco) supplemented with 1 mM sodium pyruvate, 1 mM non-essential amino acids (NEAA, GIBCO), 2% FBS, Penicillin/Streptomycin and Amphoterin. Differentiation to neuronal phenotype was induced using 2.5 μM 5Brdu (Sigma Aldrich) for 15 days with frequent change of medium every 48 h. All subsequent cell culture analysis was done ut with the 15 days differentiated IMR32 (dIMR32) cells.

### Immunocytochemistry (ICC) to confirm neuronal phenotype in differentiated IMR32

The neuronally differentiated IMR32 cells (dIMR32) were fixed in 4% paraformaldehyde at room temperature for 30 min. After PFA fixing and washing with 1xPBS, the neurons were permeabilized in permeabilization solution (1% Triton-X in 1× PBS) at room temperature for 15 min and washed again in PBS. They were then blocked in blocking solution (0.3% BSA, 1% goat serum, 0.1% Tween 20) at room temperature for 30 min. After that, the cells of each well were incubated separately with the primary antibodies of class III beta tubulin (marker for postmitotic neurons), and choline acetyltransferase / ChAT (marker for cholinergic neurons) both diluted in blocking buffer at dilution (1:200; Abcam) and incubated overnight at 4 °C. The next day, the cells were rinsed 3 times with 1× PBS and incubated with secondary antibodies, Alexa Fluor 488 goat anti-rabbit IgG (1:200; Abcam) for green fluorescence and Alexa Fluor 594 goat anti-rabbit IgG (1:200; Abcam) for red fluorescence, at room temperature in the dark for 2 h. Nuclei were counterstained with 1 µg/µl propidium iodide (PI) or DAPI (5 µg/ml, Molecular Probes) for 10 min and washed 3 times with 1× PBS. The cells were then viewed under Olympus IX51 inverted fluorescence microscope.

## Treatment of the differentiated IMR32 neurons (dIMR32) and MTT assay

Cells were seeded at $5 \times 10^4$ cells/ml in 24 well plates (Corning® CellBIND® Surface cell culture flasks) for better attachment of cells and the cells grown to 70% confluence in complete EMEM for 48 h. After 48 h, the IMR32 cells were differentiated with 2.5 µM for 15 days. On the 15th day, the differentiated cells were treated with serially diluted concentrations of PTE, starting from 250 µg/ml to 8 µg/ml for 24 h to determine the viability of differentiated (dIMR32). To study the neuroprotective effect of PTE against $H_2O_2$ cytotoxicity, the dIMR32 cells were pretreated for 24 h with the above concentrations of PTE, and then treated with the 300 µM of $H_2O_2$ for 24 h. All the treatments were done in RPMI medium without serum and sodium pyruvate. Sodium pyruvate was omitted from the medium because it is neuroprotective to dIMR32 cells and will interfere with the viability assay of the extracts. MTT assay to test the viability of the dIMR32 after treatment was carried out by adding 0.25 mg/ml MTT to the cells for 3 h. The medium was removed and the formazan formed was dissolved in DMSO and the absorbance was measured using a multiplate reader at 570 nm wavelength (Tecan, Austria). All experiments were done in triplicates. Results were expressed as percentage of the untreated cells.

$$\text{Cell Viability } (\%) = \frac{\text{OD}_{570nm}\text{treatment}}{\text{OD}_{570nm}\text{untreated}} \times 100\%$$

## Apoptosis assay using annexin V FITC/ propidium iodide assay kit

Apoptosis assay was conducted using Annexin V FITC Assay kit from Cayman Chemical, USA according to the manufacturer's protocol. Briefly after the required treatment, the dIMR32 cells were collected from each well and centrifuged at 120 0 rpm for 5 min. The pellet was then re-suspended in 200 µl binding buffer and then centrifuged again at 1200 rpm for 5 min and the supernatant removed. The pellet is re-suspended in 50 µl of the Annexin V FITC/PI staining solution and kept in

dark for 10 min. The cells were centrifuged again, supernatant discarded and the pellet was re-suspended in 150 µl of 1× binding buffer and immediately analyzed using FACS Calibur Flowcytometer and Cell Quest Pro software (BD Biosciences, USA).

## Caspase 3 activity using fluorescence assay

Caspases belong to the aspartic specific cysteinyl protease family and caspase 3 is an effector caspase and its activity is involved in both external and internal apoptosis. Caspase 3 assay is carried out using Cayman Chemical Fluorescence based assay kit. This kit utilizes a specific caspase 3 substrate N-Ac-DEVD-N'-MC-R110 which upon cleavage by active caspase 3, generates a highly fluorescent product that is measured at excitation 485 and emission 535. Briefly, after treatment cells were harvested, washed in 200 µl caspase 3 assay buffer, centrifuged at 1000 rpm for 5 min and the supernatant was discarded. The cell pellets were then lysed in ice cold 1X Cell Lysis Buffer (10 mM Tris-HCl at pH 7.5, 10 mM $NaH_2PO_4$/$NaHPO_4$, 130 mM NaCl, 1% Triton X-100, 10 mM sodium pyrophosphate) for 30 min with occasional vortexing. After centrifugation at 12,000 rpm, 4 °C for 5 min, 90 µl cell lysate was added to 10 µl of caspase assay buffer and 100 µl of caspase substrate solution. Caspase 3 substrate solution contains 100 µl of caspase 3 substrate, 400 µl dithiothreitol (DTT) and 9.5 ml Caspase 3 assay buffer. The mixture was incubated at 37 °C for 30 min and fluorescence was read at an excitation wavelength of 485 nm and an emission wavelength of 535 nm using fluorescence plate reader (Tecan). Caspase 3 activity expressed in relative fluorescence unit (RFU) was normalized against protein concentration of the cell lysates which was determined using Bradford Assay. The results are expressed as relative fluorescence unit per microgram of protein (RFU/µg protein).

## Mitochondrial membrane potential (ΔΨm) assay using JC-1 kit

The changes in Mitochondrial Membrane Potential (MMP or ΔΨm) were measured using JC-1 Mitochondrial Membrane Potential Assay Kit (Cayman Chemical. USA) as described in the manufacturer's protocol. After the required treatment, the cells were washed with the provided assay buffer and centrifuged at 1000 rpm for 5 min and the supernatant was discarded. JC1 staining solution was prepared by diluting the stock in culture medium at 1:10 dilution ratio. The cell pellet was re-suspended in 100 µl of the JC1 staining solution and incubated in the dark at 37 °C for 30 min. The cells were then centrifuged at 1200 rpm for 5 min and supernatant removed. The pellet was then re-suspended in the 100 µl assay buffer. The cells were then analyzed using black well plate and fluorescence plate reader at excitation 485 nm and emission 535 nm for green apoptotic cells and at emission 590 nm for red healthy cells using TECAN fluorescence plate reader. The ratio between healthy/apoptotic fluorescence readings was calculated. The ratio of the reading at 595 nm to the reading at 535 nm was considered as the relative $\Delta\Psi m$ value.

### Intracellular ROS detection using DCFH-DA assay

The degree of ROS generation in dIMR32 cells were measured using fluorescence assay with 2′,7′-dichlorodihydro-fluorescein diacetate (H2DCFDA, Sigma). Briefly, after treatment the cells were scraped and washed in PBS and the pellet re-suspended in 200 µl of PBS loaded with 10 µM H 2 DCFH-DA at 37 °C for 30 min and then the cells were washed twice with PBS and centrifuged at 1000 rpm for 5 min. Finally, the pellet was re-suspended in 200 µl PBS and the fluorescence's intensity of DCF was measured with BD Biosciences Accuri C6 flow cytometer.

### Western blot analysis

Briefly, after treatment as above, dIMR32 cells were harvested, cells were washed with PBS, centrifuged at 1000 rpm for 10 min, the supernatant was discarded and 200 µl of iced-cold 1xRIPA buffer was added to the cell pellet in order to lyse the cells for protein extraction. The cells in the 1× RIPA buffer were placed on ice for 30 min with occasional vortexing. The samples were centrifuged at 12000 rpm at 4 °C for 15 min. The soluble proteins that were in the supernatant were transferred to a new 1.5 ml centrifuge tubes. The protein concentration was quantified using the commercial Bradford Assay. The cell lysates samples were stored at −80 °C for further use. Proteins were separated on a 12% SDS–polyacrylamide gel, and then transferred onto a polyvinylidene difluoride transfer membrane blots (Amersham Hybond P). The blots were blocked with 5% BSA in TBST buffer (25 mM Tris-HCl, 140 mM NaCl, 2 mM KCl, 0.05% ($v/v$) Tween 20) for 1 h at room temperature. The blots were then washed 3× for 10 min each time, with TBS-T. The blots were subsequently incubated with the primary antibody (Cell Signaling) overnight at 4 °C diluted in blocking buffer (each antibody at a dilution of 1:1000; phospho-JNK (Thr183/Tyr185), JNK, phospho-p38 (Thr180/Tyr182), p38, phospho-ERK 1/2 (Thr202/Tyr204) at 1:2000 and ERK1/2 (1:1000)). Beta Actin (Cell Signaling) was used as loading control with dilution (1:1000). After overnight incubation, the blots were then washed 3× (each 10 min) with TBS-T and incubated at room temperature for 1 h with horseradish peroxidase conjugated anti-rabbit IgG secondary antibody (1:5000) diluted in TBS-T. The blots were washed again 3× each 10 min with TBS-T and developed using Amersham ECL Prime Western Blotting Detection Reagent at ratio of 1:1 (GE Healthcare Life Sciences). Protein bands were quantified by densitometric analysis using Image J software 1.46 (National Institute of Health, USA).

### Statistical analysis

Results were expressed as the mean ± SEM performed in triplicates. Graphs were plotted and data were analyzed by one-way analysis of variance ANOVA (Dunnett's test) using GraphPad Prism 6.0 software. The differences between the means of treated and untreated groups were considered significant at $p < 0.05$.

## Results

### HPLC profiling of the ethanolic extract of *Peltophorum pterocarpum* leaf (PTE)

The results in Fig. 1 show the HPLC profile of PTE and it was found that the major bioactive peak is at the retention time 8.52 min. As reported earlier the major compounds that are present in the leaves are the derivatives of quercetin among which are the (Fig. 1b) quercetin-3-O-β-D-galacto-side [9] and Quercetin-3-O-β-D-glucuronide (Fig. 1c) (identified by our group in an unpublished earlier research).

### Immunocytochemistry (ICC) of differentiated IMR32 neurons

Human neuroblastoma IMR32 cells were differentiated into neuronal-like cells by using 5-Bromo-2′-deoxyuridine (5Brdu). Undifferentiated IMR32 cells consists of two types of cells which are the N type cells consisting of small round neuroblast cells with poor cell adherence to the surface (green arrows in Fig. 2a) and large adherent fibroblast cells (red arrows in Fig. 2a). When differentiated with 2.5 µM 5Brdu in a low serum (2%) medium, the cells stops proliferating and forms extensive network of neurites (red arrows in Fig. 2b) together with connected clumps of cells (green arrow in Fig. 2b). This differentiated IMR32 (dIMR32) cells express post mitotic neuronal marker of class III β- tubulin III (Fig. 2c) and also express the ChAT (Choline Acetyltransferase) cholinergic neuronal cell marker (Fig. 2d).

### In vitro neuroprotective effect of ethanolic extract of *Peltophorum pterocarpum* leaf (PTE)

Initial experiments were conducted to determine whether PTE extract was toxic to differentiated IMR32 (dIMR32). Figure 3a shows that treatment of dIMR32 with various concentration of PTE from (8 µg/ml till 250 µg/ml) did not show any cytotoxicity in the dIMR32 cells where its viability ranges from (84, 92, 92, 94, 98 and 95%) respectively. Consequently, the neuroprotective effect of PTE against $H_2O_2$ induced neurotoxicity were investigated. Differentiated IMR32 cells (dIMR32) were pretreated with various concentrations of PTE for 24 h followed by treatment with 300 µM $H_2O_2$ for 24 h. As shown as in Fig. 3c, $H_2O_2$ induced loss of cell viability (64%) was significantly attenuated by PTE pretreatment in a dose dependent manner with cell viability of 82, 94, 116, 139, 124 and 103% at PTE concentrations of 8 µg/ml, 16 µg/ml, 31 µg/ml, 63 µg/ml, 125 µg/ml and 250 µg/ml respectively.

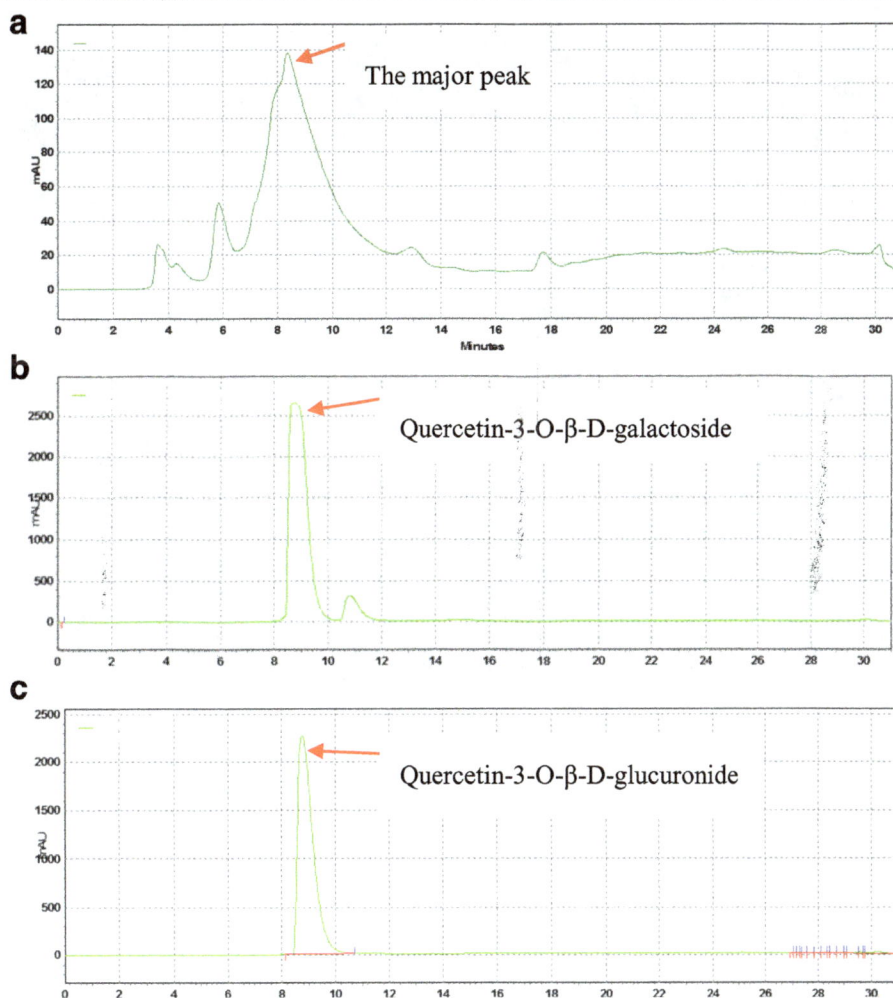

**Fig. 1 a** HPLC Profile of ethanolic extract of *Peltophorum pterocarpum* leaf (PTE) with detection at 254 nm using PDA detector. The major bioactive peak at retention time (RT) of 8.514 min that contains mainly quercetin derivatives namely **b** Quercetin-3-O-β-D-galactoside (hyperoside) and **c** Quercetin-3-O-β-Dglucuronide (Miquelianin)

### Effect of PTE against $H_2O_2$ induced apoptosis

Apoptosis study was conducted using the Annexin V FITC/PI assay where Annexin binds to the intracellular phosphatidylserine (PS) in a calcium-dependent manner. In this study, PTE treatment (Fig. 4a) alone only exhibited minimal apoptosis in dIMR32 and the viability of the cells were above 74.3% on all tested concentrations of PTE which confirms the earlier MTT results that PTE is not cytotoxic to the dIMR32. The percentage of viable cells in the untreated group was 93.4%, and from the group that was 24 h treated with PTE from concentration of 8 μg/ml, 16 μg/ml, 31 μg/ml, 63 μg/ml, 125 μg/ml and 250 μg/ml were 90.8, 93.4, 86.8, 90.6, 79.9 and 74.3%, respectively. Nevertheless, PTE treatment for 24 h increased the percentage of total apoptotic cells in a concentration dependent manner where in the untreated group total apoptotic cells (which include the early apoptotic, late apoptotic and necrotic cells) were

6.6% and the PTE treated group from concentration of 8 μg/ml, 16 μg/ml, 31 μg/ml, 63 μg/ml, 125 μg/ml and 250 μg/ml, the total apoptotic cells were 9.2, 6.6, 13.29.420.1and 25.7% respectively.

The effect of PTE pre-treatment and then subsequent treatment with 300 μM $H_2O_2$ on apoptosis status of dIMR32 were evaluated (Fig. 4b). In the absence of $H_2O_2$ or in the untreated group, the majority (93.4%) of the cells were viable and non-apoptotic (Annexin V⁻PI⁻). However, in the $H_2O_2$ treated group the viable cells were reduced to 51.9% cells and total apoptotic cells were at 48.1%. The viable cells in the PTE pre-treated cells prior to $H_2O_2$ insult, increased in a concentration dependent manner (8 μg/ml, 16 μg/ml, 31 μg/ml, 63 μg/ml, 125 μg/ml and 250 μg/ml) from 56.2, 62.7, 69.2, 79.8, 50.6 and 71.4%. PTE pre-treatment prior to 300 μM $H_2O_2$ insult significantly reduced the percentage of total apoptosis cells in a concentration dependent

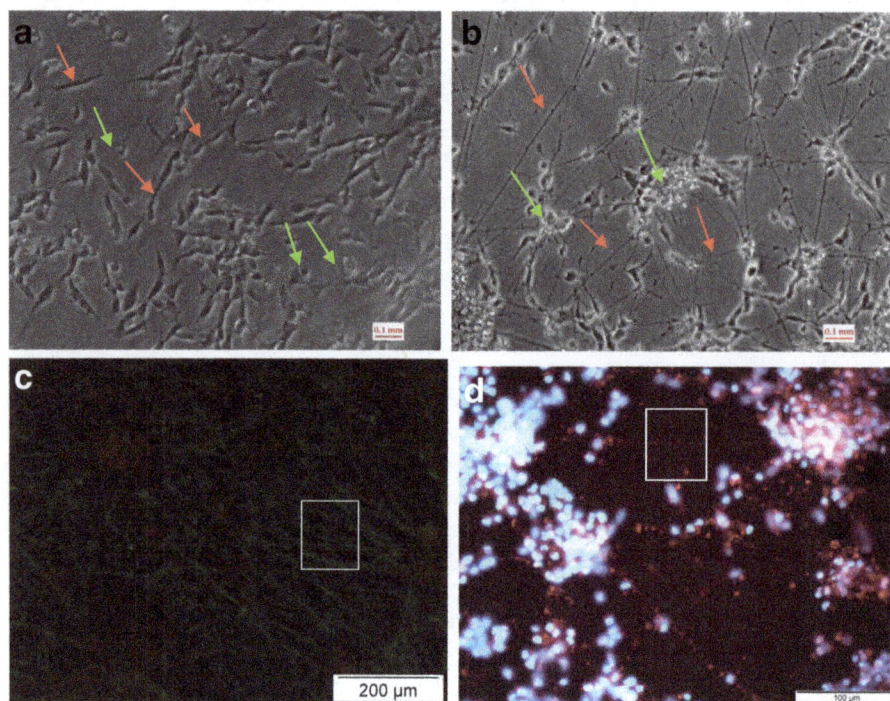

**Fig. 2** Images of IMR32 cells. **a** Phase contrast image of undifferentiated human neuroblastoma IMR32 cells. Its shows proliferating cells. The *red color arrows* indicate fibroblast type cells and *green. Color arrow* indicate neuroblast type cells. **b** 2.5 μM Brdu differentiated human IMR32 cells (Div15 days). It shows neuron like properties including neuritic outgrowth and morphological changes. *Red arrows* shows the elongated neurites, green arrows connected clumps of cells. **c** ICC image of the expression of class III Beta-tubulin neuron marker in Div15 dIMR32 cells. Nuclei stained in Propidium iodide (PI *red*) and post mitotic neurons staining with class III β-tubulin (*green*). **d** Expression of ChAT (Choline Acetyltransferase) cholinergic neuron cell marker in dIMR32 cells. Nuclei stained with DAPI (*blue*) and cholinergic neurons stained with ChAT (*red*)

manner from 8 μg/ml, 16 μg/ml, 31 μg/ml, 63 μg/ml which were 43.8, 31.2, 30.8 and 20.2% respectively as compared to the percentage total apoptotic cells of 48.1% in 300 μM $H_2O_2$ treated group (Fig. 4b). However, there was higher percentage of total apoptotic cells (40.5%) at 125 μg/ml PTE pretreated group as compared to 28.6% at 250 μg/ml PTE pre-treated group.

### Neuroprotective effect of PTE against $H_2O_2$ cytotoxicity on caspase 3 activity

Caspase 3 is the major executioner caspase that is involved both in mitochondrial mediated apoptosis and the extrinsic apoptosis. The effect of PTE pretreatment on the $H_2O_2$ induced caspase 3 activity in dIMR32 cells were evaluated. Figure 5 shows the Caspase 3 activity (in terms of RFU/μg protein) after pretreatment with PTE for 24 h and then treatment with $H_2O_2$ for 24 h. However, contrary to what was expected, $H_2O_2$ treatment (with caspase 3 activity of 420 RFU / μg protein) did not significantly increase caspase 3 activity as compared to untreated cells (with caspase 3 activity of 437 RFU / μg protein). It might be possible that $H_2O_2$ caused reversible inactivation of caspase 3 activity [10].

There was no significant decrease in the caspase 3 activity in the cells pre-treated with PTE from concentration of

8 μg/ml, 16 μg/ml, 31 μg/ml, 63 μg/ml and 125 μg/ml. The caspase 3 activity in these concentration were 487, 465, 529, 582 and 594 RFU/μg protein. The caspase 3 activity was significantly high at 250 μg/ml pre-treated cells at 931.5 RFU / μg protein as opposed to 420 RFU / μg protein in $H_2O_2$ treated cells.

### Effect of PTE pre-treatment on $H_2O_2$ induced reduction of Mitochondrial Membrane Potential (MMP) Δψм

Mitochondria is the major organelle where oxidative stress happens and it is the major source of ROS production which is produced during mitochondrial electron transport. Mitochondrial dysfunction leads to the loss of mitochondrial trans-membrane potential (MMP) which changes the permeability of mitochondrial and thus release soluble proteins such as cytochrome C or other apoptotic related proteins and activate caspase cascade [11]. Loss of MMP is an early sign of apoptosis. In this study, JC1 a cationic dye that accumulates in healthy or energized mitochondria was used. When mitochondria has low Δψм due to apoptosis, JC-1 is predominantly a monomer that yields green fluorescence with emission of (530 ± 15 nm) and when it has high Δψм and healthy the dye enters the mitochondria and aggregates, thus yielding a red to orange colored

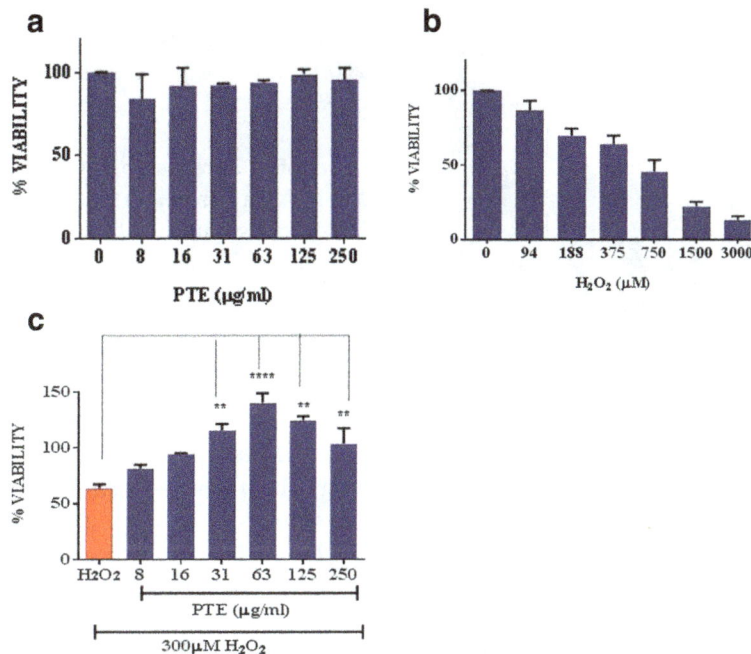

**Fig. 3 a** Effect of PTE on dIMR32 cells viability after exposure for 24 h. No statistical difference were observed between doses. **b** Effect of $H_2O_2$ on dIMR32 cells viability after exposure for 24 h. There is a dose-dependent reduction in viability of dIMR32 cells. **c** Neuroprotective effect of PTE pre-treatment (24 h) against $H_2O_2$ induced cytotoxicity in dIMR32 cells. The data are expressed as mean ± SEM, $n$ = 3. Statistical significance was analyzed with one-way analysis of variance followed by Dunnett's multiple comparison post-hoc test. Differences with $p$ value less than 0.0001 and $p$ value less than 0.05 against 300 µM $H_2O_2$ treatment were considered statistically significant. ****$p$ < 0.0001 and **$p$ < 0.05

emission (590 ± 17.5 nm). Therefore, depolarization happens when the aggregate (healthy cells) red fluorescent count decrease whereas hyperpolarization happens when the red fluorescent count increase. In this study, $H_2O_2$ induced cells have significantly lower $\Delta\psi_M$ based on the lower RFU ratio between red/green fluorescent (Fig. 6). However, pretreatment with PTE increased the $\Delta\psi_M$ by the increase in ratio (in arbitrary units) of red/green fluorescent in a dose-dependent manner where it is significantly higher at 250 and 125 µg/ml (0.91 and 0.82, respectively) as opposed to 0.46 in $H_2O_2$ treated cells.

## Effect of PTE pre-treatment on the intracellular ROS detection production

$H_2O_2$ induced cytotoxicity causes mitochondrial dysfunction and leads to the production of reactive oxidative species (ROS) which subsequently activates the apoptosis cascade. ROS generation in dIMR32 cells was determined using ROS-sensitive fluorescence indicator DCFH-DA. Figure 7 shows that exposure of dIMR32 to 300 µM of $H_2O_2$ significantly increased the ROS production to 54% as compared to the untreated cells (38%). The pre-treatment of PTE reduced the production ROS

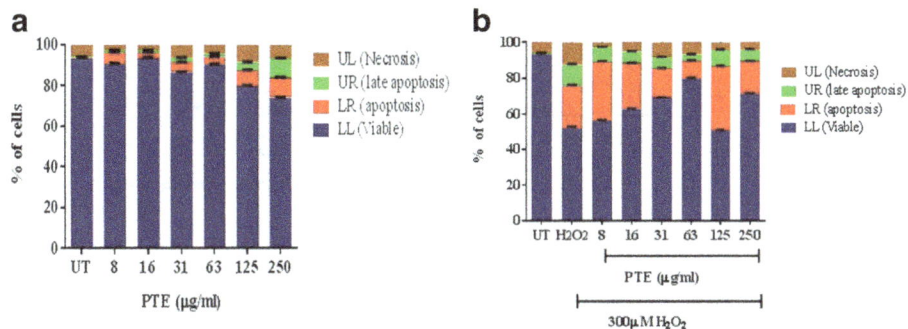

**Fig. 4 a** Effect of PTE treatment for 24 h on dIMR32 cells apoptosis. **b** Effect of PTE pre-treatment (24 h) against $H_2O_2$ induced apoptosis in dIMR32 cells. The data are expressed as mean ± SEM, $n$ = 3. The label UT = untreated control cells. Statistical significance was analyzed with one way ANOVA followed by Dunnett's multiple comparison post-hoc test. There was significant differences with the number of apoptotic cells between 300 µM $H_2O_2$ treated cells and PTE pre-treated cells for all the tested concentration with $p$ < 0.0001

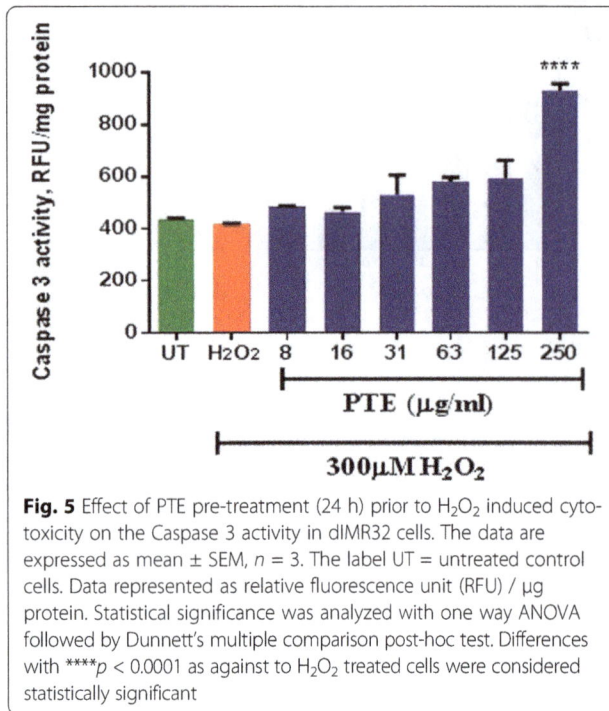

**Fig. 5** Effect of PTE pre-treatment (24 h) prior to $H_2O_2$ induced cytotoxicity on the Caspase 3 activity in dIMR32 cells. The data are expressed as mean ± SEM, $n = 3$. The label UT = untreated control cells. Data represented as relative fluorescence unit (RFU) / μg protein. Statistical significance was analyzed with one way ANOVA followed by Dunnett's multiple comparison post-hoc test. Differences with ****$p < 0.0001$ as against to $H_2O_2$ treated cells were considered statistically significant

in a dose-dependent manner from concentration of 7.8 μg/ml to 125 μg/ml of PTE. However, pre-treatment with 250 μg/ml of PTE increased the ROS production to 68%. This could be due to presence of certain compounds in the PTE that could have contributed to extra free radicals in cells on top of the oxidative stress

induced by $H_2O_2$. This was also observed in Fig. 4b, where total apoptotic cells (28.6%) were higher at 250 μg/ml PTE pre-treated cells even though the viable cells were at 71.4%.

**Effect of PTE pre-treatment on phosphorylation of MAPKs**

MAPKs play an important role in responding to various biological stimulus which includes oxidative stress in neuronal cells and thus regulate cell death or survival. Hence, western blot analysis of MAPKs protein was utilized to study the mechanism by which PTE pre-treatment protects dIMR32 cells against neuronal cell death induced by $H_2O_2$. The p38 protein is generally activated in neuronal cells via phosphorylation during oxidative stress and other extracellular stimulus. In this study, high level of phospho-p38, phospho-ERK and phospho-JNK in untreated cells as compared to 2 h $H_2O_2$ treated cells were observed as in Fig. 8a–c. This may be the result of the IMR32 neuronal differentiation, as p38, ERK and JNK also regulate differentiation [12]. However, PTE pre-treatment completely inhibited the phosphorylation of p38 as compared to 2 h $H_2O_2$ treated dIMR32 cells (Fig. 8d). PTE pre-treatment also significantly attenuated the phosphorylation of ERK1/2 as compared to $H_2O_2$ treated IMR32 cells at both the concentrations of PTE (Fig. 8e). This suggests that PTE provides protection to dIMR32 via inhibiting the p38 phosphorylation and decreasing the activation of the ERK1/2 signaling protein. PTE pre-treatment also exhibited a decreasing trend in phospho-JNK (Fig. 8f).

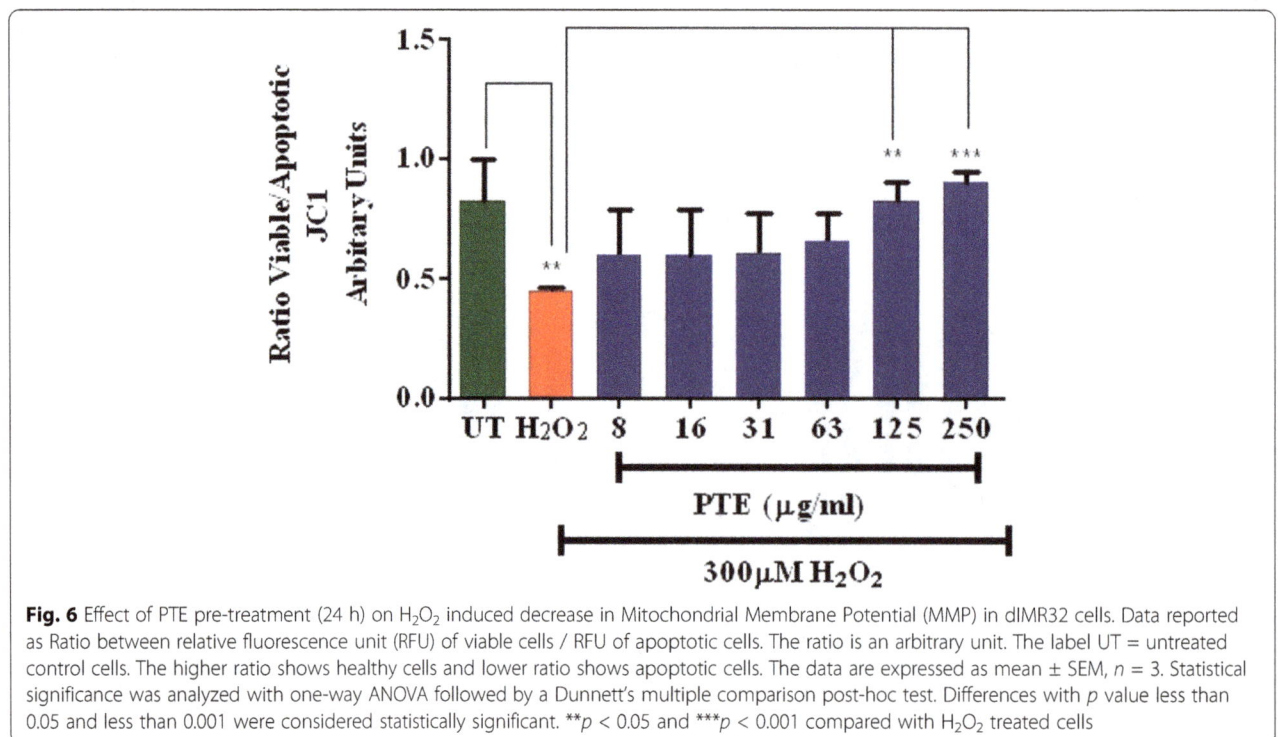

**Fig. 6** Effect of PTE pre-treatment (24 h) on $H_2O_2$ induced decrease in Mitochondrial Membrane Potential (MMP) in dIMR32 cells. Data reported as Ratio between relative fluorescence unit (RFU) of viable cells / RFU of apoptotic cells. The ratio is an arbitrary unit. The label UT = untreated control cells. The higher ratio shows healthy cells and lower ratio shows apoptotic cells. The data are expressed as mean ± SEM, $n = 3$. Statistical significance was analyzed with one-way ANOVA followed by a Dunnett's multiple comparison post-hoc test. Differences with $p$ value less than 0.05 and less than 0.001 were considered statistically significant. **$p < 0.05$ and ***$p < 0.001$ compared with $H_2O_2$ treated cells

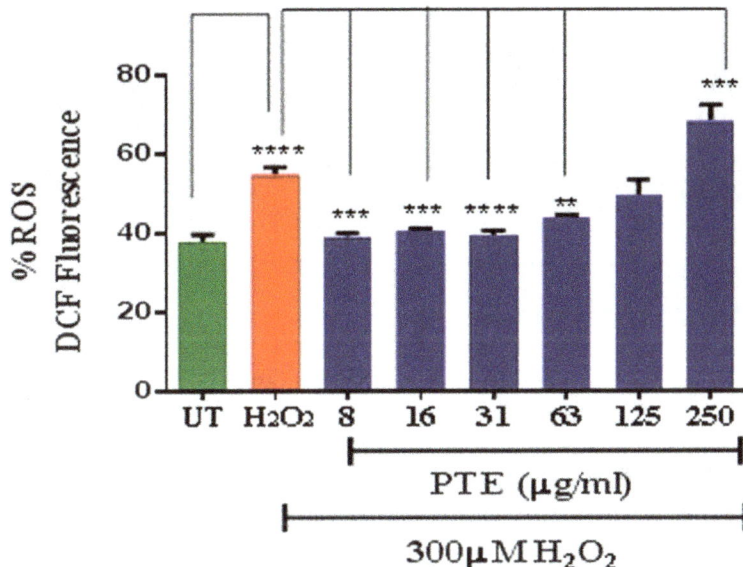

**Fig. 7** Effect of PTE pretreatment (24 h) on ROS production by $H_2O_2$ in dIMR32 cells. The data are expressed as mean ± SEM, $n = 3$. The label UT = untreated control cells. Statistical significance was analyzed with one-way ANOVA followed by Dunnett's multiple comparison post-hoc test. Differences with $p$ value less than $p < 0.0001$, $p < 0.001$ and $p < 0.05$ against 300 µM $H_2O_2$ treatment were considered statistically significant. ****$p < 0.0001$, ***$p < 0.001$ and **$p < 0.05$

## Discussion

This study used differentiated human neuroblastoma cell line IMR32 (dIMR32) as an in vitro model to study the neuroprotective effect of PTE extract against oxidative stress induced cytotoxicity (Fig. 2a and b). The results showed that IMR32 cells differentiated for 15 days (Div15) with 2.5 µM 5Brdu induced formation of extensive network of neurites which expressed the post-mitotic neuronal protein marker of class III β-tubulin and also the ChAT (choline acetyltransferase) cholinergic neuronal marker (Fig. 2c and d). Choline acetyltransferase is the enzyme that regulates the synthesis of neurotransmitter acetylcholine. It catalyzes the transfer of acetyl group from the acetyl-CoA to choline and produces acetylcholine. ChAT is produced in the body of neurons and is transported to the nerve terminal [13]. Among its other functions, acetylcholine is pivotal in the development and maintenance of memory and cognitive function in the brain [14]. Thus, this suggest that dIMR32 cells can serve an in vitro model to study neuroprotective effect of plant bioactives that affects the memory function in the brain.

*Peltophorum pterocarpum* leaves have been reported to have many anti-oxidant based bioactive compounds such as quercetin 3-O-galactoside, methyl derivatives of quercetin, naringenin, luteolin and various other anti-oxidant based compounds [9, 15]. Thus, it was used in this study as a bioactive extract to determine its neuroprotective effect against $H_2O_2$ induced oxidative stress and cytotoxicity. Based on our HPLC profiling Fig. 1b

and c we have found the presence of quercetin derivatives of Hyperoside and Miquelianin that can act as anti-oxidative neuroprotective agents against $H_2O_2$ induced cytotoxicity. The study identified that treatment with PTE extract alone did not exhibit cytotoxicity towards the dIMR32 cells and showed neuroprotection against $H_2O_2$ induced cytotoxicity (Fig. 3ac, bc & c). $H_2O_2$ is widely used an as inducer of oxidative stress in many research involving the study of neuroprotection by phytochemicals as it has high membrane permeability and can induce cytotoxicity in the cells [16, 17].

We further studied the neuroprotective mechanism of PTE against $H_2O_2$ induced oxidative stress and cytotoxicity by exploring its effect on the apoptosis in the dIMR32 cells. Apoptosis mediated cell death causes the externalization of phosphatidylserine (PS) on the plasma membrane and thus causing an increase in Annexin V and propidium iodide (PI) stained cells in Flow cytometry analysis [18]. $H_2O_2$ treatment is known to cause cell death via apoptosis [19, 20] and our results showed that PTE pre-treatment substantially attenuated the $H_2O_2$ induced apoptosis in dIMR32 cells in a dose-dependent manner (from 8 µg/ml to 250 µg/ml) except at the concentration of 125 µg/ml (Fig. 4a & b). This discrepancy in our opinion could have been attributed to the stress that might have occurred during handling of cells while harvesting the cells for the assay. Nevertheless, the results suggest that pretreatment of dIMR32 cells with PTE exerts a neuroprotective effects onto the dIMR32 through inhibition of $H_2O_2$ induced apoptotic cell death.

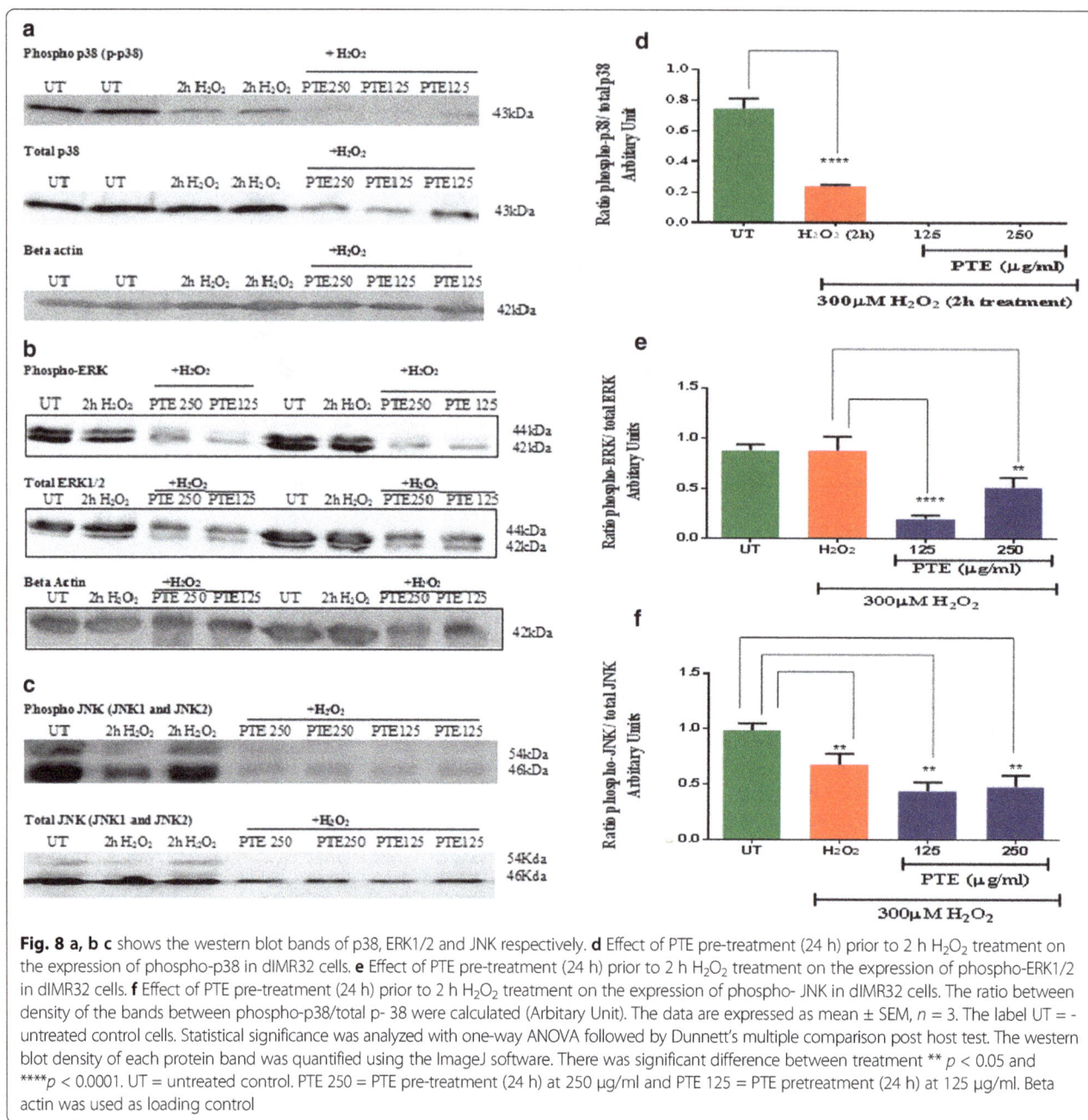

**Fig. 8 a, b c** shows the western blot bands of p38, ERK1/2 and JNK respectively. **d** Effect of PTE pre-treatment (24 h) prior to 2 h $H_2O_2$ treatment on the expression of phospho-p38 in dIMR32 cells. **e** Effect of PTE pre-treatment (24 h) prior to 2 h $H_2O_2$ treatment on the expression of phospho-ERK1/2 in dIMR32 cells. **f** Effect of PTE pre-treatment (24 h) prior to 2 h $H_2O_2$ treatment on the expression of phospho- JNK in dIMR32 cells. The ratio between density of the bands between phospho-p38/total p- 38 were calculated (Arbitary Unit). The data are expressed as mean ± SEM, $n = 3$. The label UT = - untreated control cells. Statistical significance was analyzed with one-way ANOVA followed by Dunnett's multiple comparison post host test. The western blot density of each protein band was quantified using the ImageJ software. There was significant difference between treatment ** $p < 0.05$ and **** $p < 0.0001$. UT = untreated control. PTE 250 = PTE pre-treatment (24 h) at 250 μg/ml and PTE 125 = PTE pretreatment (24 h) at 125 μg/ml. Beta actin was used as loading control

$H_2O_2$ induced apoptosis generally leads to the activation of the cysteine protease caspase cascade. Among them the caspase 3 activity is most commonly studied upon in neuronal cells [21]. Caspase 3 is the main effector caspase that is involved in both external and internal apoptosis pathway and it is the most abundant caspase in the brain [22]. Most research have shown that during $H_2O_2$ treatment of neuronal cells, the caspase 3 activity is increased and this leads to the apoptotic cell death of neurons. For example in SKNSH neuroblastoma cells, treatment with 150 μM $H_2O_2$ significantly increased the caspase 3 activity [23]. However, in our study, contrasting results were observed where treatment with 300 μM $H_2O_2$ did not increase the caspase 3 activity and PTE pre-treatment did not have any effect on the caspase 3 activity except at the highest concentration (Fig. 5). These results indicate that PTE pre-treatment does not affect the caspase 3 activity in dIMR32 cells and the mechanism of neuroprotection might be caspase independent. The possible reason why $H_2O_2$ treated dIMR32 cells did not show increase in caspase 3 activity could be because 300 μM of $H_2O_2$ might have caused necrosis to the cells. Necrotic cells do not express caspase 3 activity because caspases are sensitive to oxidative inactivation [24]. This kind of phenomena was observed in Jurkat-T-Lymphocytes where at low concentration of $H_2O_2$ (50 μM) the cells goes through apoptosis by activating caspase 3 activity starting at 3 h and peaking at 6 h [25]. However, higher concentrations of above 200 μM $H_2O_2$ decreased caspase 3 activity because cells were undergoing necrosis and high concentration of $H_2O_2$ also can directly inhibits cysteine-dependent caspase [10, 26].

Mitochondria plays an important role in $H_2O_2$ induced apoptosis and cell death. Mitochondrial dysfunction caused by $H_2O_2$ causes the collapse of the electrochemical gradient or mitochondrial membrane potential (referred to as $\Delta\Psi$m or MMP) across the mitochondrial membrane. This releases into the cytosol key apoptogenic proteins that triggers cell demise via apoptosis [27, 28]. Mitochondrial permeability transition pore (MPTP) is a voltage sensitive ion channel that resides in the inner mitochondrial membrane. This channel opens up under oxidative stress thus permitting the movement of large molecular weight solutes between the mitochondrial matrix and cytoplasm [27]. Thus, $H_2O_2$ induced oxidative stress in cells causes the inner membrane of mitochondria (which is normally impermeable) to become permeable, leading to a "large amplitude swelling" (permeability transition) and the loss of the mitochondrial membrane potential. The results in this study show that PTE pre-treatment attenuated the loss of MMP induced by $H_2O_2$ in a dose-dependent manner and the reduction was significant at the highest concentration of 125 μg/ml and 250 μg/ml of PTE (Fig. 6). The results suggest that PTE is neuroprotective against $H_2O_2$ induced oxidative stress and cytotoxicity in dIMR32 cells via the mitochondrial pathway by altering the mitochondrial membrane potential and thus reducing cascade of events that leads to apoptosis.

Oxidative stress induced by exogenous $H_2O_2$ not only causes apoptosis mediated cytotoxicity and mitochondrial dysfunction, it also leads to the generation of intracellular reactive oxygen species (ROS) in the cells. The ROS generated by the cells are determined by using the non-ionic and non-polar fluorescent dye 2,7-dichlorfluorescein-diacetate (DCFH-DA). The ROS that is produced during the oxidative stress converts the DCFH-DA into DCF which emits fluorescence that is directly proportional to the amount of ROS generated. Our studies show that PTE pre-treatment prior to $H_2O_2$ induced oxidative stress attenuated the production of ROS in dIMR32 cells in a dose-dependent manner (Fig. 7) except at the highest concentration of 250 μg/ml even though the cells did not show cytotoxicity at this concentration as reported earlier in Fig. 3a. However, based on the apoptosis results in Fig. 4a, the percentage of apoptotic cells were 28.6% at this concentration and thus could have contributed to the higher ROS production in the PTE pre-treated cells. The

higher ROS production at this concentration could also be due to the presence of certain polyphenols and antioxidants that is present in PTE which could have undergone redox recycling and thus produced more $H_2O_2$ which contribute to higher ROS [29–31]. Some compounds such as L-Dopa, dopamine, epigallocatechin, catechin, quercetin and epigallocatechin gallate can react with many cell culture medium and generate $H_2O_2$ [29, 32–34]. In fact, the results correlate with the higher caspase 3 activity at 250 μg/ml PTE pre-treated cells as shown earlier in Fig. 5.

$H_2O_2$ induced oxidative stress in cells regulates many intracellular signaling pathway and among them are the MAPKs which consist of the extra cellular signal regulated kinase (ERK1/2), stress activated p38 and JNK. $H_2O_2$ normally stimulates the activation of MAPKs via phosphorylation and thus regulate the intracellular signaling pathway, which results either in cell survival or cell death [35]. However, in this work, $H_2O_2$ treated dIMR32 cells had lower level of phospho p-38, ERK1/2 and JNK (Fig. 8 d, e and f) as compared to untreated cells. This is because MAPKs are activated during neuronal differentiation process of cells [36, 37]. ERK1/2 or p44/42 is usually activated during cell growth, cell differentiation, cell survival, and motility. ERKs are highly expressed in post-mitotic neurons and in differentiated cells and involved in adaptive responses such as long-term potentiation in post mitotic neurons and in regulating synaptic plasticity of the hippocampus [38–40]. Thus, activation of the ERK1/2 can either lead to proliferation or differentiation of cells subjected to the strength and duration of the stimulation [41, 42]. On the other hand, p38 is phosphorylated during inflammation, cell cycle, cell death, development, cell differentiation, senescence, and tumorigenesis. JNK is also activated during many cellular events, such as growth control, transformation, and apoptosis [43–45].

Our results showed (Fig. 8d, e and f) that PTE pre-treatment prior to inducing oxidative stress with $H_2O_2$, completely inhibited the activation or phosphorylation of p-38 as compared to the $H_2O_2$ treated cells. It also attenuated the phosphorylation of ERK1/2 and showed a decreasing trend of phospho-JNK, even though it was not statistically significant. The p-38 and JNK are stress activated MAPKs and they also regulate stress induced apoptosis [46]. On the contrary, ERK1/2 is a MAPKs that is generally activated for survival of cells. Nevertheless, it is also activated in some neuronal cells under $H_2O_2$ induced oxidative stress [47]. The effect of ERK1/2 activation on the pro-survival or pro-apoptotic roles in the cells depends on the kinetics, duration, stimulus and cell type [42, 48, 49].

Oxidative stress induced by $H_2O_2$ activates the phosphorylation of ERK1/2 signaling protein in many neuronal studies that leads to apoptosis of the cells. In primary cortical cells, $H_2O_2$ was reported to have activated both ERK1/2 and p-38 MAP kinase signaling protein in a concentration and time dependent manner [49]. Studies on plant bioactives such as kukoamine B and loganin in human neuroblastoma ShSy5y cells, have been reported to provide neuroprotection against $H_2O_2$ induced oxidative stress via attenuation of phospho-ERK1/2 [50, 51]. Some earlier studies in differentiated and undifferentiated Shsy5y cells have shown that treatment with $H_2O_2$ increased the phosphorylation of ERK1/2 in a time and concentration dependent manner (up to 1.25 mM $H_2O_2$) where it increased as the concentration of $H_2O_2$. This activation of ERK1/2 leads to the neuronal cell death via apoptosis [52]. In concordance to that, our study demonstrated that PTE pre-treatment prior to $H_2O_2$ injury to cells protected the dIMR32 cells by attenuating the activation of ERK1/2.

## Conclusion

In this study, it was established that the ethanolic extract of *Peltophorum pterocarpum* (PTE) did not exhibit cytotoxicity towards neuronally differentiated IMR32 cells (dIMR32) and only induced minimal apoptosis in the cells. PTE also exhibited neuroprotection in dIMR32 cells by ameliorating oxidative stress and apoptosis induced by $H_2O_2$ in a dose-dependent manner. This neuroprotection was achieved by increasing the mitochondrial membrane potential (MMP) and by attenuating the production of ROS in a dose dependent manner. However, PTE failed to reduce the caspase 3 activity suggesting caspase independent neuroprotection by PTE. Studies on the MAPKs pathway revealed that PTE was protective in dIMR32 cells by inhibiting the activation of stress activated p38 and by attenuating the phosphorylation of ERK1/2 and showed a decreasing trend in the activation of JNK. The results suggest that PTE can be further explored as an alternative preventive therapeutics for neurodegenerative diseases.

## Abbreviations

5BrdU: 5-bromodeoxyuridine; ChAT: Choline acetyltransferase; DCFDA: 2',7'-dichlorodihydrofluorescein diacetate; dIMR32: Differentiated neuroblastoma IMR32 cells; ERK: Extracellular signal-regulated kinase; $H_2O_2$: Hydrogen peroxide; ICC: Immunocytochemistry; JC1: Tetraethylbenzimidazolylcarbocyanine iodide; JNK: c-Jun N-terminal kinases; MAPK: Mitogen activated protein kinases; MMP: Mitochondrial membrane potential; MTT: 3-(4,5-dimethylthiazol-2-yl)-2,5-diphenyltetrazolium bromide; PTE: Ethanolic extract of *Peltophorum pterocarpum* leaf; ROS: Reactive oxygen species

## Acknowledgments

The authors gratefully acknowledge the Ministry of Science and Technology Innovation (MOSTI) Malaysia for the research grant (No: 02-03-02-SF0130). The authors also wish to thank Dr. Yeap Swee Keong in assisting in the use of the Flow Cytometry.

**Authors' contributions**

TM proposed the ideas, planned the experimental methods, carried out the cell based assays, analyzed the data and wrote the manuscript, TM and TS also collected the samples and carried out the extraction process and the HPLC analysis. NN and RR also contributed to the idea conception, reviewed the manuscript and gave approval for the manuscript. All authors read and approved the final manuscript.

**Competing interests**

The authors declare that they have no competing interests.

**Author details**

[1]SIRIM Bhd, Industrial Biotechnology Research Centre (IBRC), No 1, Persiaran Dato Menteri Seksyen 2, 40700 Shah Alam, Selangor, Malaysia. [2]Genetics & Regenerative Medicine Research Centre, Faculty of Medicine & Health Sciences, Universiti Putra Malaysia, 43400 Serdang, Selangor, Malaysia. [3]MAKNA-Cancer Research Laboratory, Institute Bioscience (IBS), Universiti Putra Malaysia, 43400 Serdang, Selangor, Malaysia.

**References**

1. Uttara B, Singh AV, Zamboni P, Mahajan RT. Oxidative stress and neurodegenerative diseases: a review of upstream and downstream antioxidant therapeutic options. Curr Neuropharmacol. 2009;7(1):65–74.
2. Halliwell B, Gutteridge J. Cellular response to oxidative stress: adaptation, damage, repair, senescence and death. In: Free radical in biology and medicine. 4th ed. Oxford: Oxford University Press; 2007. p. 187–267.
3. Yang F, Lim GP, Begum AN, Ubeda OJ, Simmons MR, Ambeguokar SS, Chen P, Kajed R, Glabe CG, Frautschy SA, Cole GM. Curcumin inhibits formation of amyloid beta oligomers and fibrils, binds plaques, and reduces amyloid *in vivo*. J Biol Chem. 2005;280(7):5892–901.
4. Ye J, Zhang Y. Curcumin protects against intracellular amyloid toxicity in rat primary neurons. Int J Clin Exp Med. 2012;5(1):44–9.
5. Damar U, Gersner R, Johnstone JT, Schachter S, Rotenberg A. Huperzine A as a neuroprotective and antiepileptic drug: a review of preclinical research. Expert Rev Neurother. 2016;16(6):671–80.
6. Shi C, Liu J, Wu F, Yew DT. Ginkgo biloba extract in Alzheimer's disease: from action mechanisms to medical practice. Int J Mol Sci. 2010;11(1):107–23.
7. Biswas K, Kumar A, Babaria BA, Prabhu K, Setty SR. Hepatoprotective effect of leaves of *Peltophorum pterocarpum* against paracetamol Induced acute liver damage in rats. J Basic Clin Pharm. 2009;1(1):10–5.
8. Sridharamurthy NB, Ashok B, Yogananda R. Evaluation of Antioxidant and Acetyl Cholinesterase inhibitory activity of *Peltophorum pterocarpum* in Scopolamine treated rats. Int J Drug Dev Res. 2012;4(3):115–27.
9. Manaharan T, Teng LL, Appleton D, Ming CH, Masilamani T, Palanisamy UD. Antioxidant and antiglycemic potential of *Peltophorum pterocarpum* plant parts. Food Chem. 2011;129(4):1355–61.
10. Borutaite V, Brown GC. Caspases are reversibly inactivated by hydrogen peroxide. FEBS Lett. 2001;500(3):114–8.
11. Polster BM, Fiskum G. Mitochondrial mechanisms of neural cell apoptosis. J Neurochem. 2004;90(6):1281–9.
12. Ono K, Han J. The p38 signal transduction pathway: activation and function. Cell Signal. 2000;12:1–13.
13. Strauss WL, Kemper RR, Jayakar P, Kong CF, Hersh LB, Hilt DC, Rabin M. Human choline acetyltransferase gene maps to region 10q11-q22.2 by in situ hybridization. Genomics. 1991;9(2):396–8.
14. Resende RR, Adhikari AA. Cholinergic receptor pathways involved in apoptosis, cell proliferation and neuronal differentiation. Cell Commun Signal. 2009;7:20.
15. Jash SK, Singh RK, Majhi S, Sarkar A, Gorai D. *Peltophorum pterocarpum*: chemical and pharmacological aspects. Int J Pharm Sci Res. 2014;5(1):26–36.
16. Whittermore ER, Loo DT, Watt JA, Cotman CW. Peroxide-induced cell death in primary neuronal culture. Neuroscience. 1995;67(4):921–32.
17. Gulden M, Jess A, Kammann J, Maser E& Seibert H. Cytotoxic potency of $H_2O_2$ in cell cultures: Impact of cell concentration and exposure time. Free Radic Biol Med. 2010;49(8):1298–305.
18. Vermes I, Haanen C, Nakken HS, Reutelingserger C. A novel assay for apoptosis flow cytometric detection of phosphatidylserine expression on

early apoptotic cells using fluorescein labelled Annexin V. J Immunol Methods. 1995;184(95):39–51.

19. Shaykhalishahi H, Yazdanparast R, Ha HH, Chang YT. Inhibition of $H_2O_2$-induced neuroblastoma cell cytotoxicity by a triazine derivative, AA3E2. Eur J Pharmacol. 2009;622(1-3):1–6.

20. Wang XY, He PY, Du J, Zhang JZ. Quercetin in combating $H_2O_2$ induced early cell apoptosis and mitochondrial damage to normal human keratinocytes. Chin Med J. 2010;123(5):532–6.

21. Jiang B, Liu JH, Bao Y, An LJ. Hydrogen peroxide-induced apoptosis in PC12 cells and the protective effect of puerarin. Cell Biol Int. 2003;27(12):1025–31.

22. Sanchana M, Flaskas J, Hargreaves AJ. In vitro biomarkers of developmental neurotoxicity. In: Gupta RC, editors. Reproductive and Developmental Toxicology. 1st ed. Elsevier; 2011: Chapter 19, 227–252.

23. Sattayasai J, Chaonapan P, Arkaravichie T, Saimpornkul R, Junnu S, Charoensilp P, Samar J, Jantaravinid J, Masaratara P, Suktitipat B, Manissorn J, Thongboonkerd V, Neungtom N, Moongkarndi P. Protective effects of mangosteen extract on $H_2O_2$-induced cytotoxicity in SK-N-SH cells and scopolamine-induced memory impairment in mice. PLoS One. 2013;8(12), e85053: 1–13.

24. Son YO, Jang YS, Heo JS, Chang WT, Choi KC Lee JC. Apoptosis inducing factor plays a critical role in caspase independent, pyknotic cell death in hydrogen peroxide exposed cells. Apoptosis. 2009;14:796–808.

25. Hampton MB, Orrenius S. Dual regulation of caspase activity by hydrogen peroxide: Implications for apoptosis. FEBS Lett. 1997;414(3):552–6.

26. Kim DK, Cho ES, Um HD. Caspase-dependent and -independent events in apoptosis induced by hydrogen peroxide. Exp Cell Res. 2000;257(1):82–8.

27. Ly JD, Grubb D, Lawen A. The mitochondrial membrane potential (DYm) in apoptosis; an update. Apoptosis. 2003;8:115–28.

28. Armenta MM, Ruiz CN, Rebollar DJ, Martinez E, Gomex PY. Oxidative stress associated with neuronal apoptosis in experimental models of epilepsy. Oxidative Med Cell Longev. 2014;2014:1–12.

29. Halliwell B, Clement MV, Ramalingam J, Long LH. Hydrogen peroxide. Ubiquitous in cell culture and in vivo? IUBMB Life. 2000;50(4-5):251–7.

30. Babich H, Liebling EJ, Burger RF, Zuckerbraun HL, Schuck AG. Choice of DMEM, formulated with or without pyruvate, plays an important role in assessing the in vitro cytotoxicity of oxidants and prooxidant nutraceuticals. In Vitro Cell Dev Biol Anim. 2009;45(5-6):226–33.

31. Kelts JL, Cali JJ, Duellman SJ, Shultz J. Altered cytotoxicity of ROS-inducing compounds by sodium pyruvate in cell culture medium depends on the location of ROS generation. Spring. 2015;4:269.

32. Long LH, Clement MV, Halliwell B. Artifacts in cell culture: rapid generation of hydrogen peroxide on addition of (−)-epigallocatechin, (−)-epigallocatechin gallate, (+)-catechin, and quercetin to commonly used cell culture media. Biochem Biophys Res Commun. 2000;273(1):50–3.

33. Halliwell B. Are polyphenols antioxidants or pro-oxidants? What do we learn from cell culture and in vivo studies? Arch Biochem Biophys. 2008;476(2):107–12.

34. Long LH, Halliwell B. The effects of oxaloacetate on hydrogen peroxide generation from ascorbate and epigallocatechin gallate in cell culture media: Potential for altering cell metabolism. Biochem Biophys Res Commun. 2011;406(1):20–4.

35. Chen L, Liu L, Yin J, Luo Y, Huang S. Hydrogen peroxide-induced neuronal apoptosis is associated with inhibition of protein phosphatase 2A and 5, leading to activation of MAPK pathway. Int J Biochem Cell Biol. 2009;41:1284–95.

36. Li Z, Theus MH, Wei L. Role of ERK 1/2 signaling in neuronal differentiation of cultured embryonic stem cells. Develop Growth Differ. 2006;48(8):513–23.

37. Sun Y, Liu W, Liu T, Feng X, Yang N, Zhou HF. Signaling pathway of MAPK / ERK in cell proliferation, differentiation, migration, senescence and apoptosis. J Recept Signal Transduct. 2015;9893(February):1–5.

38. English JD, Sweatt JD. Activation of p42 Mitogen- activated Protein Kinase in Hippocampal Long Term Potentiation. J Biol Chem. 1996;271(October 4):24329–32.

39. Pearson G, Robinson F, Gibson TB, Xu BE, Karandikar M, Berman K, Cobb M. Mitogen-Activated Protein (MAP) Kinase Pathways: Regulation and Physiological Functions. Endocr Rev. 2001;22(2):153–83. doi:10.1210/er.22.2.153.

40. Sweatt JD. The neuronal MAP kinase cascade: a biochemical signal integration system subserving synaptic plasticity and memory. J Neurochem. 2001;76(1):1–10.

41. Marshall C. Specificity of receptor tyrosine kinase signaling: transient versus sustained extracellular signal-regulated kinase activation. Cell. 1995;80(2):179–85.

42. Glotin AL, Calipel A, Brossas JY, Faussat AM, Tréton J, Mascarelli F. Sustained versus transient ERK1/2 signaling underlies the anti- and proapoptotic effects of oxidative stress in human RPE cells. Investig Ophthalmol Vis Sci. 2006;47(10):4614–23.

43. Spencer JPE. The interactions of flavonoids within neuronal signalling pathways. Genes Nutr. 2007;2(3):257–73.

44. Vauzour D, Vafeiadou K, Rodriguez-Mateos A, Rendeiro C, Spencer JPE. The neuroprotective potential of flavonoids: a multiplicity of effects. Genes Nutr. 2008;3(3-4):115–26.

45. Mansuri ML, Parihar P, Solanki I, Parihar MS. Flavonoids in modulation of cell survival signalling pathways. Genes Nutr. 2014;9(3):400.

46. Takeda K, Ichijo H. Neuronal p38 MAPK signalling: An emerging regulator of cell fate and function in the nervous system. Genes Cells. 2002;7(11):1099–111.

47. Crossthwaite AJ, Hasan S, William R. Hydrogen peroxide-mediated phosphorylation of ERK1/2, AKt/PKB and JNK in cortical neurones: Dependence on $Ca^{2+}$ and PI3-kinase. J Neurochem. 2002;80(1):24–35.

48. Luo Y, DeFranco DB. Opposing roles for ERK1/2 in neuronal oxidative toxicity: Distinct mechanisms of ERK1/2 action at early versus late phases of oxidative stress. J Biol Chem. 2006;281:16436–42.

49. Odaka H, Numakawa T, Adachi N, Ooshima Y, Nakajima S, Katanuma Y, Inoue T, Kanugi H. Cabergoline, dopamine D2 receptor agonist, prevents neuronal cell death under oxidative stress via reducing excitotoxicity. PLoS One. 2014;9(6):1–11.

50. Kwon SH, Kim JA, Hong SI, Jung YH, Kim HC, Lee SY, Jang CG. Loganin protects against hydrogen peroxide-induced apoptosis by inhibiting phosphorylation of JNK, p38, and ERK 1/2 MAPKs in SH-SY5Y cells. Neurochem Int. 2011;58(4):533–41.

51. Hu XL, Niu YX, Zhang Q, Tian X, Gao LY, Guo LP, Meng WH, Zhao QC. Neuroprotective effects of Kukoamine B against hydrogen peroxide-induced apoptosis and potential mechanisms in SH-SY5Y cells. Environ Toxicol Pharmacol. 2015;40(1):230–40.

52. Ruffels J, Griffin M, Dickenson JM. Activation of ERK1/2, JNK and PKB by hydrogen peroxide in human SH-SY5Y neuroblastoma cells: role of ERK1/2 in $H_2O_2$-induced cell death. Eur J Pharmacol. 2004;483(2-3):163–73.

# 13

# The effect of black tea on human cognitive performance in a cognitive test battery

Ashfique Rizwan[1], Artyom Zinchenko[2], Ceyona Özdem[3], Md. Sohel Rana[1] and Md. Mamun Al-Amin[4*]

## Abstract

**Background:** Black Tea is a widely consumed drink in the world. Evidence suggest Black Tea has stimulatory effect on humans. We investigated the effect of Black Tea on cognition using a cognitive test battery.

**Methods:** Participants ($n = 32$) were fasted overnight for 10 h and restrained from caffeine and other stimulant drugs for 14 days prior to participation. We randomly assigned participants into either an experimental ($n = 16$) or a control ($n = 16$) group. Experimental group consumed 250 ml of Black Tea (BT) while control group was received equal volume of water (W). Participants were tested on the following cognitive tasks: executive function, sustained attention, memory (memory span, immediate, delayed, working memory) and arithmetic calculation task.

**Results:** We found that BT group performed significantly ($p < 0.05$) faster in the executive function task (BT: M = 1671, SD = 319; W: M = 1935, SD = 372); simple reaction time task (BT: M = 333, SD = 87; W: M = 361, SD = 101), identification of target location in the visual search task (BT: M = 925, SD = 50; W: M = 972, SD = 115). We also showed that BT group forgotten significantly ($p < 0.05$) lower number of words in the delayed memory recall test (BT: M = 1.12, SD = 0.15; W: M = 1.37, SD = 0.33) and made significantly ($p < 0.05$) fewer errors in the trail making task (BT: M = 0.31, SD = 1.01; W: M = 1.31, SD = 1.66).

**Conclusions:** BT consumption speeded the performance, improved memory, reduced number of errors in the various cognitive tasks. Our results further showed that even in small volume of BT consumption can speed up cognitive processing.

**Keywords:** Attention, Memory, Reaction time, Cognition, Visual search

## Background

Tea is the second most extensively consumed beverages on the planet [1]. The popularity of tea could possibly be explained by its pharmacological action. For instance, the component of tea such as caffeine increases cortisol level in response to stress [2]. Drinking tea produced stimulation which further helps to overcome psychosocial stress [3], enhances cognitive performance [4] and improves attention [5]. Tea contains phenolic compounds that facilitates synaptic plasticity [6]. The principle constituents of black tea are caffeine and L-theanine. The amount of caffeine and L-theanine in one cup of tea varies. It is estimated that, 200 ml of black tea contain 35–61 mg of caffeine and 4.5–22.5 mg of L-

theanine. Caffeine is quickly absorbed (30–40 min, half-life = 3 to 6 h) [7]. Importantly, the effect of caffeine on cognitive function is not limited to a particular type of tea [8].

Previous studies investigated the effects of caffeine and L-theanine on human cognitive performances and behavior. The effect of caffeine and L-theanine on cognition are summarized in Table 1. Higher consumption of tea is associated with a lower risk of cognitive impairment [9]. In elderly people (>60 years old), Black tea consumption improves cognitive performances [10]. Importantly, caffeine improves sustained attention [5], mood and reduces fatigue [11–13], improves motor-skill performance in tasks such as a simulated driving task [14] and improves handwriting [15]. Caffeine at a dose of 200–250 mg improves attention in visual search task [16]. Functional magnetic resonance imaging (fMRI) study reported that caffeine alters neuronal activity in

* Correspondence: mamun.al-amin@northsouth.edu;
bd_pharmacy@yahoo.com; mdalaminbadal@gmail.com
[4]Department of Pharmaceutical Sciences, North South University, Plot-15, Block-B, Bashundhara, Dhaka 1229, Bangladesh
Full list of author information is available at the end of the article

**Table 1** Summary of published findings on the effect of Black Tea on cognitive process

| Study | Dose | Task type | Positive effect | Negative or No effect |
|---|---|---|---|---|
| Caffeine, ERP study [29] | 250 mg | Auditory Go/NoGo | Global increases in P1, P2 and P3b amplitudes to Go stimuli | N1 or N2 (Go stimuli), any components (NoGo stimuli) |
| Caffeine, ERP study [16] | 3 mg/kg | Visual search | Subjects reacted faster | Negative ERP deflection was unaffected |
| Caffeine [20] | 400 mg | Visual search, Simple choice reaction time | Positive effect depends on the level of caffeine use. | |
| Green tea [9] | 1 cup to 6 cups | Mini-Mental State Examination | Higher consumption is associated with a lower prevalence of cognitive impairment | |
| Breakfast cereal and caffeinated coffee [22] | | Working memory, attention and mood | | No effect on initial mood or working memory capacity |
| Caffeine [21] | | Visual information processing | | Does not affect cognition, learning & memory performance |
| Breakfast and caffeine [50] | 4 mg/kg | Free recall and recognition memory and semantic memory | | Impaired accuracy |
| Glucose & caffeine, fMRI study [53] | Glucose (75 g) + Caffeine (75 g) | Sustained attention | Increase the efficiency of the attentional system | |
| Caffeine [25] | 4 mg/kg | Delayed memory, metamemory and sustained attention | | Not affect the magnitude or accuracy of memory predictions |
| Caffeine, fMRI study [54] | 100 mg | WM maintenance task | | Detrimental effect on WM at higher levels of WM load |
| Caffeine, fMRI study[17] | 250 or 500 ml | WM | Alters brain activity in DLPFC area | |
| Caffeine [55] | 200 mg | 'N-Back' WM paradigm | Heightened WM performance | |
| Caffeine, Review paper [56] | | | | Does not improve learning and memory |
| L-theanine, caffeine [26] | L-theanine (250 mg) + caffeine (150 mg) | Simple reaction time, Numeric WM RT and sentence verification | Faster reaction time and improved sentence verification accuracy | |
| L-theanine, caffeine [28] | L-theanine (100 mg) | Target discrimination | Increase in hit rate and target discriminability (d') for the combined treatment | No effects were detected for l-theanine alone |
| L-theanine [27] | 200 mg + 100 ml water | Attention test | Improves attention and reaction time response | |

the DLPFC (dorsolateral Pre-Frontal Cortex) on working memory task [17]. Caffeine also modulates neuronal activity [18]. Caffeine improves low alertness during long drive [14]. Besides caffeine, Theanine improves attentional performance at a dose of 200 mg/100 ml water [19]. Important to notice, effect of caffeine is shown to be related to the habitual intake levels. It has been reported that higher caffeine consumers are more likely to perceive broadly positive effects of caffeine [20].

Surprisingly, caffeine does not always produces beneficial effects, especially at less than 100 mg dose. Caffeine does not affect cognition and memory performance, learning and initial mood [21, 22], long- and short term memory in a delayed recall verbal memory task [23, 24], and complex short-term memory task performance [4].

**Aim of the study**

We selected Black Tea (BT) since the principle constituent of black tea are two stimulating agents, namely caffeine and L-theanine. It is generally believed that caffeine containing black tea improves human cognitive functioning. However, previous studies reported inconsistent results. These studies used different tasks [25, 26], varied the dosage of caffeine and L-theanine in the tea [26–28], tested participants in different cognitive tasks [8, 20, 29, 30]. Therefore, we aimed to identify the influence of BT consumption on human cognitive functioning, testing the participants in a wide range of cognitive tasks with a low dose that is 50 mg and 15 mg respectively. This small dose have shown no effect on cognitive functioning due to the habitual intake level [20]. In this study, we controlled habitual black tea consumption level of each participants' prior to the experiment (i.e., consumption of tea was completely restricted for 2 weeks prior to experiment). Moreover, previous studies used relatively simple tasks [14, 30–32] (although see [4] for a more complicated task). Therefore, we used relatively complex test procedures such as trail making tests [33], card sorting test [34, 35], calculation tasks etc.

We hypothesized that BT at a low dose [caffeine (50 mg) and plus L-theanine (15 mg)] would enhance cognitive performance. This enhancement could be due to the faster bioavailablity of caffeine to the brain which is 40 min following drinking [36]. Although cerebral blood circulation may affect cognitive performance, affecting several brain regions at the same time. Therefore, the consumption of BT was expected to influence cognitive processes during the series of behavioural tasks in the cognitive test battery (PEBL) [37].

## Methods
### Participants
Thirty two healthy volunteers (12 female; mean age = 21) took part in this study. Participants were recruited and controlled for the level of IQ measured by the National Adult Reading Test (mean IQ = 110.62); [38] and were naive to the purpose of experiment. Participants fasted for 10 h overnight and restrained themselves from consumption of tea, caffeine or other stimulant drinks and drugs for 14 days prior to participation in the experiment. All participants had normal or corrected to normal vision.

### Procedure
Participants were instructed to sleep at least 8 h overnight and came at 6.30 AM to the test center (Department of Pharmacy, Jahangirnagar University, Savar, Dhaka, Bangladesh). Participants were divided into two groups; (i) experimental group consumed 250 ml of Black Tea (BT) 40 min before testing, assuming caffeine at a dose of 50 mg plus L-theanine at a dose of 15 mg while (ii) control group consumed 250 ml of water (i.e., drinking water; not boiled or distilled). Subjects were randomized to participate in this experiment. A person blind to the purpose of the experiment was involved in assigning subjects for each condition. Before starting the cognitive test battery, participants were shown the procedures for attending the battery of test by a projector as a training phase.

### Preparation of drink
BT was purchased from Kazi and Kazi tea, Dhaka, Bangladesh and added to 250 ml of drinking water.

### Immediate recall memory test
A list of 10 words was presented to the subjects at a rate of one every 2 second. At the end of the presentation, subjects were given 1 min to write down as many words as possible.

### Delayed recall memory test
At the end of the test session (average 90 min test session) subjects were given 1 min to recall as many words as possible from the list shown at the beginning of the study. The number of words forgotten was calculated by subtracting number of words reproduced correctly from the total number of words presented to participants. The difference between numbers of words remembered in the learning trial versus the delayed recall was obtained as an estimation of forgetting.

### Trail making test A and B
Participants were asked to connect circles in a specified sequence using pencil to draw lines as rapidly as possible. Condition A involved sequence for connecting the circles in a numeric sequence. Condition B involved circles with alternating numeric and alphabetic sequences.

The psychology experiment building language (PEBL) Version 0.13 [37] was used to test the performance of Visual search, Berger's card sorting test, Memory span, Sustained attention and Arithmetic calculation.

### Visual search task
Participants were asked to find the target (odd colored "X" or "O") in a randomly displayed stimulus in the screen. In some trials the target was present and in other trials it was absent. Participants responded with left click of the mouse button. Following the mouse click, the targets were replaced by a mask. Participants were instructed to 'click' on the location of the target. If the target was absent on the screen, following the mouse click, the instruction was to 'click' on the 'none' button. Each participant completed 180 trials.

### Berg's Card Sorting Test (BCST)
This is a computerized version of wisconsin card sorting test [39, 40]. Each participant had to complete 128 trials. BCST [41] assessed performance in various tasks: cognitive processing speed, concept formation, inhibition capacity and cognitive flexibility.

### Simple reaction time task
Participants were asked to press the space button as quickly as possible every time the red 'dot' was presented on the monitor in 121 trials for the PPVT (PEBL Perceptual Vigilance Task) program of PEBL. The stimuli were presented with an inter-stimulus interval that

varied randomly between 1 and 3.5 seconds. Reaction Times (RTs) were recorded in milliseconds.

### Memory span test

This test was used to measure the ability to remember a sequence of locations. In each of the trials nine blue squares were displayed on the screen and these squares lit up one at a time in different sequences. Participants were required to observe the sequence and memorize the order in which the squares lit up. After each trial, subjects were asked to replicate the sequence by clicking on corresponding squares in the right order.

### Arithmetic calculation test

It was used to examine the ability to solve a number of simple addition and subtraction problems. Participants were asked to determine whether the answer of each arithmetic operation is greater or less than 5. Each testing block is 3 min long. In separate blocks the task of participants was to do one, two and three digit addition/subtraction operations, with equal number of trials in each block. Participants were asked to perform the task as quickly and accurately as possible.

### Apparatus

Stimuli were presented on 15″ CRT (Cathode Ray Tube) screen monitor (SAMSUNG Syncmaster 794MG, made in Malaysia) with a 100 Hz refresh rate placed at a distance of 100 cm from an observer. Responses were gathered with a Logitech optical mouse (Made by Logitech Inc. in China). The whole experiment was programmed in PEBL software run on an Intel ° Core ™ 2 CPU 6700 @ 2.66 Ghz, 2CPUs) computer with Microsoft Windows XP Professional operating system.

### Data analysis

Repeated measures ANOVA was used to check for effects of BT on cognitive performance in visual search and arithmetic calculation tasks. Independent sample t-test was conducted to analyze the results of simple reaction time, BCST, memory span, immediate/delayed recall memory and verbal fluency tests. In independent sample t-test, BT and water were grouping variables and all reaction time and other interval data were dependent variable. Reaction times above 1500 ms (too slow) or below 50 ms (too fast) were excluded during the data analysis of visual search, sustained attention, simple reaction time task. In case of BCST and "mathproc" test the upper cut off value for RT was 300 ms and lowest value was 50 ms since they are complicated task and participants required more time than comparatively other tasks. Moreover mean ± 2S.D. was used to exclude odd data. All analyses were carried out with the SPSS package (version 16.0). The difference was considered

significant when $p$ value was less than 0.05. Data were represented as mean ± SD (Standard Deviation).

## Results

### Demographic information

There was no difference in between control and experimental conditions in terms of age (21.5 ± 1.26 vs 20.88 ± 0.71) and IQ level (106.29 ± 23.34 vs 100.71 ± 31.22) (Table 2).

### Immediate and delayed recall memory test

Independent samples t-test was conducted to compare the average number of words forgotten in the delayed recall test between BT and W group. There was a significant difference ($p < 0.05$) between the BT (M = 1.12, SD = 0.15) and W condition (M = 1.37, SD = 0.33); t(30) = 1.89, $p < 0.05$. Participants in W group forgot more words than BT group (Fig. 1).

### Trail making test A and B

Independent samples t-test revealed no significant difference ($p < 0.01$) between BT and W groups. Mann–Whitney test was used due to the fact that values of standard deviations (SD) were larger than the mean in each of the groups. Error rates in trail making test A were significantly lower in BT (M = 0.31; SD = 1.01) than water (M = 1.31; SD = 1.66). Moreover, participants with BT made less error ($p < 0.01$).

### Visual search task

Independent samples t-test was conducted to compare the Reaction Time for identifying the target between BT and W group. There was no difference in the RT between BT (M = 984, SD = 109) and W (M = 999, SD = 101) groups t(30) = −0.38, $p > 0.05$.

Independent samples t-test was conducted to compare the Reaction Time (RT) for identifying the location of the target between BT and W group. We found a significant difference in the RTs between BT (M = 925, SD = 50) and W (M = 972, SD = 115) condition; t(0.28) = −1.07, $p < 0.05$. Repeated measures ANOVA showed the main effect of stimulus size: a gradual increase in RTs with increase in set size for both groups $F_{(2,14)} = 5.6$, $p < 0.05$ (Fig. 2).

### Berger's card sorting test

We found no difference between the BT (M = 8.81%, SD = 5.74) and W (M = 9.38%, SD = 5.99) groups in the error rates; t(30) = −0.271, $p > 0.5$). In other words, both groups made comparable number of errors in the test. However, there was a difference in RTs. BT group (M = 1671, SD = 319) was faster relative to the W (M = 1935, SD = 372) group; t(30) = −2.155, $p < 0.05$), although participants were not instructed to give a

**Table 2** Demographic data and participant's performance in various cognitive tasks in PEBL test battery

|  |  | Black Tea (BT) | Water (W) | P value |
|---|---|---|---|---|
| Age | Year | 21.5 ± 1.26 | 20.88 ± 0.71 | >0.1 |
| IQ level |  | 106.29 ± 23.34 | 100.71 ± 31.22 | >0.1 |
| Memory Span | Average block | 5.31 ± 0.89 | 4.90 ± 0.84 | >0.1 |
| Immediate Recall Memory Test | No. of words retrieved | 8.06 ± 0.32 | 7.75 ± 0.22 | >0.1 |
| Delayed Recall Memory Test | No. of words retrieved | 7.56 ± 0.93 | 6.50 ± 0.37 | >0.1 |
|  | No. of words failed to recall | 1.12 ± 0.15 | 1.37 ± 0.32 | <0.05 |
| Berger's Card Sorting Test | Persev_error | 8.81 ± 5.74 | 9.38 ± 5.99 | >0.1 |
|  | RT (ms) | 1671 ± 319 | 1935 ± 372 | <0.05 |
| Simple Reaction Time Task to measure Sustained Attention | RT (ms) | 333 ± 2 | 361 ± 2 | <0.05 |
| Visual Search (Target identification) | RT (ms) | 984 ± 32 | 999 ± 37 | >0.1 |
| Visual Search (Target location) | RT (ms) | 925 ± 12 | 972 ± 28 | <0.05 |

Total subjects (n = 32); water (n = 16); Black Tea (n = 16); RT Reaction Time; Data were represented as Mean ± SEM; RTs were shown in millisecond (ms

speeded response. This may suggest that BT consumption could facilitate RTs in BCST task.

### Simple reaction time task

Independent samples t-test was conducted to compare the Reaction Time in the sustained attention task between BT and W group. We found a significant difference in the RT for BT condition (M = 333, SD = 87) and W condition (M = 361, SD = 101); t(30) = −8.43, $p < 0.05$.

### Memory span test

We showed no difference in the memory for BT (M = 5.31, SD = 0.89) and W conditions (M = 4.90, SD = 0.84); t(30) = −1.32, $p > 0.05$ following independent sample t-test analysis.

### Arithmetic calculation test

Repeated measure ANOVA revealed no effect of BT on neither speed nor accuracy of arithmetic calculations task F 2, 14 = 6.4, $p > 0.05$.

### Discussion

We investigated the influence of BT on the performance of a series of cognitive tasks, controlling for the habitual intake level of caffeine, complexity of the task and inter-participant differences in cognition. We used a lower amount of BT since several studies suggeste BT does not influence certain cognitive functions [28], particularly at the dosage of less than 100 mg [22, 23]. We found BT groupe sowed improved performances in a number of

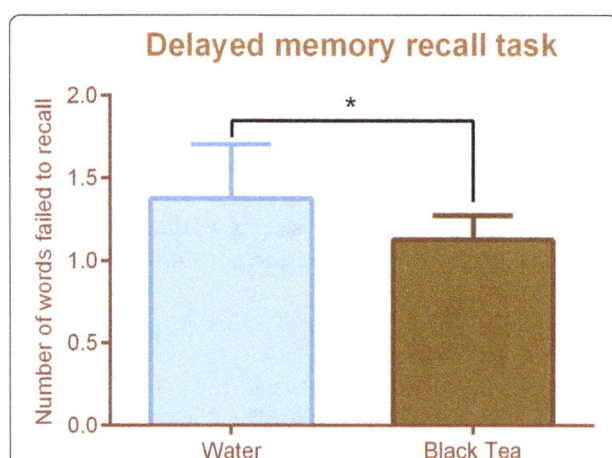

**Fig. 1** Effect of Black Tea (BT) and Water on delayed memory recall task. *Vertical axis* represents number of words failed to recall in the delayed memory recall task while *horizontal axis* represents the treatment groups (water and BT). Data is represented as Mean ± SEM (Standard Error of Mean). * indicates p value less than 0.05

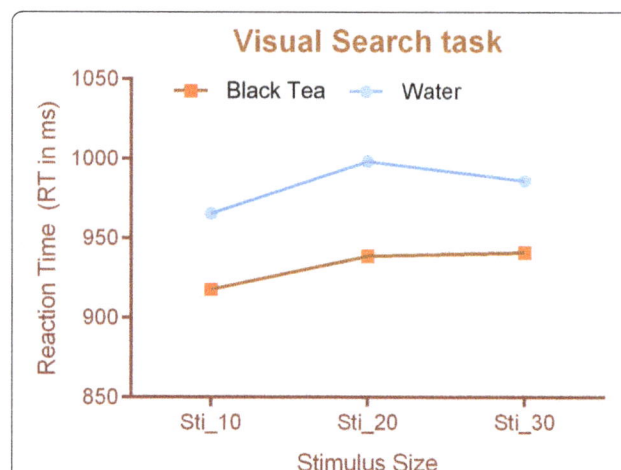

**Fig. 2** Effect of Black Tea (BT) and Water on Visual Search task. *Vertical axis* represents Reaction Time (RT) in millisecond (ms) while represents various stimulus size namely, Sti_10: Stimulus Size 10; Sti_20: Stimulus Size 20; Sti_30: Stimulus Size 30. Data is represented as Mean value

cognitive tasks. In line with previous results, we have also shown facilitation effect of BT on cognition [2].

We showed drinking of BT facilitated cognitive functions in delayed recall memory test. BT group forgotten fewer words. It is presumable that drinking of BT accelerates the consolidation [36] and retrieval of memory. The memory traces could be stabilized during the experimental sessions which helped BT consumers to retrieve the words [42]. A revious study [17] suggest that caffeine alters neuronal activity in the DLPFC (dorsolateral Pre-Frontal Cortex) during performance on a working memory task [38]. Additionally, our study showed that this effect might already had at caffeine dose of less than 70 mg.

Further, BT consumers were more accurate in performing trail making test A. Trial making is a complex task that requires sustained attention, alertness, speeded motor activity to be activated at the same time. Previous studies showed a positive effect of caffeine on sustained attention [36] alertness [25] and motor activity [43] separately. Trail making test confirms our hypothesis that a merging of facilitation events might produce a combinatory effect on cognitive processing.

Another important finding of the present study is that BT consumers were faster in identifying target location in the visual search task. This effect is only possible when a combination of higher level cognition (e.g., attention, alertness, short term memory) is involved in the task. Identifying an object in their location is a hippocampal-dependent task. It is possible that BT consumers had learned better in this spatial learning task. This finding goes in line with the caffeine related improved performance in the *Berg's Card Sorting Test* (BCST) and simple reaction time tasks and supports previous findings that showed caffeine induced facilitation of attention [32, 44] and level of alertness [13, 45]. It is also consistent with other previous studies [2, 16, 19, 38] that linked consumption of tea to robust increases in alertness and information processing capacity [4]. As cholinergic mechanisms have been shown to be a necessary condition for memory formation in rats [46], we hypothesize that BT might also be able to influence the level of cholinergic mechanisms in humans, thus improving memory formation [46].

Caffeine facilitation in visual search task raises an important issue for the cognitive psychology research that greatly relies on reaction time (RT) data in visual search tasks. Since caffeine and L-theanine in tea are a regularly consumed drink by the students, it might influence behavioral results in cognitive experiments. Therefore, it could be recommended to additionally measure the level of caffeine consumption among participants of various RT experiments and use it as an additional factor during the statistical analysis.

Visual search task is an established neuropsychological tool for testing the iconic memory [47, 48]. It measures two parameters: the reaction time (RT) necessary to either detect or determine spatial location of the target. Both groups (i.e., BT and W) performed equally well in the first task – target detection. However, BT group showed facilitated identification of target location, relative to the control group. To our knowledge, we first report that BT is able to improve iconic memory. There are several non-exclusive explanations of this effect. Possibly, caffeine is able to facilitate attention allocation that is necessary to locate a target [49]. On the other hand, caffeine could facilitate the decision making stage of visual search, which allowed BT participants to perform faster [20, 50]. Additionally, overall stimulant effect of caffeine could possibly enhance motor processes that cause the improved performance [43]. This latter point is, however, less likely since previous studies showed no effect of caffeine on human motor functioning [51]; although see [14] for a different view. Further Electroencephalographic (EEG) experiment would be necessary to identify the stage of visual processing that is influenced by caffeine: attention allocation i.e., N2PC (N200 component of posterior contralateral) [52].

Arithmetic calculation task (ACT), memory span and iconic memory (target location identification) were for the first time tested in this experiment. We showed that BT does not affect arithmetic calculation and memory span, but enhances iconic memory.

Our study has several limitations. First, the number of participants was ($n = 16$ in each groups) relatively smaller and we used a lower volume of BT. Additionally, we measured only behavioral performance. Therefore, future studies should test larger groups of participants as well as employ Event Related Potential (ERP) methodology.

## Conclusions

Tea is one of the most popular drinks because of having two stimulants, caffeine and l-theanine. Caffeine increases the level of alertness and improves cognitive functions. Previous studies showed that consumption of caffeine is able to facilitate certain cognitive processes (e.g., short term memory, simple RTs etc.). In our present study, we tested the influence of black tea on human cognitive performance in a battery of cognitive tests. We showed that BT improved the speed of attention allocation, speeded visual search and increased level of alertness. However, additional studies are required in order to identify specific stages of visual processing that are being influence by BT consumption as well as long term BT effects on human cognitive functioning.

## Abbreviations
BCST: Berg's Card Sorting Test; BT: Black Tea; PEBL: Psychology experiment building language (PEBL)

## Acknowledgements
We would like to acknowledge the contribution of the LNPR (Laboratory of Natural Product Research) team, Jahangirnagar University, Dhaka, Bangladesh. We would like to give them special thanks for providing all sorts of supports towards this study.

## Authors' contributions
AR and MMAA designed the study. AR collected the data. AR, AZ, CO and MMAA analyzed the data. MMAA and AR prepared the manuscript. AZ and MSR revised the manuscript. All authors read and approved the final manuscript.

## Competing interests
The authors declare that they have no competing interests.

## Author details
[1]Department of Pharmacy, Jahangirnagar University, Savar, Dhaka 1342, Bangladesh. [2]Max Planck Institute for Human Cognitive and Brain Sciences, Stephanstraße 1A, 04103 Leipzig, Germany. [3]Department of Psychology, Vrije Universiteit Brussel, Pleinlaan 2, B - 1050 Brussel, Belgium. [4]Department of Pharmaceutical Sciences, North South University, Plot-15, Block-B, Bashundhara, Dhaka 1229, Bangladesh.

## References
1. Matthews CM. Steep your genes in health: drink tea. Proc (Baylor Univ Med Cent). 2010;23(2):142–4.
2. Lovallo WR, Farag NH, Vincent AS, Thomas TL, Wilson MF. Cortisol responses to mental stress, exercise, and meals following caffeine intake in men and women. Pharmacol Biochem Behav. 2006;83(3):441–7.
3. Unno K, Iguchi K, Tanida N, Fujitani K, Takamori N, Yamamoto H, et al. Ingestion of theanine, an amino acid in tea, suppresses psychosocial stress in mice. Exp Physiol. 2013;98(1):290–303.
4. Hindmarch I, Quinlan PT, Moore KL, Parkin C. The effects of black tea and other beverages on aspects of cognition and psychomotor performance. Psychopharmacology. 1998;139(3):230–8.
5. Smith AP, Rusted JM, Eaton-Williams P, Savory M, Leathwood P. Effects of caffeine given before and after lunch on sustained attention. Neuropsychobiology. 1990;23(3):160–3.
6. Gomez-Pinilla F, Nguyen TTJ. Natural mood foods: the actions of polyphenols against psychiatric and cognitive disorders. Nutr Neurosci. 2012;15(3):127–33.
7. Rogers PJ. Caffeine, mood and mental performance in everyday life. Nutr Bull. 2007;32:84–9.
8. Feng L, Gwee X, Kua EH, Ng TP. Cognitive function and tea consumption in community dwelling older Chinese in Singapore. J Nutr Health Aging. 2010;14(6):433–8.
9. Kuriyama S, Hozawa A, Ohmori K, Shimazu T, Matsui T, Ebihara S, et al. Green tea consumption and cognitive function: a cross-sectional study from the Tsurugaya Project 1. Am J Clin Nutr. 2006;83(2):355–61.
10. Shen W, Xiao Y, Ying X, Li S, Zhai Y, Shang X, et al. Tea consumption and cognitive impairment: a cross-sectional study among Chinese elderly. PLoS ONE. 2015;10(9):e0137781.
11. Winston AP, Hardwick E, Jaberi N. Neuropsychiatric effects of caffeine. Adv Psychiatr Treat. 2005;11(6):432–9.
12. Rogers PJ, Dernoncourt C. Regular caffeine consumption: a balance of adverse and beneficial effects for mood and psychomotor performance. Pharmacol Biochem Behav. 1998;59(4):1039–45.
13. Smith A. Effects of caffeine on human behavior. Food Chem Toxicol. 2002;40(9):1243–55.
14. Brice C, Smith A. The effects of caffeine on simulated driving, subjective alertness and sustained attention. Hum Psychopharmacol. 2001;16(7):523–31.
15. Tucha O, Walitza S, Mecklinger L, Stasik D, Sontag TA, Lange KW. The effect of caffeine on handwriting movements in skilled writers. Hum Mov Sci. 2006;25(4–5):523–35.
16. Lorist MM, Snel J, Kok A, Mulder G. Acute effects of caffeine on selective attention and visual search processes. Psychophysiology. 1996;33(4):354–61.
17. Borgwardt S, Hammann F, Scheffler K, Kreuter M, Drewe J, Beglinger C. Neural effects of green tea extract on dorsolateral prefrontal cortex. Eur J Clin Nutr. 2012;66(11):1187–92.
18. Koppelstaetter F, Poeppel TD, Siedentopf CM, Ischebeck A, Verius M, Haala I, et al. Does caffeine modulate verbal working memory processes? An fMRI study. NeuroImage. 2008;39(1):492–9.
19. Higashiyama A, Htay HH, Ozeki M, Juneja LR, Kapoor MP. Effects of l-theanine on attention and reaction time response. J Funct Foods. 2011;3(3):171–8.
20. Attwood AS, Higgs S, Terry P. Differential responsiveness to caffeine and perceived effects of caffeine in moderate and high regular caffeine consumers. Psychopharmacology. 2007;190(4):469–77.
21. Loke WH. The effects of caffeine and automaticity on a visual information processing task. Hum Psychopharmacol Clin Exp. 1992;7(6):379–88.
22. Smith AP, Clark R, Gallagher J. Breakfast cereal and caffeinated coffee: effects on working memory, attention, mood, and cardiovascular function. Physiol Behav. 1999;67(1):9–17.
23. Herz RS. Caffeine effects on mood and memory. Behav Res Ther. 1999;37(9):869–79.
24. Warburton DM, Bersellini E, Sweeney E. An evaluation of a caffeinated taurine drink on mood, memory and information processing in healthy volunteers without caffeine abstinence. Psychopharmacology. 2001;158(3):322–8.
25. Kelemen WL, Creeley CE. Caffeine (4 mg/kg) influences sustained attention and delayed free recall but not memory predictions. Hum Psychopharmacol. 2001;16(4):309–19.
26. Haskell CF, Kennedy DO, Milne AL, Wesnes KA, Scholey AB. The effects of l-theanine, caffeine and their combination on cognition and mood. Biol Psychol. 2008;77(2):113–22.
27. Lu K, Gray MA, Oliver C, Liley DT, Harrison BJ, Bartholomeusz CF, et al. The acute effects of L-theanine in comparison with alprazolam on anticipatory anxiety in humans. Hum Psychopharmacol. 2004;19(7):457–65.
28. Kelly SP, Gomez-Ramirez M, Montesi JL, Foxe JJ. L-theanine and caffeine in combination affect human cognition as evidenced by oscillatory alpha-band activity and attention task performance. J Nutr. 2008;138(8):1572S–7.
29. Barry RJ, Johnstone SJ, Clarke AR, Rushby JA, Brown CR, McKenzie DN. Caffeine effects on ERPs and performance in an auditory Go/NoGo task. Clin Neurophysiol. 2007;118(12):2692–9.
30. Steptoe A, Gibson EL, Vuononvirta R, Williams ED, Hamer M, Rycroft JA, et al. The effects of tea on psychophysiological stress responsivity and post-stress recovery: a randomised double-blind trial. Psychopharmacology. 2007;190(1):81–9.
31. Carolyn MM. Steep your genes in health: drink tea. Proc (Bayl Univ Med Cent). 2010;23(2):142–4.
32. Henning SM, Niu Y, Lee NH, Thames GD, Minutti RR, Wang H, et al. Bioavailability and antioxidant activity of tea flavanols after consumption of green tea, black tea, or a green tea extract supplement. Am J Clin Nutr. 2004;80(6):1558–64.
33. Arbuthnott K, Frank J. Trail making test, part B as a measure of executive control: validation using a set-switching paradigm. J Clin Exp Neuropsychol. 2000;22(4):518–28.
34. Koren D, Seidman LJ, Harrison RH, Lyons MJ, Kremen WS, Caplan B, et al. Factor structure of the Wisconsin Card Sorting Test: dimensions of deficit in schizophrenia. Neuropsychology. 1998;12(2):289–302.
35. Gold JM, Carpenter C, Randolph C, Goldberg TE, Weinberger DR. Auditory working memory and Wisconsin Card Sorting Test performance in schizophrenia. Arch Gen Psychiatry. 1997;54(2):159–65.
36. Dixit A, Vaney N, Tandon OP. Evaluation of cognitive brain functions in caffeine users: a P3 evoked potential study. Indian J Physiol Pharmacol. 2006;50(2):175–80.

37. Mueller ST, Piper BJ. The Psychology Experiment Building Language (PEBL) and PEBL test battery. J Neurosci Methods. 2014;222:250–9.
38. Nelson H, Willison J. National Adult Reading Test (NART). nferNelson; 1991. https://egret.psychol.cam.ac.uk/camcops/documentation/tasks/nart.html.
39. Demakis GJ. A meta-analytic review of the sensitivity of the Wisconsin Card Sorting Test to frontal and lateralized frontal brain damage. Neuropsychology. 2003;17(2):255–64.
40. Piper BJ, Li V, Eiwaz MA, Kobel YV, Benice TS, Chu AM, et al. Executive function on the Psychology Experiment Building Language tests. Behav Res Methods. 2012;44(1):110–23.
41. Fox CJ, Mueller ST, Gray HM, Raber J, Piper BJ. Evaluation of a short-form of the Berg Card Sorting Test. PLoS One. 2013;8(5):e63885.
42. Kuchinke L, Lux V. Caffeine improves left hemisphere processing of positive words. PLoS One. 2012;7(11):e48487.
43. Lorist MM, Snel J. Caffeine effects on perceptual and motor processes. Electroencephalogr Clin Neurophysiol. 1997;102(5):401–13.
44. Ruijter J, de Ruiter MB, Snel J, Lorist MM. The influence of caffeine on spatial-selective attention: an event-related potential study. Clin Neurophysiol. 2000;111(12):2223–33.
45. Giesbrecht T, Rycroft JA, Rowson MJ, De Bruin EA. The combination of L-theanine and caffeine improves cognitive performance and increases subjective alertness. Nutr Neurosci. 2010;13(6):283–90.
46. Roussinov KS, Yonkov DI. Cholinergic mechanisms in the learning and memory facilitating effect of caffeine. Acta Physiol Pharmacol Bulg. 1976;2(3):61–8.
47. Persuh M, Genzer B, Melara RD. Iconic memory requires attention. Frontiers in Human Neuroscience. 2012;6:126.
48. Bradley C, Pearson J. The sensory components of high-capacity iconic memory and visual working memory. Front Psychol. 2012;3:355.
49. Gruber RP, Block RA. Effects of caffeine on prospective duration judgements of various intervals depend on task difficulty. Human Psychopharmacol. 2005;20(4):275–85.
50. Smith A, Kendrick A, Maben A, Salmon J. Effects of breakfast and caffeine on cognitive performance, mood and cardiovascular functioning. Appetite. 1994;22(1):39–55.
51. Valladares Lorraine CI, Bedford A. Effects of caffeine on cognitive tasks. 2009.
52. Gajewski PD, Stoerig P, Falkenstein M. ERP—Correlates of response selection in a response conflict paradigm. Brain Res. 2008;1189:127–34.
53. Serra-Grabulosa JM, Adan A, Falcón C, Bargalló N. Glucose and caffeine effects on sustained attention: an exploratory fMRI study. Hum Psychopharmacol Clin Exp. 2010;25(7–8):543–52.
54. Klaassen EB, de Groot RH, Evers EA, Snel J, Veerman EC, Ligtenberg AJ, et al. The effect of caffeine on working memory load-related brain activation in middle-aged males. Neuropharmacology. 2013;64:160–7.
55. Smillie LD, Gökçen E. Caffeine enhances working memory for extraverts. Biol Psychol. 2010;85(3):496–8.
56. Nehlig A. Is caffeine a cognitive enhancer? J Alzheimers Dis. 2010;20 Suppl 1:S85–94.

# 14

# An in vivo study regarding analgesic and anxiolytic activity of methanolic extract of *Typha elephantina* Roxb

Niloy Sen[1]* (iD), Latifa Bulbul[1], Md. Saddam Hussain[1], Sujan Banik[1] and Md. Shahbuddin Kabir Choudhuri[2]

## Abstract

**Background:** *Typha elephantina* Roxb. is a widely scattered grass like medicinal plant in Bangladesh and thus demands biological investigations to discover its therapeutic potentiality. The aim of our present study was to assess analgesic and anxiolytic properties of methanolic extract of *Typha elephantina* Roxb.

**Methods:** For evaluating analgesic activity, the methanolic extract was subjected to intraperitoneally (i.p.) administered acetic acid-induced writhing test & subcutaneously administered (s.c.) formalin-induced hind paw licking test in Swiss-albino mice. The anxiolytic activity was conducted by using elevated plus maze (EPM) and hole board models.

**Results:** For both methods of analgesic test experimental plant extract was found to have significant ($p < 0.001$) analgesia at the dose of 200 mg/kg & 400 mg/kg body weight in mice when compared to control, where acetyl salicylic acid (100 mg/kg body weight) was used as standard drug. The percentages of inhibition found in case of acetic acid-induced writhing test were 26.27%, 50.45% and 20.29% respectively for acetyl salicylic acid (100 mg/kg), 200 mg/kg extract dose and 400 mg/kg extract dose. On the other hand, during formalin-induced hind paw licking test, the percentages of inhibition also increased when the extract dose increases from 200 mg/kg to 400 mg/kg by 53.95% to 61.79% at early phase and 71.62% to 78.8% at late phase respectively while acetyl salicylic acid (100 mg/kg), responsible for 25.58% and 38.74% of inhibition at both phase sequentially. Again, the crude extract significantly ($p < 0.01$; $p < 0.001$) raised the time spent in the open arm ($149.2 \pm 27.63^{**}$ sec) & the number of head-dips ($50.00 \pm 4.66^{***}$) at the dose 400 mg/kg body weight in case anxiolytic test, while reference drug diazepam (1 mg/kg body weight) also exhibited significant ($p < 0.01$) result in case of time spent in open arm ($107.0 \pm 12^{**}$ sec) but not for head dipping ($14.83 \pm 1.6$).

**Conclusion:** Findings of the present study assure that *Typha elephantina* Roxb. may be effective for the treatment of pain and anxiety with the demands of further investigations to isolate the active compound(s).

**Keywords:** *Typha elephantina* Roxb., Analgesic, Anxiolytic, Swiss-albino mice

## Background

Pain is a kind of convoluted unsavoury phenomenon which consists of sensory experiences including time, space, intensity, emotion, cognition and motivation. The agents which are being used to attenuate pain either by acting in the central nervous system (CNS) or by peripheral pain mechanisms except altering the consciousness are called analgesic [1]. Recently attainable analgesic drugs such as non-steroidal anti-inflammatory drugs (NSAIDs) alleviate pain and edema by repressing the synthesis of prostaglandin or by blocking the action of cyclooxygenase enzymes in inflammatory pathways. On the other hand, opiates act by affecting the central nervous system [2]. But severe side effects such as gastric lesion caused by NSAIDs and tolerance, dependence introduced by opiates have been making them unsuccessful in many cases [3]. In this sense, it is exigent to investigate novel analgesic drugs as a substitute of NSAIDs and opiates with prosperous pain management capability and free from undesirable adverse effects [4].

* Correspondence: niloysen91@gmail.com
[1]Department of Pharmacy, Noakhali Science & Technology University, Noakhali-3814, Bangladesh
Full list of author information is available at the end of the article

Modern life stress linked with various tests and afflictions plays the pivotal role for the surge of a variety of psychiatric disorders [5]. Among many psychiatric disorders anxiety disorders, are the most dominant problems and about 10–30% of general population is suffering from these throughout the world [6]. Benzodiazepines are the most frequently prescribed synthetic drugs for their anxiolytic, muscle relaxant, sedative-hypnotic and anticonvulsant actions [7]. Not only impairment in cognitive functions, physical dependence and tolerance side effects, these psychoneural drugs also cause harmful effects on respiratory, digestive and immune systems of the body [5]. That's why the search for new anxiolytic agents with reduced adverse effects is still an area great interest for the researchers [6].

Generally, natural products, specifically medicinal plants are considered to be a vital arsenal of chemical substances with therapeutic potentiality [4]. In the account of this, our concentration has been focused particularly on *Typha elphantina* Roxb. belonging to the family Typhaceae, a bush like small plant which was locally known as Hogla. The plant grows plenty in the Sundarban forest as well as in other low lying areas of Sylhet, Chittagong in beels & haors [8]. *Typha elephantina* Roxb. widely scattered across northern Africa and southern Asia. It is defined as native in many countries all over the world such as Algeria, Egypt, Libya, Uzbekistan, Palestine, Israel, Saudi Arabia, Assam, Bangladesh, India, Bhutan, Nepal, Pakistan and Burma etc. [9]. It is cooling and aphrodisiac in nature; used in splenic enlargement, burning sensation and leprosy. The root-stock has astringent and diuretic properties, also useful in case of dysentery, gonorrhoea and measles and the ripe fruits and the soft and woolly floss of male spikes are used as medicated absorbent to wounds and ulcers in emergency cases [10]. Several chromatographic and spectroscopic analysis carried out on fruit extract of this plant revealed the presence of four chemical constituents named pentacosane, 1-triacontarol, β-sitosterol, β-sitostery-3-O-β glycopyranoside. These four chemical constituents are supposed to exert various pharmacological activities such as anti-inflammatory, anti-pyretic, anti-tumour activities etc. [11]. As a part of our perpetual investigations on medicinal plants of Bangladesh, the methanolic extract of *Typha elephantia* Roxb. was studied for finding its analgesic activity and anxiolytic potentiality.

## Methods
### Drugs and chemicals
Acetic acid and formalin were obtained from Sigma Chemicals, USA; while Aspirin and Sedil were purchased from Square Pharmaceuticals Ltd., Bangladesh. Both of them are internationally recognized as acetyl salicylic acid and diazepam respectively as their chemical name.

Other reagents of the analytical grade for conducting this research work were supplied from the ethno-pharmacology laboratory of Pharmacy department of Noakhali Science and Technology University.

### Plant materials
The whole plant was collected from Noakhali Science and Technology University campus, Sonapur, Noakhali, Chittagong during January 2015. The plant was ascertained by an expert of Bangladesh National Herbarium, Mirpur, Dhaka, Bangladesh (Accession number- DACB: 43,476). The plant parts were sundried in shadow type milieu for 10 days and then subjected to be grounded by the use of high capacity grinding machine to produce coarse powder using.

### Preparation of plant extracts
800 g powder of the whole plant was soaked in 4.5 l methanol in a desiccator through occasional shaking and stirring. After 15 days the solvent was removed and filtration was carried out by using sterile cotton & Whatman filter paper no. 1 (Sargent, Welch, USA). Then rotary evaporation was carried out to concentrate the filtrate and was kept at room temperature in fresh and clean air for obtaining a brownish mass.

### Pharmacological procedure
#### Animals
Healthy Swiss albino mice (25-30 g) either sex were employed for this study. These mice were collected from Pharmacy Department, Jahangir Nagar University, Savar, Dhaka, Bangladesh and were kept in polypropylene plastic cages having dimensions of $30 \times 20 \times 13$ cm and softwood shavings were employed as bedding in the cages. Feeding of the animal was done along with standard laboratory pellet diet and water at *libitum*, exposing them to an alternate cycle of 12 h dark and light, at temperature $25 \pm 2$ °C and relative humidity $55 \pm 10\%$. All the mice were allowed to acclimatize for 7 days to the laboratory conditions before conducting the experiment.

### Preparation of test samples for bioassay
In order to administer 200 mg/kg and 400 mg/kg concentrations of the sample, extract amount was calculated based on the weight of the mice and properly mixed with 10 ml distilled water using vortex mixer. Acetyl salicylic acid (ASA) at a dose 100 mg/kg was properly calculated and mixed with 10 ml distilled water with the assistance of tween-80 by subsequent used of vortex mixer and sinker for proper mixing and used as reference standard for the analgesic test. Diazepam at a dose 1 mg/kg was properly calculated and mixed properly

with 10 ml distilled water. This one was used as reference standard for the anxiolytic test.

## Acute toxicity test

Animals were intraperitoneally (i.p.) employed to a high dose (2 g/kg) of *Typha elephantina* extract. Than observed during 24 h and morbidity or mortality was recorded, it happens, for each group at the end of observation period. Hayes stated that no dose-related toxicity should be considered above 5 g/kg body weight, thus suggesting that the extract is relatively non-toxic administered [12].

## Analgesic activity

### Acetic acid induced writhing test

The analgesic activity of the extract was conducted by using acetic acid-induced writhing in mice model. Twenty mice (25–30 g) were taken for this test and they were divided into four groups named as negative control group (Group I), positive control group (Group II), and two test groups (Group III & IV) with five mice in each group. They have fasted for 18 h. Group I mice were given distilled water 10 ml/kg, i.p.; group II mice was given 100 mg/kg acetyl salicylic acid subcutaneously (s.c.) while group III and IV i.p. received 200 and 400 mg/kg per body weight of crude methanolic extract respectively. After one hour of administration of drug and extract, 0.6% glacial acetic acid (10 ml/kg) was given i.p. to all the mice to induce pain [13]. The number of writhes (characterized by contraction of the abdominal musculature and extension of the hind limbs) was then counted at 5 min interval for 30 min. The percentage of protection against abdominal writhing was used to assess the degree of analgesia and was calculated by using the formula given below [14].

For Acetic acid-induced writhing test:

$$\text{Inhibition } (\%) = \frac{\textit{Number of writhes}(\textit{control}) - \textit{number of writhes}(\textit{test})}{\textit{Number of writhes}(\textit{control})} \times 100$$

## Formalin induced hind paw licking test

Formalin-induced hind paw licking test also conducted to ascertain the analgesic property of the crude methanolic extract in mice model. Like acetic acid-induced writhing test here also twenty swiss albino mice (25–30 g) were selected and divided into four groups (Group I, II, III & IV) of five mice per group. After passing through a fasting condition of 18 h by all animals group I (negative control group) mice were given distilled water 10 ml/kg per body weight i.p. Acetyl salicylic acid 100 mg/kg per body weight were given s.c. to group II (positive control group) mice as standard drug. On the other hand, 200 and 400 mg/kg per body weight doses of crude methanolic extract were administered i.p. to group III and IV as test samples. After one hour a s.c.

injection was given beneath the plantar surface of the left hind paw of each mice to introduce 20 μL of 2.5% formalin. [15] The time (in a second) spent in licking and biting responses of the injected paw was taken as an indicator of pain response. In this test, the determination of Anti-nociceptive effect involved two phases. The early phase (phase 1) was recorded during the first 5 min, while the late phase (phase 2) was counted during the last 20–30 min after formalin injection [16, 17].

For formalin-induced hind paw licking test:

$$\text{Inhibition } (\%) = \frac{\text{Reaction time(control)-Reaction time(test)}}{\text{Reaction time(control)}} \times 100$$

## Anxiolytic activity

### Elevated plus maze test

The crude methanolic extract was assessed to determine the anxiolytic activity by the way of using an Elevated Plus Maze model (EPM). According to the description given by Lister, the EPM was constructed (1987). The EPM consisted of two open arms ($35 \times 5$ cm) crossed with two closed arms ($35 \times 5 \times 15$ cm). The arms were connected together with a central square of $5 \times 5$ cm. The apparatus was elevated to the height of 40 cm in a dimly illuminated room. Twenty Swiss albino mice (25–30 g) fasted overnight were randomly selected and categorized into four groups of five animals each denoted as negative control group (Group I), positive control group (Group II) and test groups (Group III & IV). Distilled water 10 ml/kg, diazepam 1 mg/kg, plant extracts 200 mg/kg and 400 mg/kg were administered to group I, II, III & IV mice respectively. Experimental animals of all groups were treated by i.p. route. After 1 h, mice were individually placed in the center square facing either one of the open arms. The time spent by each mouse in both the open and closed arms was counted for 5 min [18].

## Hole board test

In the present study, the anxiolytic property also evaluated by the aid of another model recognized as Hoal

**Table 1** Effects of *Typha elephantina* extract on acetic acid induced writhing in mice

| Groups | Drugs | Dose | Number of Writhes (15 min) Mean ± S.E.M | % of inhibition |
|---|---|---|---|---|
| I | Control | 10 ml/kg | 20.4 ± 4.2 | |
| II | ASA | 100 mg/kg | 15 ± 4.5* | 26.47% |
| III | Extract | 200 mg/kg | 10.2 ± 0.58*** | 50.49% |
| IV | Extract | 400 mg/kg | 6.2 ± 0.37*** | 70.29% |

Here, *ASA* Acetyl Salicylic Acid, *S.E.M* Standard Error Mean. Results are presented as mean values ± S.E.M. (*n* = 5)
*$p < 0.05$, ***$p < 0.001$ when compared to control group

**Table 2** Effects of *Typha elephantina* extract on formalin induced hind paw licking mice (Early phase: 0-5 min and late phase: 20-30 min)

| Groups | Drugs | Dose | Time of Hind Paw licking (0-5 min) Mean ± S.E.M. | % of inhibition (Early phase) | Time of Hind Paw licking Mean ± S.E.M | %of inhibition (20-30 min) |
|--------|-------|------|------|------|------|------|
| I | Control | 10 ml/kg | 43 ± 5.1 | | 74.6 ± 14.6 | |
| II | ASA | 100 mg/kg | 32 ± 7.1 | 25.58% | 45.7 ± 7.8* | 38.74% |
| III | Extract | 200 mg/kg | 19.8 ± 2.22** | 53.95% | 28.5 ± 1.58*** | 61.79% |
| IV | Extract | 400 mg/kg | 12.2 ± 0.80*** | 71.62% | 15.8 ± 0.55*** | 78.8% |

Here, *ASA* Acetyl Salicylic Acid, *S.E.M* Standard Error Mean. Results are presented as mean values ± S.E.M. (*n* = 5)
*$p < 0.05$, **$p < 0.01$, ***$p < 0.001$ when compared to control group

Board model. The hole-board consists of a wooden box (40 × 40 × 25 cm) with 16 holes (each of diameter 3 cm) evenly distributed on the floor. The apparatus was 35 cm in height. Similarly, twenty Swiss albino mice (25–30 g) were kept on fast for an overnight and again separated into four groups of five animals denoted as group I (negative control group), group II (positive control group) and group II & IV (test sample groups). These four groups of animals were treated by i.p. route with distilled water (10 ml/kg), diazepam (1 mg/kg), and plant extract (200 and 400 mg/kg) respectively. After one hour each mouse was placed in turn at one corner of the board and then renders the animal to move and dip its head into the holes. The number of head dips during a 5 min period was recorded for individual mouse [19–21].

### Statistical analysis

All the results were expressed as mean ± SEM. *P*-value was calculated by one-way ANOVA using SPSS software, version 22.0 (IBM Corporation, New York, NY, U.S.A.). Where, *$p < 0.05$, **$p < 0.01$, ***$p < 0.001$ stands for significant, more significant and most significant respectively.

### Results

The present study was an attempt to determine the analgesic and anxiolytic properties of methanolic extract of *Typha elephantina* Roxb. and the results have been circumscribed in Tables 1, 2, 3, and 4 respectively.

### Acute toxicity test

In respect of acute toxicity, the extract did not produce any mortality and visible signs of delayed toxicity administered i.p. up to 2 g/kg.

### Analgesic activity

As a part of searching drugs from natural sources having the potentiality to remove pain, the extractives of *Typha elephantina* was examined for analgesia effect and the results are presented in Tables 1 and 2 respectively for acetic acid induced writhing test and formalin induced hind paw licking test. From Table 1 it has been noticed that there was ebb in the average number of writhes in the both extract groups (Group III & IV) in a dose-dependent manner and ASA group (Group II), in comparison with the negative control group (Group I). The crude methanolic extract at the afore-mentioned two doses (200 mg/kg & 400 mg/kg body weight) was significantly susceptible in the inhibition of pain respectively by 50.49% & 70.29%. These results were statistically most significant ($p < 0.01$, $p < 0.001$) when compared to control. Standard anti-nociceptive drug, ASA, when administered at the dose of 100 mg per kg body weight, exhibited 26.47% of pain inhibition, which was also found statistically significant ($p < 0.05$) in contrast with control. Here Table 1 and Fig. 1 altogether displayed the results of acetic acid induced writhing test for anti-nociceptive activity. On the other hand, the results of formalin induced hind paw licking test were summarized in Table 2 including both the early phase and late phase. Table 2 demonstrates that both the extract doses (200 mg/kg & 400 mg/kg) were responsible for attenuating hind paw licking time

**Table 3** Effects of methanolic extract of *Typha elephantina* on mice in the open arm and closed arm of the EPM

| Groups | Drugs | Doses | Time spent in open arm (sec) Mean ± S.E.M. | Time spend in closed arm (sec) Mean ± S.E.M. |
|--------|-------|-------|------|------|
| I | Control | 10 ml/kg | 30.8 ± 6.4 | 243.5 ± 8.8 |
| II | Diazepam | 1 mg/kg | 107.0 ± 12** | 169 ± 13.1** |
| III | Extract | 200 mg/kg | 82.6 ± 13.24 | 217.6 ± 13.24 |
| IV | Extract | 400 mg/kg | 149.2 ± 27.63** | 150.8 ± 27.63* |

Results are presented as mean values ± S.E.M. (*n* = 5)
*$p < 0.05$, **$p < 0.01$ when compared to control group

**Table 4** Effects of methanolic extract of *Typha elephantina* on mice stay in the hole board

| Groups | Drugs | Doses | Number of Head Dipping Mean ± SEM |
|--------|-------|-------|------|
| I | Control | 10 ml/kg | 10.50 ± 1.3 |
| II | Diazepam | 1 mg/kg | 14.83 ± 1.6 |
| III | Extract | 200 mg/kg | 44.8 ± 2.05*** |
| IV | Extract | 400 mg/kg | 50.00 ± 4.66*** |

Results are presented as mean values ± S.E.M. (*n* = 5)
***$p < 0.001$ when compared to control group

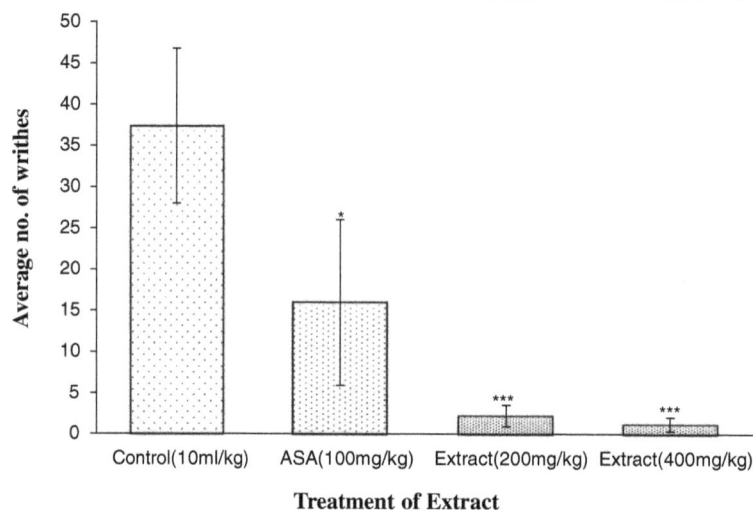

**Fig. 1** Effects of *Typha elephantina* extract on acetic acid induced writhing in mice. Results are presented as mean values ± S.E.M. ($n = 5$); *$p < 0.05$, ***$p < 0.001$ when compared to control group

significantly ($p < 0.01$, $p < 0.001$) where the percentages of inhibition of hind paw licking were 53.95% & 71.62% during early phase and 61.79% & 78.8% during late phase respectively. The reference drug acetyl salicylic acid which was administered as positive control also exerted preferable time reducing effect for hind paw licking by 25.58% and 38.74% respectively for both phases. The results of acetic acid hind paw licking test also displayed graphically in Figs. 2 and 3.

## Anxiolytic activity

The crude methanolic extract of *Typha elephantina* Roxb. was also assayed for anxiolytic activity by using EPM and hole board and the results are annexed in Tables 3 and 4 respectively. From Table 3 it can be inferred that, control group mice spent much time in the closed arm and refrain them from entering into the open arm. The average of time spent (sec) by the group IV mice treated with extract dose 400 mg/kg body weight was more significantly ($p < 0.01$) increased in open arm and decreased in closed arm by $149.2 \pm 27.63^{**}$ sec and $150.8 \pm 27.63^{**}$ sec respectively when compared to control. The other extract dose (200 mg per kg body weight) also exhibited similar attribute of effect but have no statistical significance in contrast with control. The reference drug diazepam relieved anxiety better than extract dose 200 mg/kg which was also statistically more significant

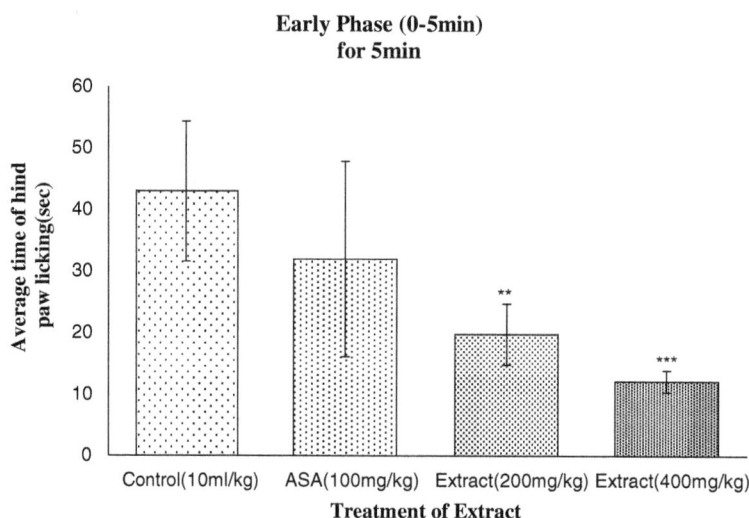

**Fig. 2** Effects of *Typha elephantina* extract on formalin induced hind paw licking mice (Early phase: 0–5 min). Results are presented as mean values ± S.E.M. ($n = 5$); *$p < 0.05$, ***$p < 0.001$ when compared to control group

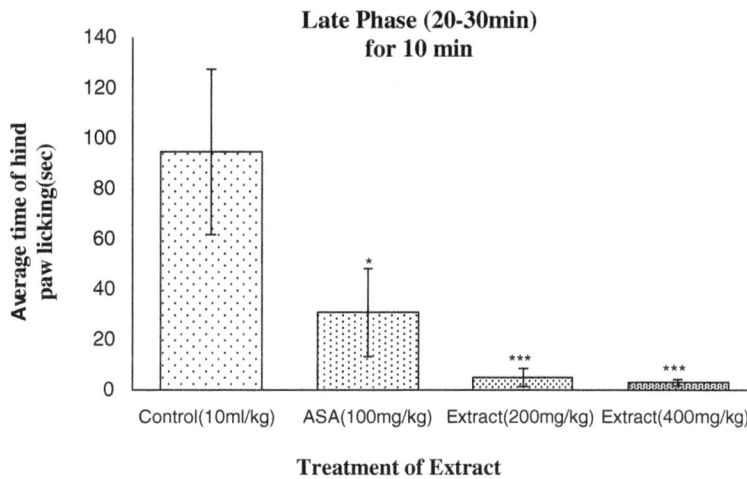

**Fig. 3** Effects of *Typha elephantina* extract on formalin induced hind paw licking mice (Late phase: 20–30 min). Results are presented as mean values ± S.E.M. ($n = 5$); **$p < 0.01$, ***$p < 0.001$ when compared to control group

($p < 0.01$) as compared to control group but less effective than 400 mg/kg body weight extract dose. The average of time spent by these positive control group mice were $107.0 \pm 12^{**}$ sec in open arm and $169 \pm 13.1^{**}$ sec in closed arm respectively. Figure 4 is used to represent these results graphically. The results of hole board test are manifested in Table 4 and Fig. 5 to represent the anxiolytic effect of a crude methanolic extract of *Typha elephantina* Roxb. Both the extract doses (200 mg/kg, 400 mg/kg) most significantly ($p < 0.001$) ameliorated the numbers of head dipping in a dose-dependent manner when compared to control. On average $44.8 \pm 2.05^{***}$ and $50.00 \pm 4.66^{***}$ head dips were performed by group III & IV mice respectively. However, no significant increases were observed in the number of head dipping in case mice treated with diazepam (1 mg/kg).

## Discussion

The present study was carried out in order to assess the analgesic and anxiolytic effects crude methanolic extract of *Typha elephantina* Roxb. on animals while the acute toxicity study provides evidence about the non-toxicity of this plant. From obtained results, it might be asserted that the plant extract possesses significant inhibition of pain and abatement of anxiety with a considerable safety profile.

Acetic acid-induced twisting of dorsoabdominal muscles constrictions [22], followed by the measurement of a number of writhing is one of the most important methods for the determination of both central and peripheral analgesia [4], as had been done in the present study. In this test, pain sensation is elicited by instigating localized inflammatory response which associated with the release of free arachidonic acid from tissue

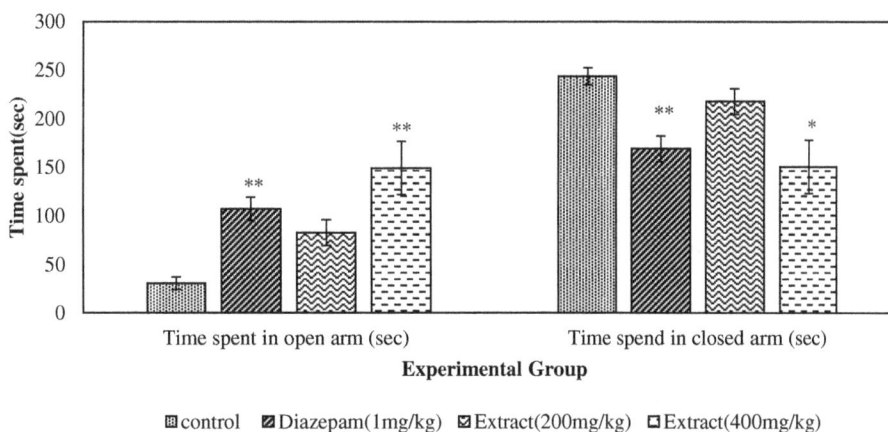

**Fig. 4** Effects of methanolic extract of *Typha elephantina* on mice in the open arm and closed arm of the EPM. Results are presented as mean values ± S.E.M. ($n = 5$); *$p < 0.05$, **$p < 0.01$ when compared to control group

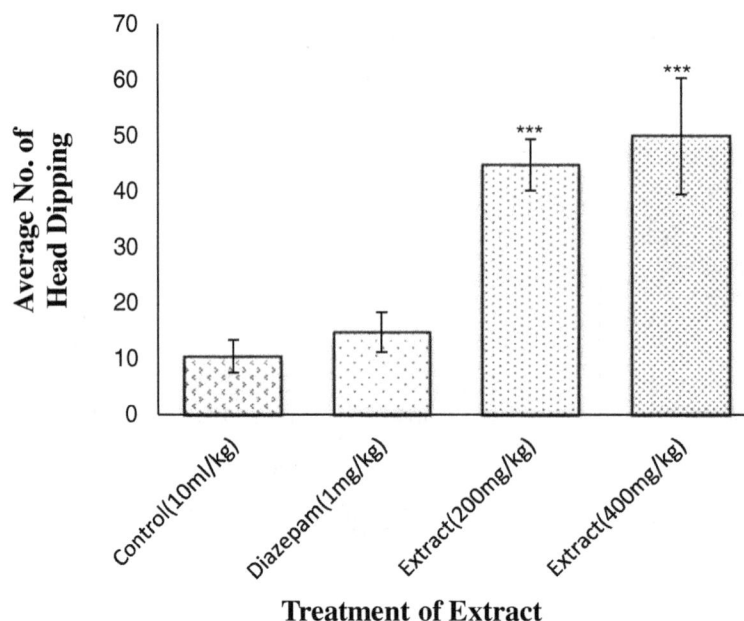

**Fig. 5** Effects of methanolic extract of *Typha elephantina* on mice stay in the hole board. Results are presented as mean values ± S.E.M. ($n = 5$); ***$p < 0.001$ when compared to control group

phospholipid via cyclooxygenase (COX), and prostaglandin biosynthesis [23, 24]. In other words, the levels of PGE2 and PGF2α, as well as lipoxygenase products are supposed to be increased in the peritoneal cavity due to acetic acid administration [25]. These excess amounts of prostaglandins within the peritoneal cavity then accelerates inflammatory pain by facilitating capillary permeability [26]. It is widely acceptable that NSAIDs serve as an inhibitor of inflammatory pain at peripheral target sites through the formation of the blockade against pin mediators such as bradykinin and prostaglandins which play important role in the generation of pain [27]. From our investigation, it was observed that methanolic extract of *Typha elephantina* at two different doses (200 mg/kg and 400 mg/kg body weight) demonstrated a significant reduction of writhes in mice in a dose-dependent manner as compared to control (distilled water). So it can be assumed that its cyclooxygenase (COX) inhibitory activity may reduce the production of free arachidonic acid from phospholipid or may inhibit the enzyme system, which is responsible for the synthesis of prostaglandins and ultimately relieve pain sensation.

As acetic acid-induced writhing test is sensitive but not selective, thus formalin-induced hind paw licking test also conducted in order to endorse the analgesic activity of the plant extract. On the other hand, previous studies have shown that formalin plays a vital role in secreting several inflammatory mediators. The formalin-induced hind paw licking test describes two types of

response, i.e. 'early response' or first phase (neurogenic pain) and 'late response' or second phase (inflammatory pain) [14, 28].

Moreover, formalin-induced nociception is also associated with direct action on a member of Transient Receptor Potential family (TRP) of cation channels denoted as TRPA1 receptor located in C fibres [29]. It is also observed from our study that both the extract doses (200 mg/kg and 400 kg/kg body weight) significantly mitigate not only neurogenic pain but also the inflammatory pain in a dose-dependent manner. So it can be assumed that *Typha elephantina* extract acts against formalin-induced nociception by interacting with the TRPA1receptor. However, previous studies on several plant extracts revealed that potential antioxidants, alkaloids, glycosides, flavonoids and saponins are reported to play role in analgesic activity primarily by targeting prostaglandin [30–33]. Since phytochemical analysis ensured the presence of flavonoids, tannin, phenols, saponin alkaloid in the crude extract of *Typha elephantina* Roxb [9] and the obtained results suggest that, methanolic extract of *Typha elephantina* possesses a significant analgesic effect in this paradigm.

The prominent inhibitory neurotransmitter in the human central nervous system is Gamma-aminobutyric acid (GABA). It has been reported that the GABAergic system substantiates a promising destination for new pharmacological techniques for the treatment of anxiety [34]. As the increment in GABAergic neurotransmission was connected with reduced anxiety; over the years, different pharmacological models have been appointed in the evaluation of medicinal plants for neuro-pharmacological activities towards the identification of botanicals and drugs with beneficial effects in the treatment of diverse CNS disorders. The choice of test methods not only determines effectiveness but in some instances also gives an indication of the mechanism(s) of the test substance [35, 36]. Models that are available for evaluating anxiolytic or anxiogenic traits of substances, hole board and EPM in rodents are most promising among them [37, 38]. On account of this, the present study was designed to investigate the anxiolytic properties of methanolic extract in EPM and hole board by using Swiss-albino mice. Moreover, it is known that anxiolytic agents raise the time spent in open arms of the EPM [37]. According to our study, administration of two different doses of plant extract (200 mg/kg & 400 mg/kg body weight, *i.p.*) significantly increased ($p < 0.05$) the permanence time in open arms, in comparison to control group. The plant extract at an increased dose (400 mg/kg body weight) likely to be more effective than diazepam (1 mg/kg) group in comparison to another experimental group (200 mg/kg body weight). Hole board test is founded on a supposition that head-dipping of animals is inversely proportional to their anxiety state in the moderately aversive environment [39]. Therefore the increased number of head dips into the holes on the board means waned anxiety state. Drugs as diazepam not significantly increase the number of head-dips in the hole-board test as compared to control. Our study revealed that, methanolic extract of *Typha elephantina* (200 and 400 mg/kg, *i.p.*) increased head-dip counts without changing locomotion in the hole-board test most significantly ($p < 0.001$) as compared with control group. Flavonoids, alkaloids, and terpenoids have been reported to be responsible for anxiolytic and sedative effects observed in different plant extracts [40–42]. On the other hand, the presence of natural flavonoids that hold anxiolytic effect not linked with myorelaxant, amnestic or sedative effects has been manifested [7]. As we stated above about the existence of flavonoids in methanolic extract of *Typha elephantina* it can be hypothesized flavonoids is responsible for its antianxiety action.

## Conclusion

Based on the above denouements it can be asserted that the methanolic extract of *Typha elephantina* Roxb. is a promising source of necessary phytochemicals having potentiality to assuage pain and anxiety. Therewith this plant could be better remedy for pain and anxiety disorders in traditional manner. Therefore it may suggest further investigations in order to disclose the underlying causes of analgesic and anxiolytic actions scientifically.

## Abbreviations

ASA: Acetyl Salicylic Acid; CNS: Central Nervous System; COX: Cyclooxygenase; EPM: Elevated Plus Maze Model; GABA: Gamma-aminobutyric acid; NSAIDS: Non-steroidal Anti-inflammatory Drugs; SC: Subcutaneously; TRP: Transient Receptor Potential family (TRP)

## Acknowledgements

The authors are grateful to Square Pharmaceuticals Ltd., Bangladesh for their generous supply of necessary drugs. The authors are also thankful to all the teachers and staffs of the Department of Pharmacy, Noakhali Science and Technology University for their cordial co-operation by providing laboratory support to carry out the research work.

## Funding

The research work was partially supported by the Department of Pharmacy, Noakhali Science and Technology University, Bangladesh. The authors have no other relevant affiliations or financial involvement with any organization.

## Authors' contributions

LB designed the experiments and conception. NS conducted the research work. Data interpretation and analysis were aided by MSH. SB critically reviews the manuscript. MSKC made the necessary corrections in the write up and gave final approval for the submission of revised version. All authors read and approved the final manuscript.

## Authors' information

Niloy Sen is a Post Graduate student of Department of Pharmacy, Noakhali Since & Technology University, Noakhali-3814, Bangladesh; Latifa Bulbul and Sujan Banik are working as Assistant Professor at Department of Pharmacy, Noakhali Science and Technology University, Noakhali-3814, Bangladesh. Md. Saddam Hussain is also a Post Graduate student of Department of Pharmacy, Noakhali Science and Technology University, Noakhali-3814, Bangladesh. Finally, Md. Shahbuddin Kabir Choudhuri is the Professor of Pharmacy Department, Jahangirnagar University, Dhaka-1342, Bangladesh.

## Competing interests

The authors declare that they have no competing interests.

## Author details

[1]Department of Pharmacy, Noakhali Science & Technology University, Noakhali-3814, Bangladesh. [2]Department of Pharmacy, Jahangirnagar University, Dhaka-1342, Bangladesh.

## References

1. Milind P, Monu Y. Laboratory Method For Sreening analgesics. Int Res J Pharm. 2013;4:15.
2. Mishra D, Ghosh G, Kumar PS, Panda PK. An Experimental study of analgesic activity of selective cox-2 inhibitor with conventional NSAIDs. Asian J Pharm Clin Res. 2011;4:78–81.
3. AHM Z, Rahman MM, Kamal M, Hossain MK, Hamid K, MEH M, Rana MS. In vivo analgesic activity of ethanolic extracts of two medicinal plants - *Scoparia dulcis* L. and Ficus Racemosa Linn. Biol Med. 2010;2:42–8.
4. Shanmugasundaram P, Venkataraman S. Anti-nociceptive activity of *Hygrophila auriculata* (SCHUM) Heine. Afr J Trad CAM. 2005;2:62–9.
5. Mishra SK, Sing PN, Dubey SD. Evaluation of CNS depressant activity of *Capparis zeylenica* Linn. Root. Res J Med Plants. 2011;5:738–46.
6. Netto SM, Warela RWB, Fechine MF, Queiroga MN, Quintans-Júnior LJ. Anxiolytic-like effect of Rauvolfia Ligustrina Willd. Ex Roem. & Schult.,

Apocynaceae, in the elevated plus-maze and hole-board tests. BJP. 2009;19:888–92.

7. Helli'on-Ibarrola MC, DAY I, Montalbetti Y, Kennedy ML, Heinichen O, Campuzano M, Tortoriello J, Tortoriello J, Fern'andez S, Wasowski C, Marder M, TCM DL, Morae S. The anxiolytic-like effects of *Aloysia polystachya* (Griseb.) Moldenke (Verbenaceae) in mice. J Ethnopharmacol. 2006;105:400–8.

8. Sen N, Bulbul L, Hussain F, Amin MT. Assessment of thrombolytic, membrane stabilizing potential and total phenolic content of *Typha elephantina* Roxb. J Med Plants Res. 2016;10:669–75.

9. Rahman MM, Chakrabarty JK, Muhit MA, Dash PR. Evaluation of analgesic activity of the different fractions of *Typha elephantina* Roxb. IJP. 2014;1:380–3.

10. Bulbul L, Kader MA, Baul S, Uddin SMN, Haque MM, Debnath PC, Kar A. In vitro anthelmintic and cytotoxic activities of the methanolic extract of *Typha elephantina* Roxb. IAJPR. 2013;3:3519–26.

11. Ruangrungsi N, Aukkanibutra A, Phadungcharoen T, Lee M. Constituents Of *Typhaelephantina*. J Sci Soc. 1987;13:57–62.

12. Hayes AW. Guidelines for acute oral toxicity testings: Principles and Methods of Toxicity, second ed. Raven Press Ltd., New York. Table. 1989; 4: 185.

13. Ezeja MI, Omeh YS, Ezeigbo II, Ekechukwu A. Evaluation of the analgesic activity of the Methanolic stem bark extract of Dialium Guineense (wild). Ann Med Health Sci Res. 2011;1:55–62.

14. Akindele AJ, Ibe IF, Adeyemi OO. Analgesic and antipyretic activities of *Drymaria Cordata* (Linn.) Willd (Caryophyllaceae) extract. Afr J Tradit Complement Altern Med. 2012;9:25–35.

15. Hunskaar S, Hole K. The formalin test in mice: dissociation between inflammatory and non-inflammatory pain. Pain. 1987;30:103–14.

16. Shibata M, Ohkubo T, Takahashi H, Inoki R. Modified Formalin test: characteristic biphasic pain response. Pain. 1989;38:347–52.

17. Ullah HMA, Zaman S, Juhara F, Akter L, Tareq SM, Masum EH, Bhattacharjee R. Evaluation of antinociceptive, in-vivo & in-vitro anti-inflammatory activity of ethanolic extract of *Curcuma zedoaria* rhizome. BMC Complement Altern Med. 2014;14:346.

18. Adeyemi OO, Yetmitan OK, Taiwo AE. Neurosedative and muscle relaxant activities of ethyl acetate extract of *Baphia nitida* AFZEL. J Ethnopharmacol. 2006;106:312–6.

19. File SE, Wardill AG. The reliability of the hole-board apparatus. Psychopharmacologia. 1975;44:47–51.

20. Yemitan OK, Ajibade AM, Adeyemi OO. Anticonvulsant activity of *Dalbergia saxatilis*. Nigerian. J Neurosci. 2001;4:33–40.

21. Dhara AK, Pal S, Nag Chaudhuri AK. Psychopharmacological studies on Tragia involucrate root extract. Phytother Res. 2002;16:326–30.

22. Raju GS, Moghal MMR, Hossain MS, Hassan MM, Billah MM, Ahamed SK, Rana SMM. Assessment of pharmacological activities of two medicinal plant of Bangladesh: Launaea Sarmentosa and Aegialitis Rotundifolia roxb in the management of pain, pyrexia and inflammation. Biol Res. 2014;47:55.

23. Ahmed F, Hossain MH, Rahman AA, Shahid IZ. Antinociceptive and sedative effects of the bark of *Cerbera odollam* Gaertn. Orient Pharm Exp Med. 2006; 6:344–8.

24. IDG D, Nakamura M, Ferreira SH. Participation Of the sympathetic system in acetic acid-induced writhing in mice. Braz J Med Biol Res. 1988;21:341–3.

25. Derardt R, Jongney S, Delvalcee F, Falhout M. Release Of prostaglandins E and F in an algogenic reaction and its inhibition. Eur J Pharmacol. 1980;51: 17–24.

26. Zakaria ZA, Gani ZDF. Antinociceptive, anti-inflammatory, and antipyretic properties of an aqueous extract of Dicranopteris Linearis leaves in experimental animal models. J Nat Med. 2008;62:179–87.

27. Kim HP, Son KH, Chang HW, Kang SS. Anti-inflammatory plant flavonoids and cellular action mechanism. J Pharmacol Sci. 2004;96:229–45.

28. Hunskaar S, Fasmer OB, Hole K. Formalin test in mice, a useful technique for evaluating mild analgesia. J Neurosci Methods. 1986;14:69–76.

29. Basak A, Uddin MMN, Sarwar MS, Mohiuddin M, Dewan SMR, Shahriar M, Islam MS. Exploration of analgesic activity of the Ethanolic extract of Erythrina variegate bark. J Therm Anal. 2014;2:37–42.

30. Bhowmick R, Sarwar MS, Dewan SMR, Das A, Das B, Uddin MMN, Islam MS, Islam MS. In vivo analgesic, antipyretic, and anti-inflammatory potential in

31. Swiss albino mice and in vitro thrombolytic activity of hydroalcoholic extract from *Litsea glutinosa* leaves. Biol Res. 2014;47:56.

31. Rajnarayana K, Reddy MS, Chaluvadi MR, Krishna DR. Biflavonoids classification, pharmacological, biochemical effects and therapeutic potential. IJP. 2001;33:2–16.

32. Ramesh M, Rao AV, Prabhakar MC, Rao CS, Muralidhar N, Reddy BM. Antinociceptive and anti-inflammatory activity of a flavonoid isolated from *Caralluma attenuata*. J Ethnopharmacol. 1998;62:63–6.

33. Brown JE, Evans CAR. Luteo-rich artichoke extract protects low density lipoprotein from oxidation in vitro. Free Radic Res. 1998;29:247–55.

34. Domschke K, Zwanzger P. GABAergic and endocannabinoid dysfunction in anxiety – future therapeutic targets? Curr Pharm Des. 2008;14:3508–17.

35. Takeda H, Tsuji M, Matsumiya T. Changes in head-dipping behavior in the hole-board test reflect the anxiogenic and/or anxiolytic state in mice. Eur J Pharmacol. 1998;350:21–9.

36. Barua CC, Roy JD, Buraguohain B, Barua AG, Borah P, Lahkar M. Anxiolytic effect of hydroethanolic extract of Drymasia cordata L wild. IJEB. 2009;47: 969–73.

37. Pellow S, Chopin P, File SE, Briley M. Validation of open: closed arm entries in an elevated plus-maze as a measure of anxiety in the rat. J Neurosci Meth. 1985;14:149–67.

38. Pellow S, File SE. Anxiolytic and anxiogenic drug effects on exploratory activity in an elevated plus-maze: a novel test of anxiety in the rat. Pharmacol Biochem Be. 1986;24:525–9.

39. Bilkei-Gorzó A, Gyertyán I. Some doubts about the basic concept of the hole-board test. Neurobiology. 1996;4:405–15.

40. Carlini EA. Plants and the central nervous system. Pharmacol Biochem Behav. 2003;75:501–12.

41. Dhawan K, Kumar S, Sharma A. Anti-anxiety studies on extracts of *Passiflora incarnata* Linneaus. J Ethnopharmacol. 2001;78:165–70.

42. Houghton PJ. The scientific basis for the reputed activity of valerian. JPP. 1999;51:505–12.

# 15

# Comprehensive evaluation of pharmacological properties of *Olea europaea* L. for Cosmeceuticals prospects

Afifa Qidwai[1], Manisha Pandey[1], Rajesh Kumar[1] and Anupam Dikshit[1,2*]

## Abstract

**Background:** *Propionibacterium acnes* (anaerobic bacteria) and *Staphylococcus epidermidis* (aerobic bacteria) have been acknowledged as key comedone forming pathological factor, eliciting an inflammation in acne. The present study was conducted to evaluate antibacterial and antioxidant activities of Olea europaea leaves extracts (OLE) of different solvents (methanol, ethanol, deionized water, and acetone) against etiologic pathogens of *acne vulgaris*.

**Methods:** The antibacterial testing against the selected pathogen *viz., P. acnes* and *S. epidermidis* were evaluated using broth micro dilution method recommended by CLSI, in duplicate. Correspondingly the total phenolic content and flavonoid content along with radicals scavenging activity by DPPH assay were also evaluated. The data of antibacterial assay demonstrated that these plant extracts differ quantitatively in their activity against the tested pathogens.

**Results:** The results (mg/ml) exhibited that *Olea europaea* leaves extracts (MIC:2.263/IC$_{50}$:1.626, MIC:0.933/IC$_{50}$:0.636, MIC: 1.054/IC$_{50}$:1.040, MIC:2.534/IC$_{50}$:2.500 of aqueous, methanol, ethanol, acetone extracts respectively) are more effective against growth of *P.acnes* as compared to *S. epidermidis* (MIC: Range (Not active at particular concentration), IC$_{50}$: Range, MIC:1.031, IC$_{50}$: 0.670, MIC:1.502, IC$_{50}$:1.234, MIC: Range, IC$_{50}$:1.890 mg/ml aqueous, methanol, ethanol, acetone extracts respectively). The readings were statically analyzed and also compared with standard drug tetracycline.

**Conclusions:** The current findings suggested *Olea europaea* L. as a promising source of potential antioxidants and antibacterial activity against *P.acnes* and *S. epidermidis* that may be an efficient therapeutic agent in the pathogenesis of *Acne vulgaris* and proves a potential source of Cosmeceuticals.

**Keywords:** *Propionibacterium acnes*, *Staphylococcus epidermidis*, CLSI, Antibacterial activities MIC, DPPH

## Background

Natural drug resources with their varied biological and pharmacological properties (due to the presence of phenolic acids, flavonoids, tannins, vitamins and terpenoids) represent a treasure for researchers, to combat problem concerning treatment of health disorders or dermal infections. In the last few years, with the increasing doses of conventional drugs, multidrug resistance of pathogens develops. To overcome these persistent dilemmas of conventional treatments an increasing interest in herbal therapy has emerged. The herbal formulations are a viable option that could be useful in reducing the side effects associated with synthetic antibiotic treatment. Emphasis has been mainly on the antibacterial, anti-inflammatory and antioxidant properties of herbal extract [1].

*Olea europaea* L. leaves are a sort of waste product, this waste product is not profitable; olive leaves are often used as animal feed or simply burned with excess branches gathered [2]. The concern in olive leaves grew in the last few years due to its high pharmacologicalproperties, presence of phenolic compound flavonoids, tannins, vitamins C and terpenoids and high concentration of phenolic compounds [3]. *O. europaea* is the most abundant phenolic compound (up to 14% of the dry weight) with numerous health benefits attributed to it [4]. It has been found to have potent antioxidant and radical scavengers with anti-tumor and anti-inflammatory,

* Correspondence: anupambplau@rediffmail.com
[1]Department of Botany, University of Allahabad, Allahabad 211002, Uttar Pradesh, India
[2]Biological Product Laboratory, Department of Botany, University of Allahabad, Allahabad 211002, Uttar Pradesh, India

antimicrobial properties and anti-atherogenic, hypoglycemic, hepatic, cardiac and neuro-protective effects [5, 6]. Oleuropein has a protective effect in counteracting low-density lipoprotein (LDL) oxidation, validated through the estimation of the decreased formation of thiobarbituric acid-reactive substances (TBARS are naturally present in organic specimens, include lipid hydroperoxides and aldehydes which increase in concentration as a response to oxidative stress) [7] and malondialdehyde (MDA, compound that results from the decomposition of polyunsaturated fatty acid lipid peroxides) and 4-hydroxynonenal (4-HNE) as lipid peroxides by-products [8]. Its anti-tumour activity has shown to inhibit proliferation and migration of a number of advanced grade human tumors cell lines in a dose dependent manner [9–11]. Its anti-inflammatory activity is also remarkable, demonstrated by decreasingthe production of monocytic inflammatory mediators, decreasing in the production of IL-1β in human whole blood cultures stimulated with monocytes-triggered by LPS [12]. Interestingly, olive oil phenolic compounds reduce the circulating concentrations of IL-6, a pro-inflammatory agent that stimulates inflammation in several pathologies. *Acne vulgaris* is a chronic inflammatory disorder of pilosebaceous unit that affects more than 85% of adolescents and young adults [13]. The increase sebum production, hypercornification of the pilosebaceous follicle, an abnormality of the microbial flora (*P. acnes* and *S. epidermidis*), and the production of inflammation are the main triggering cause of *Acne vulgaris* [14].

The present study intends to evaluate the antimicrobial properties of different solvent extracts of *Olea europaea* L. leaves (olive leaf) against most common but ticklish anaerobic bacteria of human dermal pathogen *i.e. Propionibacterium acnes* and aerobic bacteria *Staphylococcus epidermidis*, causative agent of *acne vulgaris*.

## Methods

Olive leaves were received as a gift from Riyadh, Saudi Arabia. All the chemicals and reagents used were of analytical grade, and were either purchased from Himedia.

### Preparation of extracts

Dried leaves of *O. europaea* was finely chopped and soaked overnight in 50% of different solvent *i.e.* methanol, ethanol, deionized water, acetone in 1:10 (10 g/100 ml) (Fig. 1). Subsequently, the extracts were filtered with Whatman filter paper no.1. The filtrates were subjected to evaporation under vacuum and moderate temperature in rotavapour (Advance rotatory evaporator).

### The test organisms

The test organisms *Propionibacterium acnes* (MTCC 1951) and *Staphylococcus epidermidis* (MTCC 435) were procured from Microbial Type Culture Collection, Chandigarh, India and the media were procured from Hi-Media. The culture of *P. acnes* (anaerobic bacteria) was maintained on Anaerobic Blood Agar Medium supplemented with freshsheep blood. The proper anaerobic environment was provided to the bacterial culture by the Anaxomate advance instrument after which the culture was incubated for 48 h at 37 °C in $CO_2$ incubator to provide optimum temperature for bacteria growth (Fig. 1). The culture of aerobic bacteria was maintained on Nutrient Agar and incubated in BOD incubator for their appropriate growth (Fig. 1).

### Phytochemical analysis

All four solvents were prepared separately for extracting phenolics from leaves: methanol, ethanol, acetone and deionized water (dd$H_2O$). Leaves (1 g) were ground with a mortar and pestle under liquid nitrogen. The ground leaves were supplemented to a centrifuge tube (eppendrof) containing 10 mL of solvent. The mixture was allowed to

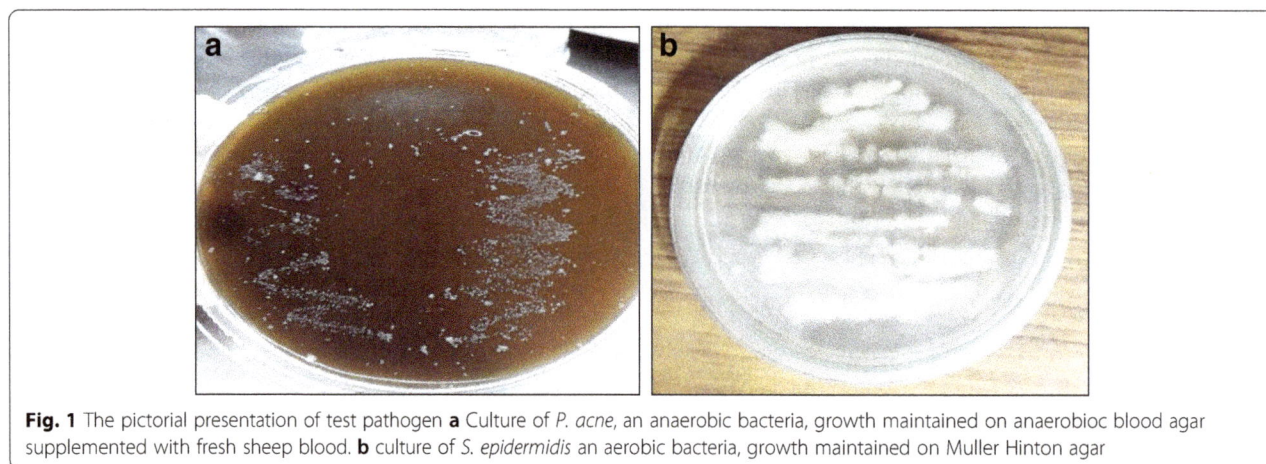

**Fig. 1** The pictorial presentation of test pathogen **a** Culture of *P. acne*, an anaerobic bacteria, growth maintained on anaerobioc blood agar supplemented with fresh sheep blood. **b** culture of *S. epidermidis* an aerobic bacteria, growth maintained on Muller Hinton agar

stand in the dark for overnight. The extract was centrifuged 5000 rpm for 10 min, at room temperature, and the supernatants were then filtered using a filter paper (Whatman No. 1). The extracts were subjected to rotary evaporator to make thick slurryunder vacuum at operating temperature below 45 °C. Thereafter, the thick slurry was kept at -20 °C for further usage.

1. **Phenolic content**: 20 μl of each extract solution and standard (tannic acid) were mixed with 1 ml of ddH2O and 100 μl of Folin-Ciocalteu reagent, followed by the addition of 300 μl of 20%$Na_2CO3$ solution after 1 minutethe resulted mixture now incubated in shaker incubator (temp 40 °C, 30 min). The phenolic content was determined as milligram tannic acid equivalents (TAE)/g of dry weight powder (DW) [15].

2. **Flavonoidscontent**: 4 ml of ddH$_2$O was mixed with1ml of each olive extract. Subsequently, 5% sodium nitrite solution (0.3 mL) and 10% aluminum chloride solution (0.3 mL) was added and incubated at room temp for 5-10 min. Then 2 mL of 1 M NaOH was added to the mixture, the volume makes upto 10 ml with ddH$_2$O and subjected to vortex thoroughly. The pink colour developed and show absorbance at 510 nm. Total flavonoids content was determined as mg catechin equivalents per g of dry weight powder (mg CE g-1 DW) [16].

3. **DPPH**: it is a method to measure the antioxidant/ free radical scavenging activity of extracts. The antioxidant activity/radical scavenging of leaf extracts were evaluated using 1, 1-Diphenyl-2-Picrylhydrazyl. For this purpose 0.1 mM solution of DPPH in methanol was prepared. 30 μL of extracts in different concentration (10, 50, 100, 500, and 1000 μg/mL) were mixed with DPPH solution and thoroughly vortex and incubated for 30 min at 25 °C, decrease in absorbance was measured at A = 517 nm against blank. The standard (butylhydroxyl toluene) was used as synthetic antioxidant positive control. The scavenging ability of the plant on DPPH was calculated using the equation:

$$\text{DPPH scavenging activity } (\%) = \frac{\text{Abs control} - \text{Abs sample}}{\text{Abs control}} \times 100$$

Where Abs control is the absorbance of DPPH + methanol; Abs sample is the absorbance of DPPH radical + sample extract or standard [17].

## Antibacterial assay-

The susceptibility of the *P. acnes* and *S. epidermidis* was assayed against *Oleo europaea*L. leaf solvents extracts using the broth micro dilution method recommended by the Clinical and Laboratory Standards Institute (CLSI) [18]. Freshly prepared Muller Hinton Broth (MHB) medium was used as a base medium for the assay. Stock solutions of all the extracts and standard (Tetracycline) were prepared (50 mg/ml) in Dimethyl Sulfoxide (DMSO) and homogenized by using vortex for 4–5 min. The bacterial inocula suspension was prepared as per 0.5 McFarland standards. The experiment was performed according to CLSI guidelines in flat bottom sterile 96-well microtitre plates. Initial dispensing of 100 μl medium (MHB) in all the wells, followed by the addition of 100 μl, 90 μl and 80 μl of MHB in columns 2, 3 and 4 respectively. Further, 10 μl and 20 μl of drugs (each solvent extract in duplicate wells) were added to each well of columns 3 (sample control) and 4 (dilution well) respectively. Further, serial dilution was done from 4th column wells (2.5 mg/ml) to 11thcolumn wells (0.02 mg/ml) and after dilution, and content dragged from 11th well was discarded so as to maintain 100 μl from 4–11 wells [19] (Fig. 2).

After the serial dilution, 100 μl of bacterial inoculums was added to each well of column 4 to column 12, to make up final volume of 200 μl. Column 1 contained media and formaldehyde to serve as a negative control. Column 12 was taken as the positive control (O. D. control), which contains 100 μl medium and 100 μl inocula (Fig. 3). This is how, set of all extracts were maintained (in triplet). Thesecultured 96 well plate of anaerobic bacteria incubated in CO$_2$incubator (Galaxy 170 S New Brunswick, USA) for 48 h and aerobic bacterium 96 well plates were placed in BOD incubator for 24 h.

## Determination of minimum inhibitory concentrations (MICs) and IC$_{50}$

For extracts the MIC was determined as the lowest drug concentration showing absence of growth visually or 80% growth inhibition compared with the growth in the drug-free well. IC$_{50}$ defined as the drug concentration that produces 50% of growth inhibition compared to the growth in the drug-free well. Comparative inhibition percent of bacteria inoculum in media treated with extracts were calculated by using formula [20].

$$\%\,\text{Inhibition} = \frac{\text{O.D. Control} - \text{O.D. treatment}}{\text{O.D. control}} \times 100$$

## Statistical analysis

All experiments were carried out in duplicate. The data were analyzed using analysis of variance (ANOVA) and significant differences ($p < 0.05$) among means were determined by R commander software.

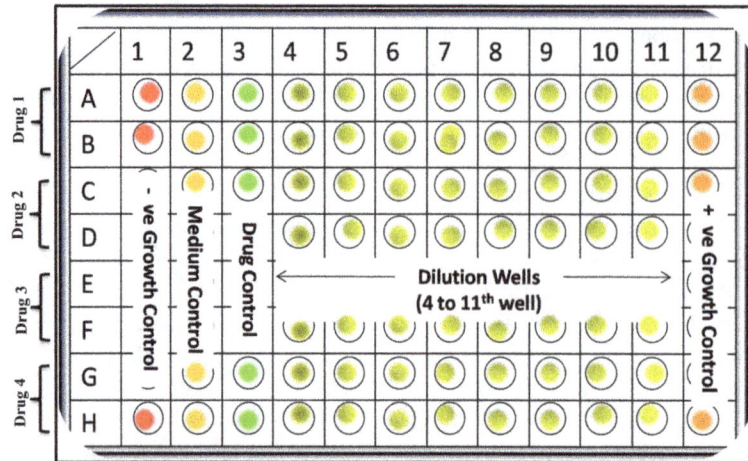

**Fig. 2** Pictorial representation of CLSI recommended broth micro-dilution protocol. *a–h* contains drugs (50mg/ml) in duplicated: *a, b* contains *Drug 1 i.e. Olea europaea* ethanolic extract, *c, d* contains *Drug 2 i.e. O europaea* methanolic extracts, *e, f* Drug 3 *i.e.* acetone extract, *g, h* Drug 4 contain aqueous extracts [36]

## Results and discussion

In present study the preliminary qualitative and quantitative analyses of the *Olea europaea* L. leaves extracts (methanol, ethanol, acetone and aqueous) were executed to analyze antibacterial and antioxidant properties against *P. acnes* and *S epidermidis*. The results of our study clearly portray significant antibacterial and antioxidant properties with reference to the MICs as well as IC$_{50}$ (mg/ml) values through 96 well microtitre plates (CLSI recommended broth micro dilution method). The leaves extracts were found to be more effective against anaerobic bacteria *P. acnes* (methanolic extracts MIC: 0.933/IC$_{50}$:0.636, ethanolic extracts MIC: 1.050/IC$_{50}$: 1.040, aqueous MIC: 2.263/IC$_{50}$:1.626 and

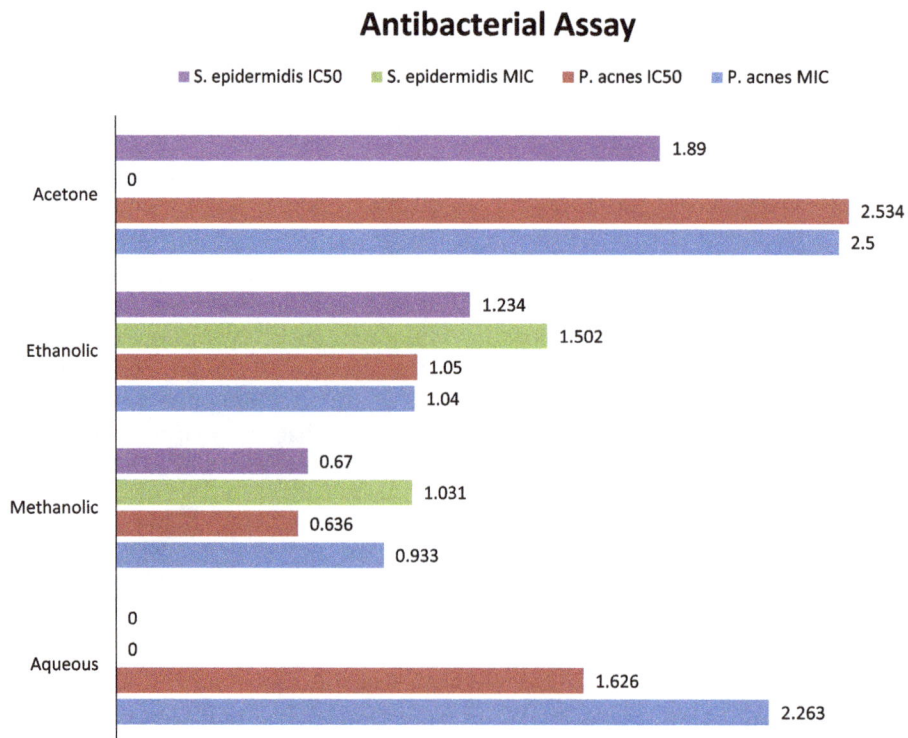

**Fig. 3** Graphical presentation of activity of *Olea europaea* leaf extracts (acetone, ethanol, methanol and aqueous) in IC50 and MIC (mg/ml) against *S. epidermidis* and *P. acnes*

**Table 1** Antibacterial activity of *Olea europaea* leaf extracts of different solvent along with standard against *P. acnes* and *S. epidermidis*

| Pathogenic microbe | Bactericidal activity (IC50 and MIC mg/ml) | | | | | | | | | |
|---|---|---|---|---|---|---|---|---|---|---|
| P. acnes | Olea europaea | | | | | | | | Standard drug (Tetracycline) | |
| | Aqueous | | Methanolic | | Ethanolic | | Acetone | | | |
| | IC50 | MIC | IC50 | MIC | IC50 | MIC | IC50 | MIC | IC50 | MIC |
| | 1.626 | 2.263 | 0.636 | 0.933 | 1.040 | 1.050 | 2.500 | 2.534 | 0.013 | 0.028 |
| S. epidermidis | Range (NA) | Range (NA) | 0.670 | 1.031 | 1.234 | 1.502 | 1.890 | Range (NA) | 0.106 | 0.159 |

NA not active at particular concentration

acetone MIC: 2.534/IC$_{50}$:2.500) as compared to aerobic bacteria *S. epidermidis* (methanolic extracts MIC: 1.031, IC$_{50}$:0.670, ethanolic extracts MIC: 1.502/IC$_{50}$: 1.234, aqueous extracts MIC: Range/IC$_{50}$: Range and acetone extracts MIC: Range/IC$_{50}$:1.890). These quantitative value were compared by standard (tetracycline) against *P.acnes* (MIC: 0.028, IC$_{50}$: 0.013) and *S. epidermidis* (MIC: 0.159, IC$_{50}$:0.106) (Table 1).

The *Olea europaea* L. leaves have a tremendous history of traditional therapeutic uses (antimicrobial and antioxidant) [21]. Olive leaves are acknowledged for the secondary metabolites such as oleacein oleuropein [22, 23] Flavonoids and tannins etc. were among the major phenolic contents present in plant extracts [24]. The phenolic radicals were testified to be less reactive and retain lower electron reduction potential than the oxygen radicals [25]. Owing to these properties, the phenolic compounds are reflected as excellent radical scavengers. Thus our study, correspondingly evaluates the total phenolic content and flavonoid content along with radicals scavenging activity by DPPH assay. Our data have validated that the mean phenolic content (PC) in olive leaf extracts in terms of mg dispense from 16.9 to 25.6 mg and flavonoid content (FC) from 9.5 to 24.1 respectively (Table 2). Our results showed that methanolic, ethanolic and acetone extracts had the highest amount of phenolic content as well as flavonoid than aqueous extract [26, 27]. In general, the obtained data showed a statistical significant correlation between leaves extracts (of all the solvents) phytoconstituents analyses, *i.e.* total phenols and total flavonoids.

Higher the antioxidant concentration (in solvent) higher will be the percentage of DPPH scavenging activity of a compound and better will be the antioxidant activity. Further, DPPH radical scavenging activity was found to agree with total phenolics and total flavonoids outcomes. The present data revealed methanolic extracts of olive leaves exhibited appreciative higher free radical scavenging activity, followed by ethanolic ≥ acetone ≥ aqueous respectively, using DPPH. Free radical scavenging DPPH assay data dispensed from 14.7 to 92.5 (Table 2). These values were compared to the value obtained using standard (91.8 μg/ml). These data were also in statistical significant correlation with the data of total phenols and flavonoids. The hight free radical scavenging activity would be due to the high content of phenolic compounds in methanolic extractof *O. europaea* leaf especially oleuropein and hydroxytyrosol [28]. The reducing properties of polyphenols as hydrogen or electron-donating agents relay their potential for free-radical scavengers (antioxidants). Polyphenols holds an ideal chemical structure for free radical-scavenging activities and most of them have been shown to be strong antioxidants in vitro than vitamin E [29]. It has been demonstrated that hydroxytyrosol is empowered with a potent antioxidant activity due to the ortho diphenol function. Thus, the high antioxidant activities of oleuropein can be described by

**Table 2** Phenolic content, Flavonoid content and DPPH radical scavenging activity of *Olea europaea* L. leaf extracts along with standard

| Extraction solvent | Phenolic content | Total Flavonoid | DPPH radical scavenging activity (μg/ml) | | | | |
|---|---|---|---|---|---|---|---|
| | | | 10 | 50 | 100 | 500 | 1000 |
| Methanolic extracts | 25.6 | 24.1 | 14.7 | 23.5 | 66.1 | 75.2 | 92.5 |
| Ethanolic extracts | 24.0 | 19.5 | 14.1 | 22.9 | 64.6 | 70.2 | 86.8 |
| Acetone extracts | 24.8 | 17.3 | 11.9 | 17.6 | 45.2 | 60.5 | 80.8 |
| Aqueous extracts | 16.9 | 9.5 | 10.5 | 11.6 | 24.3 | 35.2 | 70.5 |
| Standard | | | | | | | 91.2 |

the presence of hydroxytyrosol unit in its structure [30, 31].

Regarding antimicrobial properties, OLE exhibits high antibacterial activity against anaerobic and aerobic bacteria causing *acne vulgaris*, this activity isalso in correlation with the data of above discussed results. The presence of phenolic content confers *O. europaea* L. natural resistance to microbe (Gram negative, Gram positive) outbreak [32]. Studies have demonstrated that the phenolic compounds may also stimulates anti-inflammatory effects of lipoxygenase activity, leukotriene B4 production [33] and hindering biosynthesis of pro-inflammatory cytokines [34] or tempering inflammatory parameters [35]. Likewise COX-2, an enzyme involved in the generation of some inflammatory mediators (TNF-αand IL-1β mediated enzyme) and the expression of these inflammation inducing enzymes, interleukins and tumor necrosis factors were reported to be attenuated significantly with the treatment of Olive-derived phenolic compounds [36, 37]. All these activities of OLE confer antibacterial activity against pathogens of *Acne vulgaris*.

## Conclusions

The developing natural therapies encase naturally derived drugs from active plant extracts, essential oilsand phytomolecules. The antibacterial and antioxidant potential of the olive leaf extracts can be attributed to its high contents of phenols, flavonoids and vitamin C that act synergistically. Although there is an observed significant variation in chemical constituents and biological activities of olive leaf extracts treated with different solvents, the current findings support that this medicinal plant *Olea europaea* L. is a promising source of potential antibacterial and antioxidants that may be efficient therapeutic agent in the pathogenesis of *acne vulgaris* and proves potential source of Cosmeceuticals.

### Acknowledgement
The authors would like to expresstheir gratitude to Head, Department of Botany, and University of Allahabad to providing research facilities, UGC, New Delhi for financial support, Mr. Rick Z for providing anaerobic jar and Moti Lal Nehru Medical College, Allahabad for providing the anaerobic culturing facilities.

### Authors' contributions
AQ conducted the experiments and design conception and conduction of research. Data interpretation and analysis were done by MP participated in drafting the manuscript revised the manuscript critically for important intellectual content. RK critically reviews the manuscript. AD made the necessary corrections in the write up and gave final approval for the submission of revised version. All authors read and approved the final manuscript.

### Competing interests
The authors declare that they have no competing interests.

### References

1. Kumar R, Shukla SK, Pandey A, Pandey H, Pathak A and Dikshit A: Dermatophytosis: Infection and Prevention -A Review. Int J Pharm Sci Res 2016;7(8):3218-25.
2. Tsatsanis C, Androulidaki A, Venihaki M, Margioris AN. Signalling networks regulating cyclooxygenase-2. Int J Biochem Cell Biol. 2006;38:1654-61.
3. Makari H, Haraprasad N, Patil H, Ravi k. In vitro antioxidant activity of the hexane and methanolic extracts of Cordia Wallichii and Celastrus paniculata. The Internet J. Aesthetic and Antiaging Med.. 2008; 1: 1-10
4. Ghanbari R, Anwar F, Alkharfy KM, Gilani AH, Saari N. Valuable nutrients and functional bioactives in different parts of olive (Olea europaea L.)-A review. Int J Mol Sci. 2012;13:3291-340.
5. Cicerale S, Conlan XA, Sinclair AJ, Keast RS. Chemistry and health of olive oil phenolics. Crit Rev Food Sci Nutr. 2009;49:218-36.
6. Cicerale S, Lucas L, Keast R. Biological activities of phenolic compounds present in virgin olive oil. Int J Mol Sci. 2010;11:458-79.
7. Armstrong D, Browne R. Free Rad. Diag Med. 1994;366:43-58.
8. Visioli F, Bellomo G, Montedoro G, Galli C. Low density lipoprotein oxidation is inhibited in vitro by olive oil constituents. Atherosclerosis. 1995;117:25-32.
9. Chimento A, Casaburi I, Rosano C, Avena P, De Luca A, Campana C, Martire E, Santolla MF, et al. Oleuropein and hydroxytyrosol activate gper/gpr30dependent pathways leading to apoptosis of er-negative skbr3 breast cancer cells. Mol Nutr Food Res. 2013;58:478-9.
10. Carrera-González MP, Ramírez-Expósito MJ, Mayas MD, Martínez-Martos JM. Protective role of oleuropein and its metabolite hydroxytyrosol on cancer. Trends Food Sci Technol. 2013;31:92-9.
11. Cardeno A, Sanchez-Hidalgo M, Rosillo MA, AlarcondelaLastra C. Oleuropein, a secoiridoid derived from olive tree, inhibits the proliferation of human colorectal cancer cell through downregulation of hif-1alpha. Nutr Cancer. 2013;65:147-56.
12. Miles EA, Zoubouli P, Calder PC. Differential anti-inflammatory effects of phenolic compounds from extra virgin olive oil identified in human whole blood cultures. Nutrition. 2005;21:389-94.
13. Qidwai A, Pandey M, Shukla SK, Pandey A, Kumar R, Dikshit A. Risk factor assessment for Acne vulgaris in human and implications for public health interventions in north central India: A survey based study. 2017;10(5):404-409.
14. Qidwai A, Pandey M, Pathak S, Kumar R, Dikshit A. The emerging principles for acne biogenesis: A dermatological problem of puberty. Human Microbiome Journal. 2017;4:7-13.
15. Arabshahi S, Urooj A. Antioxidant properties of various solvent extracts of mulberry (Morusindica L.) leaves. Food Chem. 2007;102:1233-40.
16. Kim D, Jeong S, Lee C. Antioxidant capacity of phenolic phytochemicals from various cultivars of plums. Food Chem. 2003;81:321-26.
17. Shimada K, Fujikawa K, Yahara K, Nakamura T. Antioxidative properties of xanthone on the auto oxidation of soybean in cylcodextrin emulsion. J Agr Food Chem. 1992;40:945-8.
18. Methods for dilution antimicrobial susceptibility tests for bacteria that grow aerobically (5th Ed.). Approved standard, M7-A5. Pennsylvania: Wayne. NCCLS, 2003.
19. Qidwai A, Pandey M, Shukla SK, Kumar R, Pandey A, Dikshit A. Antibacterial activity of mentha piperita and citrus limetta against *Propionibacterium acnes* (anaerobic bacteria). Int J Pharma Sci Res. 2016;7(7):2917-24.
20. Pathak A, Shukla SK, Pandey A, Mishra RK, Kumar R, Dikshit A. In vitro antibacterial activity of Ethno medicinally used lichens against three wound infecting genera of Enterobacteriaceae. Proc. Natl. Acad. Sci. India B Biol. 2015;86:1-2.
21. Soni MG, Burdock GA, Christian MS, Bitler CM, Crea R. Safety assessment of aqueous olive pulp extract as an antioxidant or antimicrobial agent in foods. Food ChemToxicol. 2006;44:903-15.
22. Pereira AP, Ferreira ICFR, Marcelino F, et al. Phenolic compounds and antimicrobial activity of olive (Olea europaea L. Cv. Cobrançosa) leaves. Molecules. 2007;12:1153-62.
23. Sato H, Genet C, Strehle A, et al. Anti-hyperglycemic activity of a TGR5 agonist isolated from Olea europaea. BiochemBiophys Res Commun. 2007; 362:793-8.
24. Kaur C, Kapoor HC. Anti-oxidant activity and total phenolic content of some Asian vegetables. Int. J. Food Sci. Technol., 2002;37:pp.153-161.

25. Gillespie KM, Chae JM, Ainsworth EA. Rapid measurement of total antioxidant capacity in plants. Nat Protocols. 2007;2(4):867–70.
26. Ali MA, Nancy SR, Aboubaker MG, Said KA. Antibacterial effect of olive (Olea europaea L.) leaves extract in raw peeled undeveined shrimp (Penaeus semisulcatus). Int J. of Veterin Sci and Med . 2014;2(1):53–56.
27. Ainsworth EA, Gillespie KM. Estimation of total phenolic content and other oxidation substrates in plant tissues using Folin-Ciocalteu reagent. Nat Protocols. 2007;2(4):875–7.
28. Khlif I, Jellali K, Michel T, Halabalaki M, Skaltsounis AL, Allouche N. Characteristics, phytochemical analysis and biological activities of extracts from Tunisian chetoui olea europaeaVariety. J Chem. 2015;2015:11.
29. Goldsmith CD, Vuong QV, Stathopoulos CE, Roach PD, Scarlett CJ. Optimization of the aqueous extraction of phenolic compounds from olive leaves. Antioxidants. 2014;3(4):700–12.
30. Allouche N, Fki I, Sayadi S. Toward a high yield recovery of antioxidants and purified hydroxytyrosol from olive mill wastewaters. J Agri Food Chem. 2004;52(2):267–73.
31. Cicerale S, Lucas LJ, Keast RS. Antimicrobial, antioxidant and anti-inflammatory phenolic activities in extra virgin olive oil. Curr Opin Biotechnol. 2012;23:129–35.
32. Sousa A, Ferreira IC, Barros L, Bento A, Pereira JA. Effect of solvent and extraction temperatures on the antioxidant potential of traditional stoned table olives "alcaparras". LWT-Food Sci Tech. 2008;41(4):739–45.
33. Lee OH, Lee BY, Lee J, Lee HB, Son JY, Park CS, Shetty K, Kim YC. Assessment of phenolics-enriched extract and fractions of olive leaves and their antioxidant activities. Biores tech. 2009;100(23):6107–13.
34. Lihu Y, Yueming J, Datta N. HPLC analyses of flavanol and phenolic acids in the fresh young shoots of tea (Camellia sinesis) grown in Australia. Food Chem. 2004;84:253–63.
35. Manian R, Anusuya N, Siddhuraju P, Manian S. The antioxidant activity and free radical scavenging potential of two different solvent extracts of Camellia sinensis (L.) O. Kuntz, Ficusbengalensis L. and Ficusracemosa L. Food Chem. 2008;107:1000–7.
36. Pandey M, Pandey A, Kumar R, Pathak A, Dikshit A. A Comparative antimicrobial analysis of Tridaxprocumbens L. various extracts on waterborne bacterial pathogens. Int Cur Pharma J. 2016;5(3):22–6.
37. Goldsmith CD, Vuong QV, Sadeqzadeh E, Stathopoulos CE, Roach DE, Scarlett CJ. Phytochemical Properties and Anti-Proliferative Activity of Olea europaea L. Leaf Extracts against Pancreatic Cancer Cells. Molecules. 2015;20:12992-13004.

# 16

# Caffeic acid rich *Citrus macroptera* peel powder supplementation prevented oxidative stress, fibrosis and hepatic damage in CCl$_4$ treated rats

Md Ashraful Alam[1*†], Abu Taher Sagor[1†], Nabila Tabassum[1], Anayt Ulla[1], Manik Chandra Shill[1], Ghazi Muhammad Sayedur Rahman[1], Hemayet Hossain[2] and Hasan Mahmud Reza[1*]

## Abstract

**Background:** *Citrus macroptera* has been used as a culinary fruit and medicinal plant in traditional medicine system in Bangladesh. The aim of the present study was to evaluate the presence of phenolic compounds in *Citrus macroptera* peel powder and the protective effect of *Citrus macroptera* against carbon tetrachloride (CCl$_4$)-induced liver injury in rats.

**Methods:** The hepatoprotective activity was assessed using various biochemical parameters such as liver marker enzymes (alanine aminotransferase (ALT), aspartate aminotransferase (AST), alkaline phosphatase (ALP)) and oxidative stress parameters. Histopathological changes in the liver of different groups were also studied.

**Results:** Administration of CCl$_4$ increased the serum ALT, AST, ALP enzymatic activities and lipid peroxidation products but decreased the cellular antioxidant activities and reduced glutathione (GSH) levels in rats which were brought back to near normal levels by the treatment with *Citrus macroptera*. *Citrus macroptera* administration has also shown to decrease the necrotic zones, fibrosis and inflammatory cell infiltration in CCl$_4$ treated rats. HPLC-DAD analysis of *Citrus macroptera* extract showed the great presence of caffeic acid and (−) epicatechin.

**Conclusion:** The results of this study suggest that *Citrus macroptera* exerts hepatoprotective activity via promoting the antioxidant defense against CCl$_4$-induced oxidative liver damage.

**Keywords:** *Citrus macroptera*, Oxidative stress, Fibrosis, Inflammation, Caffeic acid

## Background

Hepatotoxicity is a growing public health concern in modern society due to the increasing incidence of alcoholism, cigarette smoking, drug abuse and other unhealthy lifestyle options such as consuming high fructose-containing beverages and high fat containing foods. Liver damage is characterized by a progressive development of steatosis to chronic hepatitis, fibrosis, cirrhosis, and hepatocellular carcinoma [1, 2]. Oxidative stress plays a central role in the development of liver diseases. Carbon tetrachloride (CCl$_4$) is a widely used solvent in chemical industries and well known for its hepatic and renal toxic actions. It is also used to establish experimental animal model of hepatic dysfunction in the laboratory [3, 4]. The metabolism of CCl$_4$ occurs mainly in the liver by CYP450 enzyme system into trichloromethyl ($^{\cdot}$CCl$_3$) and peroxy trichloromethyl ($^{\cdot}$OOCCl$_3$) free radicals which have been reported to cause hepatotoxic effects, like fibrosis, steatosis, necrosis, and hepatocarcinoma [3, 5]. Chronic insult to the liver due to hepatotoxins, alcohol consumption and high-calorie diet triggers inflammation and fibrosis [4]. Liver fibrosis is a dynamic process where oxidative stresses are responsible for the activation of hepatic stellate cells (HSCs) [6]. HSCs are the major cell types responsible for the deposition of a large amount of extracellular matrix

* Correspondence: sonaliagun@yahoo.com; ashraful.alam@northsouth.edu; hasan.reza@northsouth.edu
†Equal contributors
[1]Department of Pharmaceutical Sciences, North South University, Dhaka, Bangladesh
Full list of author information is available at the end of the article

(ECM) and collagen in liver [7]. CCl₄-mediated liver fibrosis is characterized by activation of Kupffer cells and induction of an inflammatory response by secreting cytokines, chemokines and other pro-inflammatory factors [8]. CCl₄ treatment also attracts more inflammatory cells in liver apart from Kuffer cells and further contributes to liver necrosis [8]. High level of lipid peroxidation products and decreased antioxidant levels were also noted in CCl₄ mediated hepatic dysfunction in animal [9]. As oxidative stress plays a central role in liver pathologies and their progression, the use of antioxidants would have been an alternative therapeutic approach to counteract the liver damage. Citrus fruits are a rich source of natural antioxidants and showed beneficial role in various degenerative diseases [10]. Caffeic acid was found in high amount compared to other phenolic compounds in *Citrus macroptera* peel which is a strong antioxidant compound [11]. Caffeic acid also showed hepatic protection and prevented fibrosis in various experimental animal models [12–14]. This hepatoprotective activity of caffeic acid is linked to improved antioxidant defense and inflammatory state in liver [11, 15].

*Citrus macroptera* is known as 'Satkara' in Bengali and 'Wild orange' in English. It is a semi-wild species of citrus fruits which is native to the regions of Southeast Asia and found in large amount in Sylhet Division of Bangladesh. The fruit is used as a cooking ingredient in different kinds of meats and as an aromatic vegetable in Bangladesh. Meats cooked with satkara are now served in many Bangladeshi/Indian restaurants in the United Kingdom. *Citrus macroptera* (Satkara) fruit is also used as an appetite stimulant and in the treatment of fever as reported in the traditional system of medicine in Bangladesh. The previous report suggested that *Citrus macroptera* contains mainly lupeol and stigmasterol [16]. Other studies conducted on the bark and leaves of the *Citrus macroptera* reported the antioxidant and antimicrobial activities [16, 17]. A recent investigation also suggests that *Citrus macroptera* extract showed in-vitro α-amylase inhibitory activity and hypoglycemic activity in normal rats [18]. We recently reported the hepatoprotective activity of *Citrus maxima* peel powder in CCl₄ treated rats [19]. However, limited data and few scientific literatures are available on any therapeutic effect of *Citrus macroptera* in liver diseases. Therefore, this current research was designed to understand the possible anti-inflammatory and anti-fibrotic activity of *Citrus macroptera* peel powder in hepatic dysfunction in CCl₄ treated rats.

## Methods

### Chemicals

Arbutin (AR), gallic acid (GA), hydroquinone (HQ), (+)-catechin hydrate (CH), vanillic acid (VA), caffeic acid (CA), Syringic acid (SA), (–)-epicatechin (EC), vanillin (VL), *p*-coumaric acid (PCA), *trans*-ferulic acid (FA), rutin hydrate (RH), ellagic acid (EA), benzoic acid (BA), rosmarinic acid (RA), myricetin (MC), quercetin (QU), *trans*-cinnamic acid (TCA), and kaempferol (KF) were purchased from Sigma–Aldrich (St. Louis, MO, USA). Acetonitrile (HPLC), methanol (HPLC), acetic acid (HPLC), and ethanol were obtained from Merck (Darmstadt, Germany).

### Plant material

*Citrus macroptera* fruits were collected from Sylhet, Bangladesh and authenticated by Sarker Nasir Uddin, Senior Scientific Officer, National Herbarium, Mirpur, Dhaka. A voucher specimen (Acc. No. 40847) was deposited in the herbarium for future reference. The peels were removed and dried for further processing. The dried peels were grinded to fine powder using an electric grinder machine and mixed with the food directly as supplementation. A portion of the dried peel powder was used to prepare crude ethanol extract and used for polyphenol detection and quantification.

### High performance liquid Chromatograpgy (HPLC) detection and quantification of polyphenolic compounds

Detection and quantification of selected phenolic compounds in the ethanol extract were determined by HPLC-DAD analysis as described by Ismet et al. [20] with some modifications. It was carried out on a Dionex UltiMate 3000 system equipped with quaternary rapid separation pump (LPG-3400RS) and photodiode array detector (DAD-3000RS). Separation was performed using Acclaim® C₁₈ (5 µm) Dionex column (4.6 × 250 mm) at 30 °C with a flow rate of 1 ml/min and an injection volume of 20 µl. For the preparation of calibration curve, a standard stock solution was prepared in methanol containing arbutin, (–)-epicatechin (5 µg/ml each), gallic acid, hydroquinone, vanillic acid, rosmarinic acid, myricetin (4 µg/ml each), caffeic acid, Syringic acid, vanillin, *trans*-ferulic acid (3 µg/ml each), *p*-coumaric acid, quercetin, kaempferol (2 µg/ml each), (+)-catechin hydrate, ellagic acid (10 µg/ml each), *trans*-cinnamic acid (1 µg/ml), rutin hydrate (6 µg/ml) and benzoic acid (8 µg/ml). The UV detector was set to 280 nm for 22.0 min, changed to 320 nm for 28.0 min, again change to 280 nm for 35 min and finally to 380 nm for 36 min and held for the rest of the analysis period while the diode array detector was set at an acquisition range from 200 nm to 700 nm.

### Animals and treatment

Ten to 12 weeks old, 24 Long Evans female rats (150–170 g) were obtained from Animal breeding unit of Animal House at the Department of Pharmaceutical Sciences, North South University and were kept in individual cages at room temperature of $25 \pm 3$ °C with a 12 h dark/light cycles. They had free access to standard laboratory feed and water, according to the study protocol approved by Ethical Committee of Department of Pharmaceutical Sciences, North South University for animal care and experimentation. To evaluate the hepatoprotective effect of *Citrus macroptera*, rats were equally divided into four groups (six rats in each group). The groups are as follows-

Group I- Animals were treated with 1 ml/kg of saline (0.85%) and olive oil (1 ml/kg) intragastrically twice a week for 2 weeks

Group II- Animals were treated with 1 ml/kg of saline (0.85%) and olive oil (1 ml/kg) intragastrically twice a week for 2 weeks. Animals of group II also received *Citrus macroptera* fruit peel powder supplementation mixed with food (0.5% of the diet, *w/w*).

Group III – Animals were treated with $CCl_4$ (1:3 in olive oil) at a dose of 1 ml/kg intragastrically twice a week for 2 weeks.

Group IV- Animals were treated with $CCl_4$ (1:3 in olive oil) at a dose of 1 ml/kg intragastrically twice a week for 2 weeks. Animals of group IV also received *Citrus macroptera* fruit peel powder mixed in food (0.5% of the diet, w/w) respectively, in addition to $CCl_4$ treatment, twice a week for 2 weeks.

Animals of group I were served as control animals. Animals were checked for the body weight, food and water intake on a daily basis. After 14 days, all animals were weighted and sacrificed, collected the blood in citrate buffer containing tubes and all the organs such as heart, kidney, spleen, and liver were havested. Immediately after collection of the organs, they are weighted and one part was stored in neutral buffered formalin (pH 7.4) for histological analysis and another part was kept in the refrigerator at – 20 °C for further studies. The collected blood was centrifuged at 8000 rpm and separated the plasma and stored in a refrigerator at – 20 °C for further analysis.

## Assessment of hepatotoxicity

Liver marker enzymes (alanine aminotransferase (ALT), aspartate aminotransferase (AST), and alkaline phosphatase (ALP)) were estimated in plasma by using Diatec diagnostic kits (Hungary) according to the manufacturer's protocol.

## Preparation of tissue sample for the assessment of oxidative stress markers

For determination of oxidative stress markers, 0.2 g of liver tissue was homogenized in 1.8 mL Phosphate buffer (pH 7.4) and centrifuged at 10000 rpm for 30 min at 4 °C.

The supernatant was collected and used for the determination of protein and enzymatic studies as described below.

## Estimation of lipid peroxidation

Lipid peroxidation in liver was estimated colorimetrically measuring thiobarbituric acid reactive substances (TBARS) followed by previously described method [21].

## Assay of nitric oxide (NO)

Nitric oxide (NO) was determined according to the method described by Tracey et al. as nitrate [22]. In this study, Griess-Illosvoy reagent was modified by using naphthyl ethylenediamine dihydrochloride (0.1% *w/v*) instead of 1-naphthylamine (5%).

## Advanced protein oxidation products (APOP) assay:

APOP levels were measured by a modification of the method of Witko-Sarsat et al. [23] and Tiwari et al. [24]. APOP concentrations were expressed as $nmol \cdot mL^{-1}$ chloramine-T equivalents.

## Catalase assay (CAT)

CAT activities were determined using previously described the method by Chance and Maehly [25]. One unit of CAT activity was defined as an absorbance change of 0.01 as units/min.

## Reduced glutathione assay (GSH)

Reduced glutathione was estimated by the method of Jollow et al. [26]. 1.0 ml sample of 10% homogenate was precipitated with 1.0 ml of (4%) sulfosalicylic acid. The samples were kept at 4 °C for 1 h and then centrifuged at 4000 rpm for 20 min at 4 °C. The total volume of 3. 0 ml assay mixture composed of 0.1 ml filtered aliquot, 2.7 ml phosphate buffer (0.1 M, pH 7.4) and 0.2 ml DTNB (5,5-dithiobis-2-nitrobenzoic acid), (100 mM). The mixture which was developed as yellow color, UV absorbance was taken immediately at 412 nm on a Smart SpecTM plus Spectrophotometer and the content of GSH was expressed as ng/mg protein.

## Histopathological determination

For microscopic evaluation, liver tissues were fixed in neutral buffered formalin and embedded in paraffin, sectioned at 5 μm and subsequently stained with hematoxylin/eosin to see the architecture of hepatic tissue and inflammatory cell infiltration. Liver injury score in the Hematoxylin/ eosin stained sections were evaluated as follows: 0, minimal or no evidence of injury; 1, mild injury consisting of cytoplasmic vacuolation and focal nuclear pyknosis; 2, moderate to severe injury with extensive nuclear pyknosis and loss of intercellular borders and 3, severe necrosis with disintegration of hepatic cords, hemorrhage and neutrophil infiltration. All evaluations were made in 3 fields per section and 3 sections per liver.

Sirius red staining for fibrosis and Prussian blue staining for iron deposition were also done in liver sections. Sections were then studied and photographed under a light microscope (Zeiss Axioscope) at 40 magnifications. Collagen deposition was semiquantitatively measured using NIH Image J free software (Version 1.48v).

## Statistical analysis

All values are expressed as a mean ± standard error of the mean (SEM). The results were evaluated by using the One-way ANOVA followed by Bonferroni test using Graph Pad Prism Software, version 6. Statistical significance was considered $p < 0.05$ in all cases.

## Results
### Effect on body weight, food, and water intake

Body weight of each rat was recorded every day during the experiment, and % change was calculated for all groups. It was found that the body weight decreased significantly in $CCl_4$-intoxicated rat group, which is a typical feature of chronic liver intoxication. On the other hand, treatment of $CCl_4$ treated group with Citrus macroptera markedly improved the weight loss of rats (Table 1). $CCl_4$ treated rats group showed significant decrease in food, and water intake compared to control rats. Reduction of food and water intake in $CCl_4$ treated rats group was further improved in Citrus macroptera treated group (Table 1).

### Effect on organ wet weight

Table 1 shows the effect of various treatments on the rats' organs weight. The spleen wet weight was significantly ($p = 0.012$) increased in the $CCl_4$-treated rats compared to control rats. Citrus macroptera (0.5% per kg of diet) treatment did not significantly attenuate the wet weight of the spleen in the $CCl_4$-treated rats. $CCl_4$-

treated rats also showed decreased in liver wet weight; however, Citrus macroptera supplementation did not change the wet weight of the liver compared to the control. Another crucial finding in this study was the reduction of kidney wet weight due to $CCl_4$ intoxication which was normalized by Citrus macroptera supplementation (Table 1). Wet weights of the heart were relatively unchanged among the groups tested in this study (Table 1).

### Effect on biochemical parameter of liver functions

Biochemical assay of liver function markers revealed that $CCl_4$ administration in rats induced a significant ($p < 0.05$) increase in plasma AST ($p = 0.036$), ALT ($p < 0.0001$), and ALP ($p < 0.0001$) activity compared to control rats, respectively (Table 2). Citrus macroptera (0.5% of diet) supplementation concurrently with $CCl_4$ significantly ($p < 0.05$) counteracted the alteration in all hepatotoxicity indices compared to the $CCl_4$-treated group. In addition, supplementation with Citrus macroptera alone in the diet for 2 weeks in normal control rats did not show any significant change in liver enzymes compared to the control rats (Table 2).

### Oxidative stress markers and antioxidant enzymes

To determine the oxidative stress in our study, we evaluated the MDA, nitric oxide and APOP concentration in plasma and liver homogenates. $CCl_4$ administration in rats showed an increased lipid peroxidation product, MDA concentration both in plasma ($p < 0.0001$) and in liver ($p = 0.0004$) homogenates significantly ($p < 0.05$) (Table 2). Additionally, Citrus macroptera (0.5% of diet) supplementation significantly (p < 0.05) reduced the level of lipid peroxides compared to $CCl_4$ intoxicated group.

$CCl_4$ administration in rats also increased APOP development in plasma and in liver compared to control rats significantly ($p < 0.0001$). Citrus macroptera (0.5% of diet) supplementation in $CCl_4$ intoxicated rats significantly ($p <$

**Table 1** Effect of Citrus macroptera peel powder supplementation on body weight, food and water intake and organ weight of $CCl_4$ treated rats

| Parameters | Control | Control+Citrus macroptera | $CCl_4$ | $CCl_4$ + Citrus macroptera |
|---|---|---|---|---|
| Initial Bodyweight (g) | 156.07 ± 2.38 | 165.63 ± 2.99 ns | 162.92 ± 4.81nss | 162.67 ± 1.52 ns |
| Final Bodyweight (g) | 167.37 ± 4.05 | 182.40 ± 5.95 ns | 165.92 ± 5.23 ns | 174.20 ± 3.16 ns |
| Food intake/d (g/day) | 16.49 ± 0.88 | 15.68 ± 0.97a | 12.21 ± 0.54a | 15.03 ± 0.57b |
| Water intake/d (ml/day) | 18.85 ± 0.62 | 20.11 ± 1.20 ns | 13.44 ± 0.73a | 15.20 ± 0.78b |
| Liver wet weight (g/100 g of body weight) | 3.67 ± 0.15 | 3.68 ± 0.06 ns | 3.32 ± 0.09 ns | 3.47 ± 0.05 ns |
| Kidneys wet weight (g/100 g of body weight) | 0.62 ± 0.02 | 0.56 ± 0.04 ns | 0.53 ± 0.02a | 0.62 ± 0.01b |
| Heart wet weight (g/100 g of body weight) | 0.34 ± 0.01 | 0.28 ± 0.00 | 0.31 ± 0.02 | 0.30 ± 0.01 |
| Spleen wet weight (g/100 g of body weight) | 0.31 ± 0.03 | 0.39 ± 0.02 ns | 0.46 ± 0.04a | 0.41 ± 0.02 ns |

Values are presented as mean ± SEM. N = 6 in each group or otherwise specified. One way ANOVA with Bonferoni tests were done as post hoc test. Values are considered significance at $p < 0.05$. control vs $CCl_4$ significanltly different at a < 0.05. $CCl_4$ vs Citrus macroptera treatment which are significantly different at b < 0.05. ns- non significant

**Table 2** Effect of *Citrus macroptera* peel powder supplementation on biochemical parameters in plasma and liver of CCl$_4$ treated rats

| Parameters | Groups | | | |
|---|---|---|---|---|
| | Control | Control+*Citrus macroptera* | CCl$_4$ | CCl$_4$ + *Citrus macroptera* |
| Plasma | | | | |
| AST(U/L) | 34.45 ± 3.85 | 35.89 ± 3.46 ns | 65.46 ± 8.87a | 47.37 ± 4.85b |
| ALT(U/L) | 30.15 ± 2.94 | 31.58 ± 2.87 ns | 66.04 ± 2.87a | 43.07 ± 5.88b |
| ALP(U/L) | 57.60 ± 1.38 | 33.76 ± 4.95b | 80.35 ± 5.58a | 37.57 ± 7.21b |
| MDA(nmol/mL) | 7.27 ± 0.19 | 11.01 ± 0.47 ns | 17.27 ± 1.79a | 9.81 ± 0.42b |
| NO (nmol/mL) | 3.87 ± 0.27 | 4.43 ± 0.70 ns | 6.80 ± 0.65a | 3.42 ± 0.61b |
| APOP (nmol/mL equivalent to Chloramine-T) | 228.33 ± 10.66 | 326.35 ± 56.23 ns | 736.27 ± 54.83a | 347.38 ± 26.18b |
| GSH (ng/mg protein) | 11.85 ± 0.51 | 11.25 ± 0.74 ns | 7.50 ± 0.40a | 13.63 ± 1.22b |
| Catalase (U/min) | 7.17 ± 0.79 | 10.50 ± 1.20 ns | 5.33 ± 1.05 ns | 7.00 ± 1.06 ns |
| Liver | | | | |
| NO (nmol/mL) | 14.12 ± 0.91 | 12.35 ± 0.92 ns | 15.87 ± 2.23 ns | 12.47 ± 1.20 ns |
| MDA (nmol/mL) | 38.77 ± 1.84 | 40.31 ± 2.02 ns | 64.41 ± 4.89ba | 51.33 ± 5.13 ns |
| APOP (nmol/mL equivalent to Chloramine-T) | 632.06 ± 33.84 | 497.78 ± 29.20 ns | 968.57 ± 70.27a | 566.43 ± 48.60b |
| Catalase (U/min) | 20.83 ± 3.52 | 24.17 ± 3.00 ns | 14.17 ± 2.01a | 23.33 ± 2.47b |

Values are presented as mean ± SEM. N = 6 in each group or otherwise specified. One way ANOVA with Bonferroni tests were done as post hoc test. Values are considered significant at $p < 0.05$. Values are considered significance at $p < 0.05$. control vs CCl$_4$ significanltly different a < 0.05. CCl$_4$ vs *Citrus macroptera* treatment which are significantly different at b < 0.05. ns- non significant. APOP-Advanced protein oxidation product expressed as nmol/mL equivalent to Chloramine-T

0.05) reduced the APOP concentration in plasma and liver tissue homogenates significantly (Table 2).

NO measured as nitrate was also increased significantly ($p = 0.0027$) in plasma of CCl$_4$ administered rats compared to control rats (Table 2). *Citrus macroptera* (0.5% of diet) supplementation (Table 2) in CCl$_4$ administered rats normalized the elevated the NO level in plasma. However, NO level was not changed significantly in liver homogenates of CCl$_4$ administered rats compared to control rats. This effect could be attributed to the rapid excretion of nitrate into the plasma from liver tissues.

CCl$_4$ administration also decreased plasma antioxidant such as GSH concentration ($p = 0.0002$) compared to the control rats (Table 2). *Citrus macroptera* (0.5% of diet) supplementation in CCl$_4$ administered rat significantly counteracted the oxidative stress by restoring the antioxidant GSH concentration compared to the CCl$_4$ administered rats (Table 2). Moreover, catalase activity was decreased in CCl$_4$ administered rats compared to control rats. However, the changes were not statistically significant. *Citrus macroptera* (0.5% of diet) supplementation in CCl$_4$ administered rat increased the catalase activity compared to the CCl$_4$ administered rats (Table 2). *Citrus macroptera* (0.5% of diet) supplementation in control rats did not alter the catalase activity compared to control rats (Table 2).

**Inflammation, fibrosis iron deposition in liver**
Figure 1a showed the well-formed hepatocytes in an intact hepatic lobule of normal rat liver. However, inflammation

was seen in rats treated with CCl$_4$. A massive surge of inflammatory cells was found in the centrilobular part of liver sections stained Researchers are still working on natural plants to discover new compounds of high biological activitystaining in CCl$_4$ treated rats group (Fig. 1c). Necrotized tissue scar in liver was also seen in the liver of CCl$_4$ treated rats (Fig. 1c). *Citrus macroptera* (0.5% of diet) supplementation attenuated the inflammatory cell infiltration and necrosis in the liver tissues of CCl$_4$ treated rats (Fig. 1d). Liver fibrosis was evaluated histologically by visualizing the red color of collagen fibers using Sirius red stain. No collagen deposition was observed in control rats (Fig. 2a). Collagen fibers were heavily deposited around portal tracts and central veins in CCl$_4$-intoxicated rat's liver and extended from central vein to portal tract resulting in the formation of pseudolobules (Fig. 2c). *Citrus macroptera* (0.5% of diet) supplementation prevented the deposition of collagen fibers in the liver of CCl$_4$ treated rats (Fig. 2d).

Histological staining also revealed that no free iron was deposited in the liver of control rats (Fig. 3a) whereas high amount iron deposition was found in liver section stained for the free iron depot in CCl$_4$ treated rats (Fig. 3c). *Citrus macroptera* supplementation decreased iron deposition in CCl$_4$ treated rats (Fig. 3d).

**Analysis of ethanol extract of *Citrus macroptera* by HPLC-DAD**
Identification and quantification of individual phenolic compounds in the ethanol extract of *Citrus macroptera*

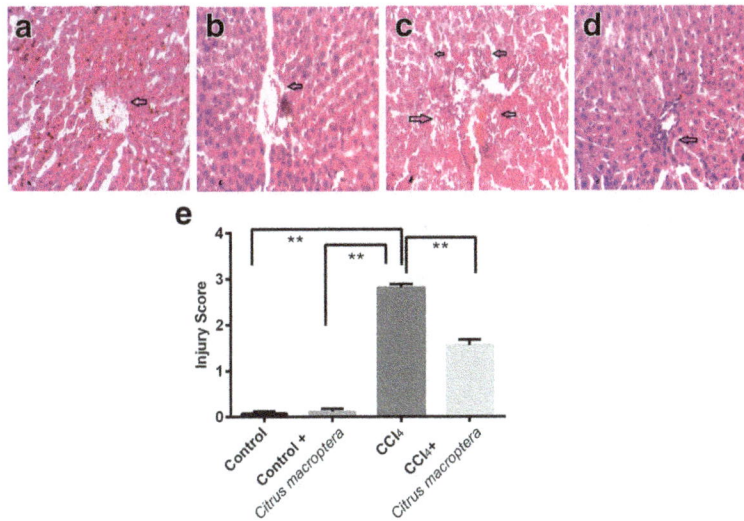

**Fig. 1** Effect of *Citrus macroptera* peel powder on hepatic inflammation in CCl$_4$ treated rats. **a**, Control, showed normal architecture of hepatocyte with no nuclear pyknosis; **b**, Control + *C macroptera*, showed normal architecture of hepatocyte with no nuclear pyknosis; **c** CCl$_4$, showed severe necrosis with disintegration of hepatic cords, hemorrhage and neutrophil infiltration and **d**, CCl$_4$+ *C macroptera*, showed reduced necrosis, less hemorrhage and minimized neutrophil infiltration. Magnification 40×. *ic*-inflammatory cells. **e**, shows the injury scores in different experimental groups after CCl$_4$ chalenge and treatment

*were* analyzed by HPLC-DAD. The chromatographic separations of polyphenols in ethanol extract are shown in Fig. 4. The content of each phenolic compound was calculated from the corresponding calibration curve and presented as the mean of five determinations as shown in Table 3. Caffeic acid was detected as the most abundant phenolic compound (428.36 mg/100 g of dry extract) found in the ethanol extract.

## Discussion

Currently, public awareness program against liver diseases such as fibrosis and cirrhosis are being aggressively focused [27]. The liver is the main organ where almost all kinds of toxins, foods as well as drugs are detoxified [28]. CCl$_4$ is metabolized in phase-I reaction and activates the ROS producing system [29]. In the current study, CCl$_4$ administration in rats developed hepatic damage by increasing lipid peroxidation and oxidative stress. CCl$_4$ administration in rats also increased

inflammatory cells infiltration and fibrosis in liver tissues. Our investigation also suggests that *Citrus macroptera* peel powder supplementation ameliorated most of the deleterious effects developed in CCl$_4$ administered rats.

The active metabolite of CCl$_4$ lead to hepatocyte damage and may initiate the leakage of a lot of hepatic enzymes (AST, ALT, and ALP) in blood circulation which was associated with immune cells infiltration, massive centrilobular apoptosis, ballooning degeneration and finally cell death [30]. Elevated liver marker enzymes activities (AST, ALP, and ALT) indicate the dysfunction and damage in the liver during disease condition [31]. This study also revealed the increased liver marker enzymes (AST, ALP, and ALT) activities in CCl$_4$ administered rats which were decreased or normalized by *Citrus macroptera* supplementation. The previous study reported that reduction of liver enzyme activity would be beneficial in case of hepatic damage protection [32]. Earlier investigations also showed that derivative of

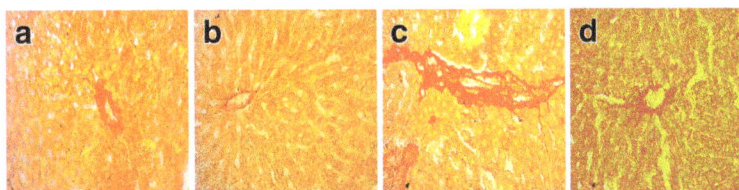

**Fig. 2** Effect of *Citrus macroptera* peel powder on hepatic fibrosis in CCl$_4$ treated rats. **a**, Control, showed baseline collagen around the hepatic duct, no fibrosis developed; **b**, Control + *C macroptera*, showed baseline collgen around the hepatic duct, no fibrosis developed; **c**, CCl$_4$, Collagen deposition and fibrosis occured around the central vein and hepatic duct. **d**, CCl$_4$+ *C macroptera*, Collagen deposition was reduced significantly around the central vein and bile duct. Magnification 40×. *fb*- fibrosis

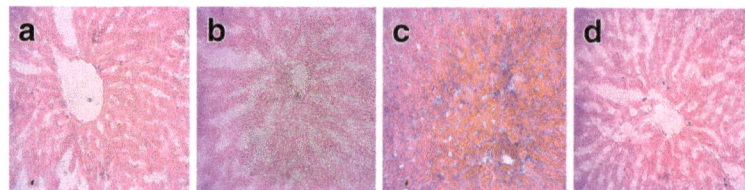

**Fig. 3** Effect of *Citrus macroptera* peel powder on hepatic iron deposition in $CCl_4$ treated rats. **a**, Control, showed no free iron deposition as seen as blue color stain; **b**, Control + *C macroptera*, showed no free iron deposition as seen as blue color stain; **c**, $CCl_4$, showed free iron deposition as seen as blue color stain and **d**, $CCl_4$ + *C macroptera*. Magnification 40×

caffeic acid also prevented the liver damage and decreased the liver marker enzymes activities [33, 34].

One of the major markers of hepatic damage is oxidative stress-mediated lipid peroxidation which plays irreversible damage to hepatocellular components. MDA is the outcome of lipid peroxidation in cell membranes and damages the integrity of cells. MDA development also causes an imbalance to lysosomes and helps to oxidize the protein [35]. Our study showed that *Citrus macroptera* supplementation decreased lipid peroxidation level in plasma and liver tissue compared to $CCl_4$ administered rats. The strong antioxidant can scavenge the free radical and superoxide anions from a biological system. Caffeic acid is a strong antioxidant showed protection against free radical-mediated lipid peroxidation in experimental animals reported previously [34].

Previous studies also reported that anti-oxidant system can reduce inflammatory, pro-inflammatory signaling by inhibiting inducible nitric oxide synthase (iNOS) which is a key factor for immunity responder [36, 37]. iNOS is considered as the major source of NO in stress condition and generates nitrosative stress. NO is a vasodilator which maintains regular vascular tone in blood vessels. It also works as a signaling molecule to produce immunological substances when the body needed [38]. However, increased production of NO in oxidative stress may turn into peroxynitrite ($^-$ONOO•) radical formation which further initiate nitrosative stress in tissues. In this study, we found that $CCl_4$ increased the level of NO in plasma but not in tissue, which was normalized by the supplementation of *Citrus macroptera* peel powder. These findings are also supported by a recent investigation, suggested that derivative of caffeic acid prevents NO production in liver [39].

Furthermore, free radicals-mediated oxidative stress also reduces the amount of natural anti-oxidant like SOD, catalase, and GSH which fights against any free radicals-mediated damage in tissues. It is well reported that superoxide radicals ($O_2^{•-}$) are removed by SOD which produces hydrogen peroxide ($H_2O_2$) [40]. $H_2O_2$ then further converted into water by another antioxidant enzyme known as catalase [40]. Moreover, $CCl_4$ administration also depleted intracellular-reduced GSH levels, suggesting that GSH loss might result from detoxification of $CCl_4$ by GSH conjugation [40]. GSH also breaks $H_2O_2$, ROOH and helps against protein oxidation [41]. Our study revealed that administration of oral $CCl_4$ reduced the amount of anti-

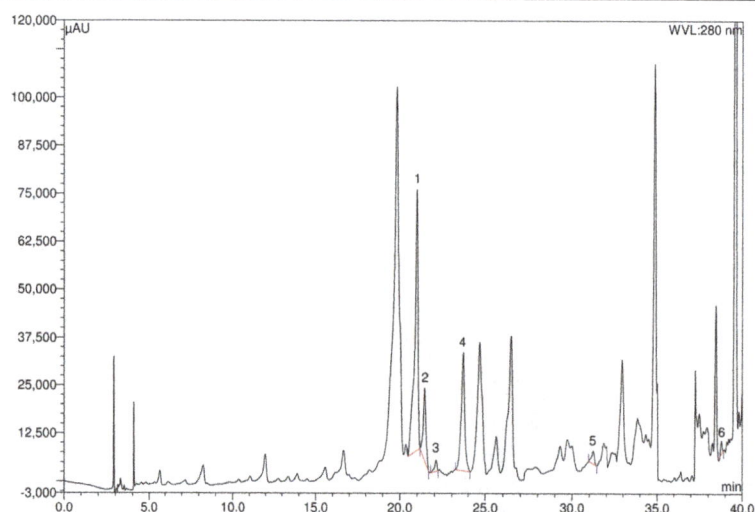

**Fig. 4** HPLC chromatogram of *Citrus macroptera*. Peaks: 1, caffeic acid; 2, syringic acid; 3, (−)-epicatechin; 4, vanillin; 5, benzoic acid; 6, kaempferol

**Table 3** Contents of polyphenolic compounds in the ethanol extract of Citrus (n = 5)

| Polyphenolic compound | Ethanol extract of Citrus macroptera | |
|---|---|---|
| | Content (mg/100 g of dry extract) | % RSD |
| Caffeic Acid | 428.36 | 1.91 |
| Syringic Acid | 81.91 | 0.53 |
| (−)-epicatechin | 33.87 | 0.16 |
| vanillin | 52.46 | 0.27 |
| benzoic acid | 47.84 | 0.36 |
| kaempferol | 2.12 | 0.03 |

oxidant capacity in both plasma and liver tissue which was restored by Citrus macroptera supplementation. Our previous study also demonstrated that iron overload could lead to cause hepatic damage. Free iron in tissues may start Fenton like reaction resulted in a hydroxyl free radicals generation [42]. Supplementation with Citrus macroptera peel powder supplementation reduced iron deposition in the liver of $CCl_4$ treated rats.

The most noteworthy pathological characteristics of $CCl_4$ intoxicated hepatotoxicity are inflammation and fibrosis. Hepatic fibrosis is usually initiated by hepatocyte damage, leading to the recruitment of inflammatory cells and platelets with the subsequent release of cytokines, chemokines, and growth factors [7]. Inflammatory cells infiltration further lead to activation of HSCs and their transformation into myofibroblast-like cells [43]. Chronically activated HSCs produce large amounts of ECM proteins and enhance fibrosis followed by TGF-β1 mediated signaling pathways [1]. Free radicals may also activate HSC which further help to secret collagenase-1 from local fibroblast [1, 44]. Our investigation showed that $CCl_4$ administration significantly enhanced inflammatory cell infiltration and fibrosis in the liver of rats. These findings are in agreement with previously published literature which showed that $CCl_4$ mediated oxidative stress is responsible for the inflammation and fibrosis in liver [45, 46]. Moreover, Citrus macroptera peel powder supplementation reduced inflammatory cells infiltration and fibrosis in the liver of $CCl_4$ treated rats. This antifibrotic activity of Citrus macroptera peel powder could be attributed to the presence of the antioxidant and anti-inflammatory compound, caffeic acid. Recent findings also suggested that caffeic acid administration in experimental animals may prevent hepatic fibrosis [14, 39].

Researchers are still working on natural plants to discover new compounds of high biological activity. It is reported by World Health Organization (WHO) that more than 80% people in developing countries basically depends on herbal medicines [47]. Researchers are

more focusing on plant-derived polyphenols, seeing that the synthetic anti-oxidants have several adverse effects [48]. Our investigation showed that caffeic acid; syringic acid and vanillic acid are present in Citrus macroptera peel powder. The previous report also suggests that syringic acid and vanillic acid which are important polyphenols showed anti-oxidants, anti-inflammatory, anti-fibrogenic and hepatoprotective activities in $CCl_4$ induced rats [49]. Citrus macroptera or wild orange is occasionally used for increasing appetite, reducing fever and making meat preparation [50]. A recent investigation also suggests that Citrus macroptera is extremely safe, even methanolic extract at a dose of 1000 mg/kg did not produce toxic effects in rats considering biochemical as well as histological assessment [51]. Our investigation also supports this notions that Citrus macroptera peel powder supplementation in normal rats did not alter any of the biochemical as well as histological parameters compared to control rats.

## Conclusion

The current study showed that Citrus macroptera peel powder possesses a good number of polyphenols such as vanillic acid, caffeic acid and syringic acid and benzoic acid. This study also pointed out that oxidative stress can be reduced by Citrus macroptera peel powder supplementation in $CCl_4$ treated rats. Citrus macroptera peel powder was able to reduce iron deposition, inflammation and fibrosis in the liver of $CCl_4$ treated rats. Further studies are required to assess efficacy in the clinical condition of liver damage.

**Abbreviations**
ALP: Alkaline phosphatase; ALT: Alanine aminotransferase; APOP: Advanced protein oxidation product; AST: Aspartate aminotransferase; CAT: Catalase; $CCl_3$: Trichloromethyl free radical; $CCl_3O_2$: Trichloroperoxyl radical; $CCl_4$: Carbon tetrachloride; DTNB: 5,5-dithiobis-2-nitrobenzoic acid; ECM: Extracellular matrix; GSH: Reduced glutathione; $H_2O_2$: Hydrogen peroxide; HPLC-DAD: High performance liquid choromatography diod array ditector; HSCs: Hepatic stellate cells; iNOS: Inducible nitric oxide synthase; MDA: Malondialdehyde; MPO: Myeloperoxidase; NO: Nitric oxide; ONOO: Peroxynitrate; ROS: Reactive oxygen species; SOD: superoxide dismutase; TBA: Thiobarbituric acid; TCA: Trichloroacetic acid; TGF-β: Transforming growth factor-β; TNF-α: Tumor necrosis factor-alpha

**Acknowledgements**
Research was conducted in Department of Pharmaceutical Sciences, North South University, Bangladesh. The authors gratefully acknowledge the logistic support provided by the Department of Pharmaceutical Sciences, North South University Bangladesh.

**Funding**
This research received no specific grant from any funding agency in the public, commercial, or not-for-profit sectors.

## Authors' contributions

MAA, MATS, and HMR designed the experimental design. MATS and NT carried out the animal care, treatment and data acquisition from the experiment. MAA, MATS, and NT performed all the biochemical analysis. MAA, MATS, and AU also performed the histological staining and analysis of tissues. MHH analyzed the extract for phenolic contents through HPLC-DAD system. MAA, AU, GMR and HMR took part in data analysis and manuscript writing. MAA, GMR and HMR checked and finalized the manuscript for submission. The contribution of MCS should be incorporated. All authors read and approved the final manuscript.

## Author details

[1]Department of Pharmaceutical Sciences, North South University, Dhaka, Bangladesh. [2]BCSIR Laboratories, Bangladesh Council of Scientific and Industrial Research (BCSIR), Dhaka, Bangladesh.

## References

1. Lee UE, Friedman SL. Mechanisms of hepatic fibrogenesis. Best Pract Res Clin Gastroenterol. 2011;25(2):195–206.
2. Novo E, Parola M. The role of redox mechanisms in hepatic chronic wound healing and fibrogenesis. Fibrogenesis Tissue Repair. 2012;5:1.
3. Constandinou C, Henderson N, Iredale JP. Modeling liver fibrosis in rodents. Methods Mol Med. 2005;117:237–50.
4. Liedtke C, Luedde T, Sauerbruch T, Scholten D, Streetz K, Tacke F, et al. Experimental liver fibrosis research: update on animal models, legal issues and translational aspects. Fibrogenesis Tissue Repair. 2013;6(1):19.
5. Weber LW, Boll M, Stampfl A. Hepatotoxicity and mechanism of action of haloalkanes: carbon tetrachloride as a toxicological model. Critical. Rev Toxicol. 2003;33(2):105–36.
6. Elpek GÖ. Cellular and molecular mechanisms in the pathogenesis of liver fibrosis: an update. World J Gastroenterol. 2014;20(23):7260–76.
7. Friedman SL. Liver fibrosis – from bench to bedside. J Hepatol. 2003; 38(Suppl 1):S38–53.
8. Luster MI, Simeonova PP, Gallucci RM, Matheson JM, Yucesoy B. Immunotoxicology: role of inflammation in chemical-induced hepatotoxicity. Int J Immunopharmacol. 2000;22(12):1143–7.
9. Yang J, Li Y, Wang F, Wu C. Hepatoprotective effects of apple polyphenols on CCl4-induced acute liver damage in mice. J Agric Food Chem. 2010; 58(10):6525–31.
10. Alam MA, Subhan N, Rahman MM, Uddin SJ, Reza HM, Sarker SD. Effect of citrus flavonoids, naringin and naringenin, on metabolic syndrome and their mechanisms of action. Adv Nutr. 2014;5(4):404–17.
11. Tsai T-H, Yu C-H, Chang Y-P, Lin Y-T, Huang C-J, Kuo Y-H, et al. Protective effect of caffeic acid derivatives on tert-butyl hydroperoxide-induced oxidative hepato-toxicity and mitochondrial dysfunction in HepG2 cells. Molecules 2017;22(5):702.
12. Bocco BM, Fernandes GW, Lorena FB, Cysneiros RM, Christoffolete MA, Grecco SS, et al. Combined treatment with caffeic and ferulic acid from Baccharis uncinella C. DC. (Asteraceae) protects against metabolic syndrome in mice. Braz J Med Biol Res 2016;49.
13. Pari L, Karthikesan K. Protective role of caffeic acid against alcohol-induced biochemical changes in rats. Fundam Clin Pharmacol. 2007;21(4):355–61.
14. Li M, Wang X-F, Shi J-J, Li Y-P, Yang N, Zhai S, et al. Caffeic acid phenethyl ester inhibits liver fibrosis in rats. World J Gastroenterol. 2015;21(13):3893–903.
15. Zhao WX, Wang L, Yang JL, Li LZ, Xu WM, Li T. Caffeic acid phenethyl ester attenuates pro-inflammatory and fibrogenic phenotypes of LPS-stimulated hepatic stellate cells through the inhibition of NF-kappaB signaling. Int J Mol Med. 2014;33(3):687–94.
16. Chowdhury SAHS, Datta BK, Choudhury MH. Chemical and antioxidant studies of Citrus macroptera. Bangladesh J Sci Ind Res. 2008;43(4):449–54.
17. Waikedre J, Dugay A, Barrachina I, Herrenknecht C, Cabalion P, Fournet A. Chemical composition and antimicrobial activity of the essential oils from new Caledonian Citrus macroptera and Citrus hystrix. Chem Biodivers. 2010; 7(4):871–7.
18. Uddin N, Hasan MR, Hossain MM, Sarker A, Hasan AHMN, Islam AFMM, et al. In vitro α-amylase inhibitory activity and in vivo hypoglycemic effect of

19. methanol extract of Citrus macroptera. Montr. Fruit. Asian Pac J Trop Biomed. 2014;4(6):473–9.
19. Chowdhury MRH, Sagor MAT, Tabassum N, Potol MA, Hossain H, Alam MA. Supplementation of Citrus maxima peel powder prevented oxidative stress, fibrosis, and hepatic damage in carbon tetrachloride (CCl4) treated rats. Evid Based Complement Alternat Med. 2015;2015:10.
20. Jahan I, Akbar P, Khan N, Khan T, Rahman M, Arpona H, et al. Comparative study of anti-nociceptive activity and phenolic content of the ethanol extracts of Piper nigrum and Piper longum fruits. Int J Pharm Sci Rev Res. 2014;27:47–52.
21. Niehaus WG, Samuelsson B. Formation of malonaldehyde from phospholipid arachidonate during microsomal lipid peroxidation. Eur J Biochem. 1968;6(1): 126–30.
22. Tracey WR, Tse J, Carter G. Lipopolysaccharide-induced changes in plasma nitrite and nitrate concentrations in rats and mice: pharmacological evaluation of nitric oxide synthase inhibitors. J Pharmacol Exp Ther. 1995; 272(3):1011–5.
23. Witko-Sarsat V, Friedlander M, Capeillère-Blandin C, Nguyen-Khoa T, Nguyen A, Zingraff J, et al. Advanced oxidation protein products as a novel marker of oxidative stress in uremia. Kidney Int. 1996;49:1304–13.
24. Tiwari BK, Kumar D, Abidi AB, Rizvi SI. Efficacy of composite extract from leaves and fruits of medicinal plants used in traditional diabetic therapy against oxidative stress in Alloxan-induced diabetic rats. ISRN Pharmacol. 2014;2014:7.
25. Khan RA. Protective effects of Sonchus asper (L.) hill, (Asteraceae) against CCl4-induced oxidative stress in the thyroid tissue of rats. BMC Complement Altern Med. 2012;12(1):181.
26. Jollow D, Mitchell J, Zampaglione N, Gillette J. Bromobenzene-induced liver necrosis. Protective role of glutathione and evidence for 3,4-bromobenzene oxide as the hepatotoxic metabolite. Pharmacology. 1974;11:151–69.
27. Heron M. Deaths: leading causes for 2009. Natl Vital Stat Rep. 2012;61(7):1–94.
28. Singh BN, Singh BR, Singh RL, Prakash D, Sarma BK, Singh HB. Antioxidant and anti-quorum sensing activities of green pod of Acacia nilotica L. Food Chem Toxicol. 2009;47(4):778–86.
29. Singh P, Singh U, Shukla M, Singh R. Antioxidant activity imparting biomolecules in Cassia fistula. Adv Life Sci 2008a. 2008;2:23–8.
30. Gowri Shankar NL, Manavalan R, Venkappayya D, David Raj C. Hepatoprotective and antioxidant effects of Commiphora berry (Arn) Engl bark extract against CCl4-induced oxidative damage in rats. Food Chem Toxicol. 2008;46(9):3182–5.
31. Bolanle JD, Adetoro KO, Balarabe SA, Adeyemi OO. Hepatocurative potential of Vitex doniana root bark, stem bark and leaves extracts against CCl4-induced liver damage in rats. Asian Pac J Trop Biomed. 2014;4(6):480–5.
32. Huo HZ, Wang B, Liang YK, Bao YY, Gu Y. Hepatoprotective and antioxidant effects of licorice extract against CCl4-induced oxidative damage in rats. Int J Mol Sci. 2011;12(10):6529–43.
33. Janbaz KH, Saeed SA, Gilani AH. Studies on the protective effects of caffeic acid and quercetin on chemical-induced hepatotoxicity in rodents. Phytomedicine. 2004;11(5):424–30.
34. Kus I, Colakoglu N, Pekmez H, Seckin D, Ogeturk M, Sarsilmaz M. Protective effects of caffeic acid phenethyl ester (CAPE) on carbon tetrachloride-induced hepatotoxicity in rats. Acta Histochem. 2004;106(4):289–97.
35. Gressner OA, Weiskirchen R, Gressner AM. Biomarkers of liver fibrosis: clinical translation of molecular pathogenesis or based on liver-dependent malfunction tests. Clin Chim Acta. 2007;381(2):107–13.
36. Shim JY, Kim MH, Kim HD, Ahn JY, Yun YS, Song JY. Protective action of the immunomodulator ginsan against carbon tetrachloride-induced liver injury via control of oxidative stress and the inflammatory response. Toxicol Appl Pharmacol. 2010;242(3):318–25.
37. Qiao Y, Bai XF, Du YG. Chitosan oligosaccharides protect mice from LPS challenge by attenuation of inflammation and oxidative stress. Int Immunopharmacol. 2011;11(1):121–7.
38. Quan J, Piao L, Wang X, Li T, Yin X. Rossicaside B protects against carbon tetrachloride-induced hepatotoxicity in mice. Basic Clin Pharmacol Toxicol. 2009;105(6):380–6.
39. Shi Y, Guo L, Shi L, Yu J, Song M, Li Y. Caffeic acid phenethyl ester inhibit hepatic fibrosis by nitric oxide synthase and cystathionine gamma-lyase in rats. Med Sci Monit. 2015;21:2774–80.
40. Lee J, Koo N, Min DB. Reactive oxygen species, aging, and antioxidative nutraceuticals. Compr Rev Food Sci Food Saf. 2004;3(1):21–33.

41. Yin G, Cao L, Xu P, Jeney G, Nakao M, Lu C. Hepatoprotective and antioxidant effects of Glycyrrhiza glabra extract against carbon tetrachloride (CCl$_4$)-induced hepatocyte damage in common carp (*Cyprinus carpio*). Fish Physiol Biochem. 2011;37(1):209–16.

42. Reza HM, Sagor MAT, Alam MA. Iron deposition causes oxidative stress, inflammation and fibrosis in carbon tetrachloride-induced liver dysfunction in rats. Bangladesh. Aust J Pharm. 2015;10(1):152–9.

43. Liu C, Tao Q, Sun M, Wu JZ, Yang W, Jian P, et al. Kupffer cells are associated with apoptosis, inflammation and fibrotic effects in hepatic fibrosis in rats. Lab Investig. 2010;90(12):1805–16.

44. Urtasun R, de la Rosa LC, Nieto N. Oxidative and nitrosative stress and fibrogenic response. Clin Liver Dis. 2008;12(4):769–viii.

45. Jang JH, Kang KJ, Kim YH, Kang YN, Lee IS. Reevaluation of experimental model of hepatic fibrosis induced by hepatotoxic drugs: an easy, applicable, and reproducible model. Transplant Proc. 2008;40(8):2700–3.

46. Sebastiani G, Gkouvatsos K, Maffettone C, Busatto G, Guido M, Pantopoulos K. Accelerated CCl$_4$-induced liver fibrosis in Hjv−/− mice, associated with an oxidative burst and precocious profibrogenic gene expression. PLoS One. 2011;6(9):e25138.

47. Canter PH, Thomas H, Ernst E. Bringing medicinal plants into cultivation: opportunities and challenges for biotechnology. Trends Biotechnol. 2005;23(4):180–5.

48. Aggarwal S, Ichikawa H, Takada Y, Sandur SK, Shishodia S, Aggarwal BB. Curcumin (diferuloylmethane) down-regulates expression of cell proliferation and antiapoptotic and metastatic gene products through suppression of I kappaB alpha kinase and Akt activation. Mol Pharmacol. 2006;69(1):195–206.

49. Itoh A, Isoda K, Kondoh M, Kawase M, Watari A, Kobayashi M, et al. Hepatoprotective effect of syringic acid and vanillic acid on the CCl$_4$-induced liver injury. Biol Pharm Bull. 2010;33(6):983–7.

50. Rahmatullah M, Khatun MA, Morshed N, Neogi PK, Khan SUA, Hossan MS, et al. A randomized survey of medicinal plants used by folk medicinal healers of Sylhet division, Bangladesh. Adv in Nat. Appl Sci. 2010;4(1):52–62.

51. Uddin N, Hasan MR, Hasan MM, Hossain MM, Alam MR, Hasan MR, et al. Assessment of toxic effects of the methanol extract of *Citrus macroptera* Montr. Fruit via biochemical and hematological evaluation in female Sprague-Dawley rats. PLoS One. 2014;9(11):e111101.

# 17

# Evaluation of aphrodisiac activity of ethanol extract of *Ganoderma lucidum* in male Wistar rats

Hammad Ahmed[1] and Muhammad Aslam[1,2]* (iD)

## Abstract

**Background:** *Ganoderma lucidum* was traditionally used to manage male sexual dysfunction. This study was designed to investigate and establish the traditional aphrodisiac potential of the herb.

**Methods:** Aphrodisiac potential was evaluated following the oral administration of two different doses (150 and 300 mg/kg) of ethanol extract of *Ganoderma lucidum*. Sildenafil citrate (Viagra) and distilled water were used as positive and negative controls respectively. Mounting, intromission and ejaculation frequencies, mating performance, and orientation activities towards females, towards the environment, and towards self were observed. Serum testosterone levels were also evaluated.

**Results:** The results of the study show that the extract has significantly increased the mounting behavior and mating performance of the rats. There was also significant increase in the number of intromissions and ejaculations. The rats treated with extract were more interested in female rats as indicated by significant increase in the number of anogenital sniffing and climbing. Serum testosterone levels were also significantly increased in the treatment groups.

**Conclusion:** Ethanol extract of *Ganoderma lucidum* possesses aphrodisiac activity in male Wistar rats. The lower dose of 150 mg/kg was more effective in terms of aphrodisiac potential of the extract.

**Keywords:** *Ganoderma lucidum*, Sildenafil citrate, Aphrodisiac, Testosterone

## Background

Male infertility is due to any problem in the male reproductive system, including: decreased sexual desire, barrenness, premature ejaculation and erectile dysfunction [1]. Sex is a highly important aspect of living organisms which plays a key role in their survival. Substances that increase the sexual desire are called aphrodisiac agents. The term aphrodisiac is derived from "Aphrodite", that means the "Greek goddess of sexuality and love" [2]. In allopathic medicine, there are various drugs which can increase the sexual craving in both male and female, although these drugs have numerous harmful effects [3]. Phosphodiesterase type 5 inhibitors, like tadalafil (Cialis) and sildenafil (Viagra) are the most commonly used

aphrodisiac agents, but these drugs cause dizziness, headache, visual disturbance, pulse irregularities, dyspepsia, priapism, diarrhoea and flushing [4].

Mushrooms have been one of the major sources of several medicinal products. There are around 10,000 varieties of mushrooms, out of which 2000 have nonpoisonous effects and around 300 of them have shown important medicinal effects [5]. Studies show that mushroom extracts are advantageous for the human body, as they have shown several pharmacological activities such as anti-bacterial, anti-inflammatory, anti-viral and anti-hyperglycemic activity [6].

*Ganoderma lucidum* (reishi) is denoted as a sacred mushroom in Chinese culture [7]. These days, reishi has gained a great value in medicinal product development because of its medicinal properties [8]. *Ganoderma lucidum* is not only used to treat common health problems,

* Correspondence: Pharmacologist1@yahoo.com
[1]Department of Pharmacology, Faculty of Pharmacy, Ziauddin University, Karachi 75600, Pakistan
[2]Department of Pharmacology, Faculty of Pharmacy, University of Sindh, Jamshoro 76080, Pakistan

[9] but it has also been used as an anti-cancer agent alone or with western chemotherapy medications [10].

From the fruiting bodies, spores, and mycelia of reishi, various types of bioactive compounds have been identified which commonly consist of proteins, peptides, triterpenoids, sterols, polysaccharides, steroids, nucleotides and trace elements [11, 12]. *Ganoderma lucidum* has shown various pharmacological activities which include antiviral (anti-HIV), hepatoprotective, anti-ulcer antibacterial, anti-tumour, anti-inflammatory, radio-protective, age promoting, analgesic, hypolipidemic, sleep promoting, cytotoxic, chemopreventive, antifibrotic, antiatherosclerotic, antidiabetic, radical scavenging and antioxidative properties [8, 11, 13–16]. In this study, we have evaluated the potential aphrodisiac activity of ethanol extract of *Ganoderma lucidum* (GLE) in male Wistar rats.

## Methods
### Drugs and chemicals
*Ganoderma lucidum* extract composed of cracked spores and fruiting bodies, branded ReishiMaxGLpTM, was procured from Pharmanex Inc. (United States of America). Sildenafil was purchased from Pfizer, USA, while progesterone and estradiol benzoate were procured from Sigma Aldrich, Pakistan.

### Animals
Healthy adult rats (Wistar strain) bearing weight of 150–200 g were purchased from the animal house of Dow University of Health Sciences, Pakistan. Polypropylene cages have been used for keeping the animals under controlled conditions at room temperature (25–30 °C) with light-dark cycle of 12\12 h. Standard diet and water ad libitum were given to the rats. Handling of the animals was done according to the requirements mentioned in "Guidelines for the care and use of laboratory animals 8$^{th}$ edition" [17]. Prior approval of the ethical review committee of Ziauddin University was taken before starting this research study.

### Animal groups
Male rats were divided into four groups ($n = 6$):

Group I: Control group, given distilled water (10 ml/kg) orally for 40 days.
Group II: Treatment group, given extract (150 mg/kg) for 40 days.
Group III: Treatment group, given extract (300 mg/kg) for 40 days.
Group IV: Standard drug group, given sildenafil citrate (5 mg/kg) for 40 days.

### Preparation of male rats
Sexual behaviour training was given to male rats for 10 days. The animal that did not show any sexual interest was replaced by another sexually active rat [18, 19].

### Preparation of female rats
Oestrus (heat) was developed artificially in female rats by giving progesterone (0.5 mg / 100 g body weight) and estradiol benzoate (10 microgram/100 g body weight) over the subcutaneous route sequentially before mating. Before conducting the experiment the receptivity of female rats was ensured [18, 19].

A number of parameters such as mounting behaviour, mating performance, orientation activities of male rats towards the surrounding, towards female and towards themselves were observed for the assessment of aphrodisiac activity of the extract.

### Mounting behaviour test
The climbing property of male rats onto the female rats is known as "Mounting". To assess the number of mounts, the mounting behaviour test was performed. Males, treated with the extract, were paired with non-oestrus female rats. The behaviour of the animals was noted for 3 h on the 10th, 20th and 40th day of the study. Male rats were placed individually in each cage. After 15 min of acclimation, non-oestrus female was introduced into each cage and number of mounts were noted at the beginning of 1st hour for next 15 min. Every female was then given a resting period of 105 min by pulling it from each cage. The females were again introduced into the cages and the number of mounts were again noted for 15 min before the end of 3rd hour of the test. The test was performed at room temperature of 25–27 °C between 9 a.m. to 12 p.m. [18, 19].

### Determination of mating performance
In this test every male rat was settled separately in a glass cage. After the acclimation period of 15 min, five oestrus females were admitted into each cage and they cohabited overnight. For the detection of any sperms in females, microscopic investigation of the vaginal smear of every female rat was performed. Sperm positive females were noted in every group [18, 19].

### Test for libido
In this test sexually experienced male rats demonstrating vigorous sexual performance were selected. Mounting Frequency (MF) was observed in these rats in the evening of 10th, 20th and 40th day. Before initiating the observation, the sheath of the penis was retracted to expose the penis of rats and xylocaine 5% ointment (AstraZeneca Pharma) was applied at the interval of 5, 15 and 30 min. Each male rat was allocated separately in

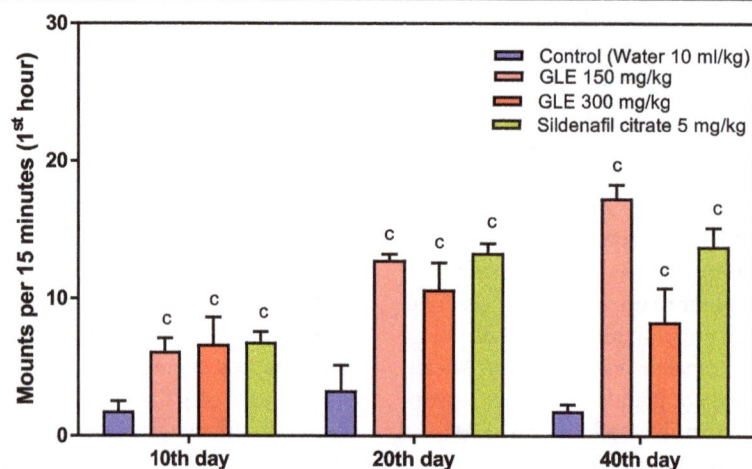

**Fig. 1** Effect of *Ganoderma lucidum on* mounting behavior (1st hour) in male rats. Animals per group (n) = 6. The values are mean ± S.E.M.; [a]p < 0.05; [b]p < 0.01; [c]p < 0.001 when compared with control group. (One-way ANOVA followed by Tukey's post hoc test)

a cage and female rats were admitted in the similar cage. The total number of intromissions and ejaculations were observed [20].

### Determination of the orientation activities of male rats

In this test the behavioural activities of the male rats, towards the surrounding, towards themselves and towards females were examined. The rats were observed and the number of climbings, genital groomings, lickings and anogenital sniffings were counted for one hour [21].

### Preparation of serum for testosterone analysis

The blood was collected via cardiac puncture using chloroform anaesthesia. Using sterilized syringe, 5 ml of blood was collected in appropriately labelled blank tubes containing no anti-coagulant. The tubes

were given 5 to 10 min for coagulation before they were subjected to centrifugation. The needles were changed for every single animal. After coagulation these tubes were centrifuged at 3000 rpm for 10 min. The supernatant formed after centrifugation was sucked and collected in a clean, empty tube for testosterone assay [22].

### Testosterone analysis

Quantitative determination of total testosterone was done by the competitive imunoenzymatic colorimetric method mentioned in the manufacturer's test procedure (Diametra testosterone ELISA kit). The absorbance was noted at 420 nm against a reference wavelength of 620–630 nm.

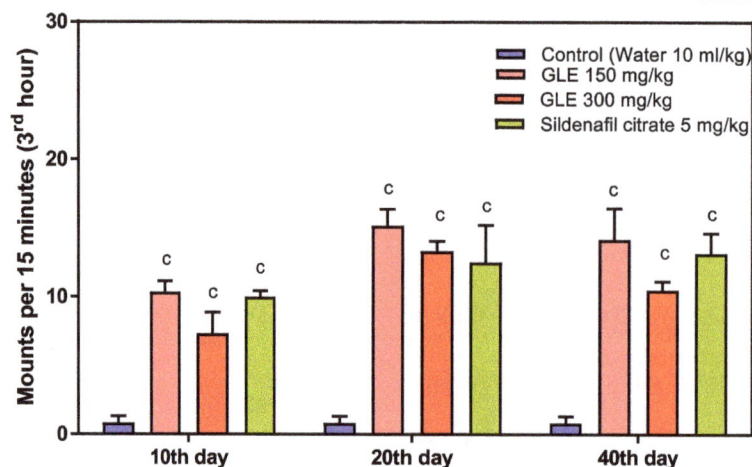

**Fig. 2** Effect of *Ganoderma lucidum* on mounting behavior (3rd hour) in male rats. Animals per group (n) = 6. The values are mean ± S.E.M.; [a]p < 0.05; [b]p < 0.01; [c]p < 0.001 when compared with control group. (One-way ANOVA followed by Tukey's post hoc test)

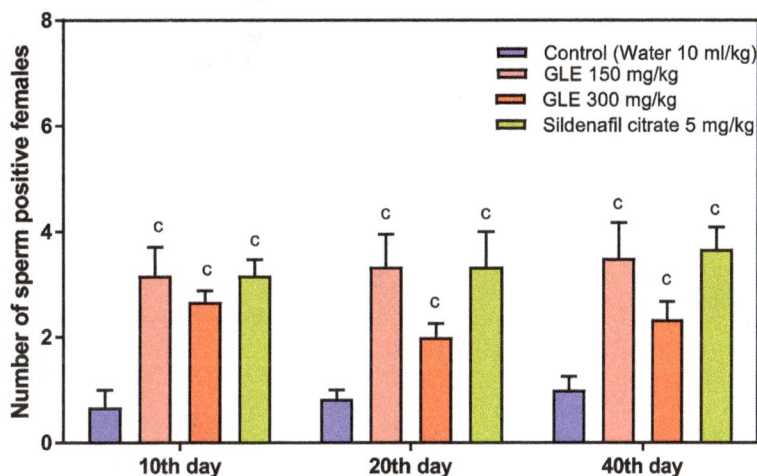

**Fig. 3** Effect of *Ganoderma lucidum* on mating performance test in male rats. Animals per group (n) = 6. The values are mean ± S.E.M.; $^a p < 0.05$; $^b p < 0.01$; $^c p < 0.001$ when compared with control group. (One-way ANOVA followed by Tukey's post hoc test)

## Statistical analysis

One-way ANOVA followed by Tukey's test was used for analysing the data. Data were expressed as mean ± standard error of mean. A statistical level of 0.05 or less was accepted as significant.

## Results

In mounting behavior test, during 1st and 3rd hour of the test, GLE showed extremely significant effect at both doses viz. 150 mg/kg and 300 mg/kg when compared with control group. However, 150 mg/kg GLE was noted as the most effective aphrodisiac dose (Figs. 1 and 2).

An extremely significant difference was recorded in mating performance test. The results show that there were more sperm positive females in GLE (150 mg/kg and 300 mg/kg) groups in comparison to normal control group on 10th, 20th and 40th day of the study. Our results suggest that 150 mg/kg dose is more effective than 300 mg/kg dose in terms of mating performance test. The results of 150 mg/kg are comparable to sildenafil citrate, positive control (Fig. 3).

The results of libido test show that the number of intromissions and ejaculations in GLE groups was significantly high when compared with control group. We observed very promising results of GLE in terms of the number of intromissions and ejaculations. The effect of GLE (150 mg/kg) was greater than sildenafil citrate in libido test (Figs. 4 and 5).

The results of orientation activities show significant increase in the activities of male rats in terms of anogenital sniffing, licking, climbing and genital grooming. There was extremely significant increase in the orientation

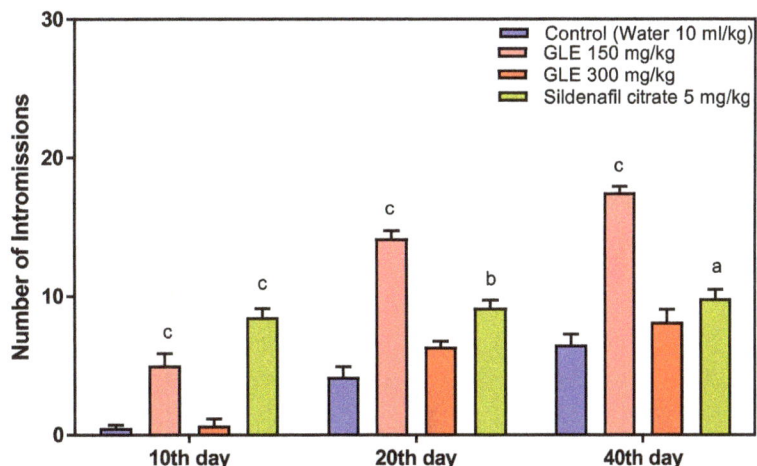

**Fig. 4** Effect of *Ganoderma lucidum* on number of intromissions in male rats. Animals per group (n) = 6. The values are mean ± S.E.M.; $^a p < 0.05$; $^b p < 0.01$; $^c p < 0.001$ when compared with control group. (One-way ANOVA followed by Tukey's post hoc test)

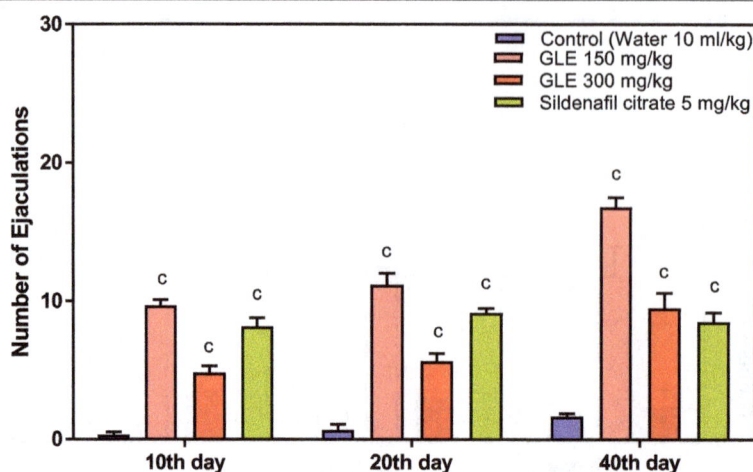

**Fig. 5** Effect of *Ganoderma lucidum* on number of ejaculations in male rats. Animals per group (n) = 6. The values are mean ± S.E.M.; $^{a}p < 0.05$; $^{b}p < 0.01$; $^{c}p < 0.001$ when compared with control group. (One-way ANOVA followed by Tukey's post hoc test)

activities of GLE (150 mg/kg) when compared with control group (Figs. 6, 7, 8 and 9).

*Ganoderma lucidum* significantly increased the serum testosterone levels in male rats when compared with control group (Fig. 10).

## Discussion

Mounting and intromission frequencies are the important indicators of libido. Mounting frequency shows the increase in sexual desire and increase in intromission frequency reflects the ability of penile erection, penile introduction, and the responses which trigger ejaculation [23, 24].

In this study, the results show that *Ganoderma lucidum* increases the number of mounts which represents that continuous administration of the extract significantly increases the sexual desire when compared with control group and sildenafil citrate 5 mg/kg group.

The ability of doing sex is not only dependent on sexual desire but it also depends on erectile function. If an individual is suffering from erectile dysfunction, it can cause a major barrier in sexual performance even in presence of strong sexual desire. Sexual performance depends on neurovascular occasions by means of hemodynamic mechanism of penile erection [25]. Therefore, the increase in the intromission and ejaculation frequencies with the administration of GLE indicates that extract significantly increases the sexual performance of male rats. The increase in the intromission frequency proposed that adequate penile erection was accomplished by this extract [26]. Hence, GLE may be investigated for the treatment of erectile dysfunction.

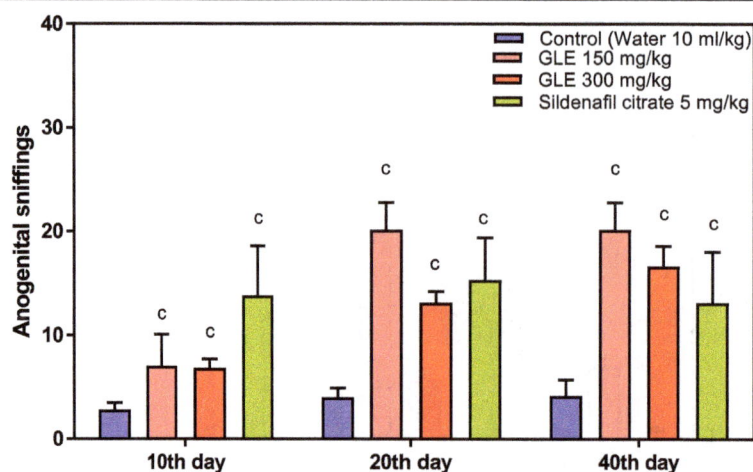

**Fig. 6** Effect of *Ganoderma lucidum* on anogenital sniffing. Animals per group (n) = 6. The values are mean ± S.E.M.; $^{a}p < 0.05$; $^{b}p < 0.01$; $^{c}p < 0.001$ when compared with control group. (One-way ANOVA followed by Tukey's post hoc test)

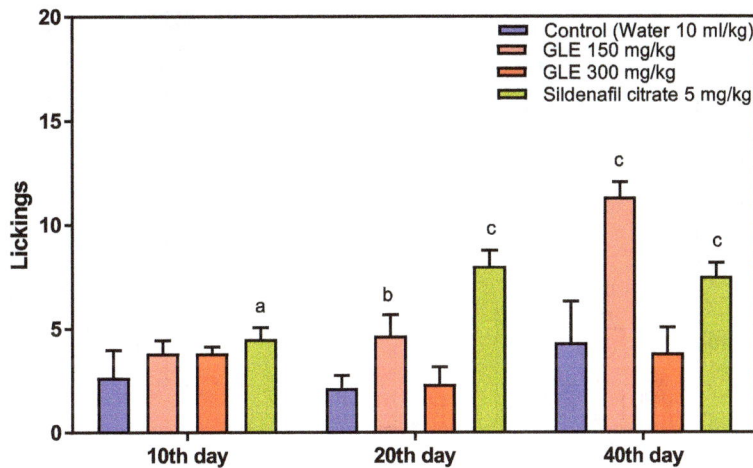

**Fig. 7** Effect of *Ganoderma lucidum* on lickings. Animals per group (n) = 6. The values are mean ± S.E.M.; $^{a}p < 0.05$; $^{b}p < 0.01$; $^{c}p < 0.001$ when compared with control group. (One-way ANOVA followed by Tukey's post hoc test)

Moreover, there were more sperm positive females in the mating performance test which also supports the aphrodisiac potential of the extract. The similarity in the results of mating performance test of ethanol extract of *Ganoderma lucidum* and sildenafil citrate reveals identical aphrodisiac activity of both agents. However, in mating performance test a reverse inhibition of sexual performance was seen at the dose of 300 mg/kg of the extract on 10th and 40th day of the study which may be because of sedation in the form of negative sexual interest among the rats. The same result of sexual inhibition was shown with the findings of Afolayan and Yakubu and Ratnasooriya and Dharmasiri which supports the results of our study [24, 26].

The orientation activity of the male rat is one of the very important parameters to evaluate the aphrodisiac activity in rodents. Results of orientation activity tests of male rats showed that GLE, at the dose of 150 mg/kg; significantly increased the attention of male rats towards female rats when compared with control group and sildenafil citrate 5 mg/kg group.

Many research studies have reported that increase in the sexual desire may be due to an increment in the levels of serum testosterone and anterior pituitary hormones. These hormones are considered as major stimulators of neurotransmitters such as dopamine which helps in conducting the actions related to sexual behavior and copulation [24, 27, 28]. Testosterone is an important steroidal hormone secreted from the leydig cells of the testes [29]. It has been reported that the use of testosterone significantly increases the sexual desire and function. Testosterone

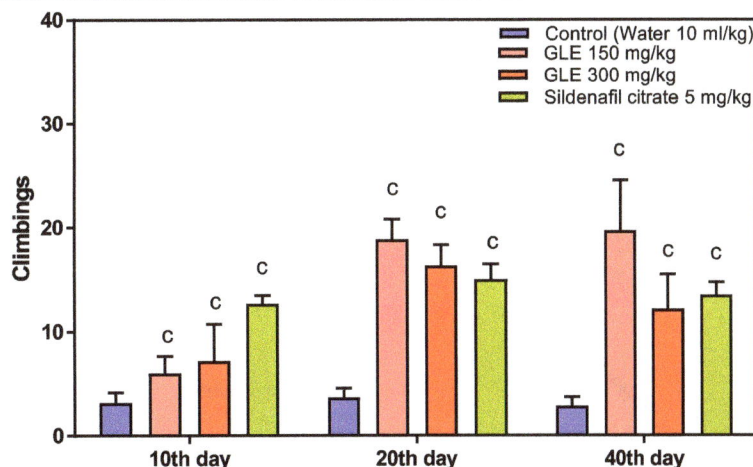

**Fig. 8** Effect of *Ganoderma lucidum* on climbing. Animals per group (n) = 6. The values are mean ± S.E.M.; $^{a}p < 0.05$; $^{b}p < 0.01$; $^{c}p < 0.001$ when compared with control group. (One-way ANOVA followed by Tukey's post hoc test)

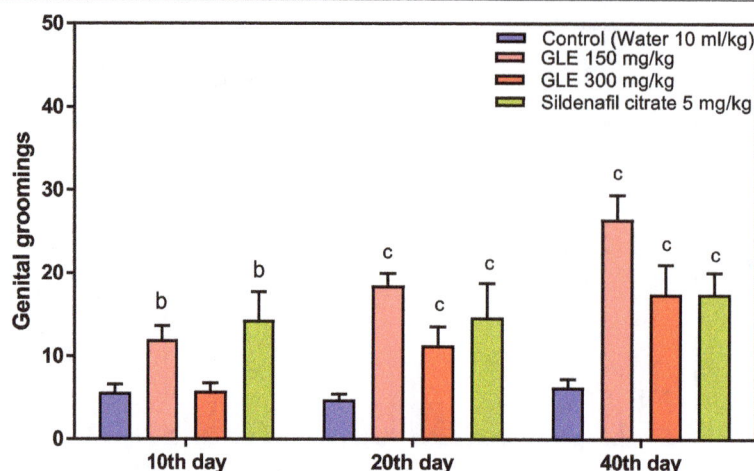

**Fig. 9** Effect of *Ganoderma lucidum* on genital grooming. Animals per group (n) = 6. The values are mean ± S.E.M.; $^ap < 0.05$; $^bp < 0.01$; $^cp < 0.001$ when compared with control group. (One-way ANOVA followed by Tukey's post hoc test)

also increases the climax of sexual excitement and ejaculation [30, 31].

The results of our study show that *Ganoderma lucidum* significantly elevated the testosterone level in male rats. This increase in the testosterone level is the most important parameter to establish the aphrodisiac potential of the GLE.

Certain bioactive compounds play the major role in enhancing testosterone levels endogenously and for boosting the sexual behavior in males. These compounds work by special mechanism which includes: steroids by promoting androgen production [32, 33] alkaloids through widening the blood vessels in the reproductive organs, saponins through stimulating gonadal tissue and CNS by means of NO based mechanism [34] flavonoids by increasing testosterone synthesis or by preventing its metabolic deterioration [35, 36] Steroids are one of the dominant

components of *Ganoderma lucidum* [11]. Thus, the enhancement in sexual activity exhibited in the present study may be due to the presence of steroids in GLE.

## Conclusion

According to Solomon P. Wasser [37], *Ganoderma lucidum* was traditionally used to manage male sexual dysfunction. This study was designed to investigate and establish the traditional aphrodisiac potential of the herb. The results of this study show that the parameters of mounting behavior test, mating performance test, orientation activities and the test for libido were increased in the animals treated with GLE when compared with the animals treated with distilled water. The increase in above mentioned parameters may due to enhancing effect of GLE on the testosterone levels. Hence, we conclude that GLE may be a new promising aphrodisiac agent, which can be used to promote the sexual performance of many troubled men.

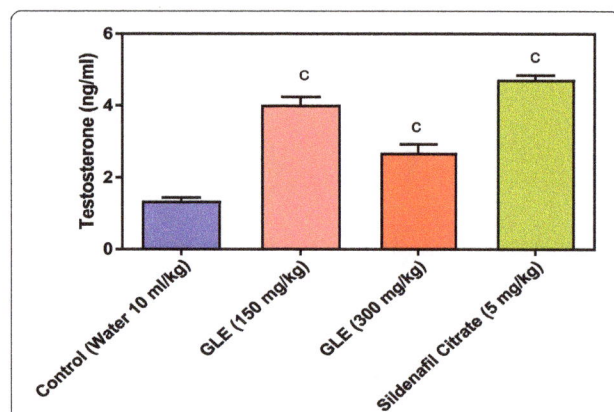

**Fig. 10** Effect of *Ganoderma lucidum* on testosterone levels. Animals per group (n) = 6. The values are mean ± S.E.M.; $^ap < 0.05$; $^bp < 0.01$; $^cp < 0.001$ when compared with control group. (One-way ANOVA followed by Tukey's post hoc test)

### Abbreviations
ANOVA: Analysis of variance; CNS: Central nervous system; ELISA: Enzyme linked immunosorbent assay; GLE: *Ganoderma lucidum* extract; kg: Kilogram; MF: Mounting frequency; mg: Milligram; NO: Nitric oxide; rpm: Rotations per minute; SEM: Standard error of mean

### Funding
This research study was not granted any specific fund.

### Authors' contributions
Study design and supervision, analysis of data, graphical representation, interpretation of results and drafting manuscript were done by MA. Sample collection and laboratory experiments were performed by HA. Both authors read and approved the final manuscript.

## Competing interests
The authors declare that they have no competing interests.

## References

1. Kothari P. Common sexual problems - solutions. 2nd ed. New Delhi: UBS Publishers Distributors (P), Limited; 1994.
2. Kulkarni SK, Reddy DS. Pharmacotherapy of male erectile dysfunction with sildenafil. Indian J Pharmacol. 1998;30(6):367–8.
3. Aagaard L, Hansen E. Side effects reported by European consumers for medications for erectile dysfunction. J Res Pharm Pract. 2013;2(2):93.
4. Hammoud MA, Jin F, Lea T, Maher L, Grierson J, Prestage G. Off-label use of phosphodiesterase type 5 inhibitor erectile dysfunction medication to enhance sex among gay and bisexual men in Australia: results from the FLUX study. J Sex Med. 2017;14(6):774–84.
5. Wasser SP, Weis AL. Therapeutic effects of substances occurring in higher Basidiomycetes mushrooms: a modern perspective. Critc Rev Immunol. 1999;19(1):1–32.
6. De Silva DD, Rapior S, Fons F, Bahkali AH, Hyde KD. Medicinal mushrooms in supportive cancer therapies: an approach to anti-cancer effects and putative mechanisms of action. Fungal Divers. 2012;55(1):1–35.
7. Babu PD, Subhasree RS. The sacred mushroom "Reishi"-a review. American-Euras. J Bot. 2008;1(3):107–10.
8. Chang ST, Buswell JA. Ganoderma lucidum (Curt.: Fr.) P. Karst. (Aphyllophoromycetideae)– a mushrooming medicinal mushroom. Int J Med Mushrooms. 1999;1(2):139–46.
9. Shiao MS. Natural products of the medicinal fungus Ganoderma lucidum: occurrence, biological activities, and pharmacological functions. The Chem Record. 2003;3(3):172–80.
10. Gordan JD, Chay WY, Kelley RK, Ko AH, Choo SP, Venook AP. And what other medications are you taking? J Clin Oncol. 2011;29(11):e288–91.
11. McKenna D, Jones K, Hughes K. Botanical Medicines. New York: Routledge; 2011.
12. Gao Y, Zhou S, Chen G, Dai X, Ye J. A phase I/II study of a Ganoderma lucidum (Curt.: Fr.) P. Karst. Extract (Ganopofy) in patients with advanced cancer. Int J Med Mushrooms. 2002;4(3):1–8.
13. Zhao XL, Campos AR. Insulin signalling in mushroom body neurons regulates feeding behaviour in Drosophila larvae. J Exp Biol. 2012; 215(15):2696–702.
14. Batra P, Sharma AK, Khajuria R. Probing Lingzhi or Reishi medicinal mushroom Ganoderma lucidum (higher Basidiomycetes): a bitter mushroom with amazing health benefits. Int J Med Mushrooms. 2013;15(2):127–43.
15. Yuen JW, Gohel MD, Ng CF. Synergistic cytotoxic effects of Ganoderma lucidum and bacillus calmette guérin on premalignant urothelial HUC-PC cells and its regulation on proinflammatory cytokine secretion. Evid Based Complement Alternat Med. 2012;2012:1–9.
16. Li F, Zhang Y, Zhong Z. Antihyperglycemic effect of Ganoderma lucidum polysaccharides on streptozotocin-induced diabetic mice. Int J Mol Sci. 2011;12(9):6135–45.
17. Garber J, Barbee W, Bielitzki J, Clayton L, Donovan J, Kohn D, Lipman N, Locke P, Melcher J, Quimby F, Turner P, Wood G, Würbel H. Guidelines for care and use of laboratory animals. 8 Ed. Washington, D.C: The National Academies Press; 2011.
18. Aslam M, Sial AA. Effect of hydroalcoholic extract of Cydonia oblonga miller (quince) on sexual behaviour of Wistar rats. Adv Pharmacol Sci. 2014;2014:1–6.
19. Ahmad S, Latif A, Qasmi IA. Aphrodisiac activity of 50% ethanolic extracts of Myristica fragrans Houtt. (nutmeg) and Syzygium aromaticum (L) Merr. & Perry. (clove) in male mice: a comparative study. BMC Complement Altern Med. 2003;3(1):1–6.
20. Zade V, Dabhadkar D, Thakare V, Pare S. Evaluation of potential aphrodisiac activity of Moringa oleifera seed in male albino rats. Int J Pharm Pharm Sci. 2013;5(4):683–9.
21. Pande M, Pathak A. Aphrodisiac activity of roots of Mimosa pudica Linn. Ethanolic extract in mice. Int J Pharm Sci Nanotechnol. 2009;2(1):477–86.
22. Yakubu MT, Akanji MA, Oladiji AT. Aphrodisiac potentials of the aqueous extract of Fadogia agrestis (Schweinf. Ex Hiern) stem in male albino rats. Asian J Androl. 2005;7(4):399–404.
23. Yakubu MT, Akanji MA. Effect of aqueous extract of Massularia acuminata stem on sexual behaviour of male Wistar rats. Ev-Based Compl and Alter Med. 2011;2011:1–10.
24. Ratnasooriya WD, Dharmasiri MG. Effects of Terminalia catappa seeds on sexual behaviour and fertility of male rats. Asian J Androl. 2000;2(3):213–20.
25. Andersson KE. Mechanisms of penile erection and basis for pharmacological treatment of erectile dysfunction. Pharmacol Rev. 2011;63(4):811–59.
26. Afolayan AJ, Yakubu MT. Effect of Bulbine natalensis baker stem extract on the functional indices and histology of the liver and kidney of male Wistar rats. J Med Food. 2009;12(4):814–20.
27. Giuliano F, Allard J. Dopamine and male sexual function. Europ Urol. 2001; 40(6):601–8.
28. Bahmanpour S, Talaei T, Vojdani Z, Panjehshahin MR, Poostpasand A, Zareei S, Ghaeminia M. Effect of Phoenix dactylifera pollen on sperm parameters and reproductive system of adult male rats. Iran J Med Sci. 2015;31(4):208–12.
29. Cao L, Leers-Sucheta S, Azhar S. Aging alters the functional expression of enzymatic and non-enzymatic anti-oxidant defense systems in testicular rat Leydig cells. J Steroid Biochem Mol Biol. 2004;88(1):61–7.
30. Aversa A, Fabbri A. New oral agents for erectile dysfunction: what is changing in our practice. Asian J Androl. 2001;3(3):175–9.
31. Morales AJ, Laughlin GA, Bützow T, Maheshwari H, Baumann G, Yen SS. Insulin, somatotropic, and luteinizing hormone axes in lean and obese women with polycystic ovary syndrome: common and distinct features. J Clin Endocrinol Metabol. 1996;81(8):2854–64.
32. Drewes SE, George J, Khan F. Recent findings on natural products with erectile-dysfunction activity. Phytochemistry. 2003;62(7):1019–25.
33. Gauthaman K, Ganesan AP. The hormonal effects of Tribulus terrestris and its role in the management of male erectile dysfunction–an evaluation using primates, rabbit and rat. Phytomed. 2008;15(1–2):44–54.
34. Murphy LL, Ginseng LEETJ. Sex behavior, and nitric oxide. Annal New York Acad Sci. 2002;962(1):372–7.
35. Ratnasooriya WD, Fernando TS. Effect of black tea brew of Camellia sinensis on sexual competence of male rats. J Ethnopharmacol. 2008;118(3):373–7.
36. Yang NY, Kaphle K, Wang PH, Jong DS, Wu LS, Lin JH. Effects of aqueous extracts of" betel quid" and its constituents on testosterone production by dispersed mouse interstitial cells. American J Chinese Med. 2004;32(5):705–15.
37. Wasser SP. Reishi or Ling Zhi (Ganoderma lucidum). Encycl Diet Suppl. 2005; 1:603–22.

# 18

# Anthelmintic activity of *Piper sylvaticum* Roxb. (family: Piperaceae): In vitro and in silico studies

Arkajyoti Paul[1,2*] [ID], Md. Adnan[3], Mohuya Majumder[1,6], Niloy Kar[4], Muntasir Meem[4], Mohammed Shahariar Rahman[5], Akash Kumar Rauniyar[7], Nishat Rahman[1,6], Md. Nazim Uddin Chy[1,3] and Mohammad Shah Hafez Kabir[1,3]

## Abstract

**Background:** The present study was conducted to investigate the anthelmintic activity of methanol extract of *Piper sylvaticum* stem (MEPSS) in experimental model followed by in silico molecular docking study and ADME/T analysis.

**Methods:** Anthelmintic activity was determined by an aquarium worm (*Tubifex tubifex*). Then, molecular docking study was performed to identify compounds having maximum activity against TUBULIN-COLCHICINE enzymes by using Schrödinger-Maestro v 10.1 docking fitness. Additionally, ADME/T profiles were checked by Swiss ADME Analysis and Molinspiration Cheminformatics software.

**Results:** A preliminary phytochemical analysis of MEPSS revealed that it contained alkaloids, carbohydrates, flavonoids, tannins, and saponins. MEPSS exhibited a dose-dependent and statistically significant anthelmintic activity on aquarium worm (*Tubifex tubifex*).The best concentration of MEPSS for anthelmintic activity on *Tubifex tubifex* compare with reference standard Levamisole (1 mg/mL) is 11.90 mg/mL. On the other hand, our molecular docking study shows that piperine has the best fitness score of − 6.22 kcal/mol with TUBULIN-COLCHICINE enzyme among three major compounds of *Piper sylvaticum*. Moreover, predicted properties of all compounds were in the range to satisfy the Lipinski's rule of five to be recognized as drug like potential.

**Conclusion:** Results of the present study confirmed potential anthelmintic activity of *Piper sylvaticum* stem extract and all compounds were found to be effective in computer aided drug design models.

**Keywords:** *Piper sylvaticum*, Tannins, Anthelmintic, Molecular docking, Toxicity prediction

## Background

Helminths such as roundworm, tapeworm, flukes are soil transmitting parasitic nematodes generally found in the human intestine causing infection to one-third of the humanity and further resulting in great losses of livestock and crops [1]. The last fifty years research has provided few drugs used to cure human helminthiases infection however in long-term use; many parasites are showing resistance to these drugs. This is becoming a foremost problem for environmental and agriculture sector; for example, multiple varieties of drugs containing macrocyclic lactones, benzimidazoles, praziquantel, and imidathiazoles are used to treat helminthic diseases but one of the studies revealed resistance counter to antihelmintics occurs as soon as their introduction. The reason provided for the decreased response can be either because of heritable changes (genetic or epigenetic) inability of anthelmintic against a population of parasites or reduction in time to which drug treatment applies its effect. Therefore, the use of plant can play a pivotal role in antihelmintic drug target identification [2, 3].

The Piperaceae family of genus Piper has 700 species in the form of herbs, shrubs or infrequently trees. Many of the Piper species have high medicinal and commercial importance [4]. Commercially, these species can be found in the spice markets. The therapeutic application

* Correspondence: arka.bgctub@gmail.com
[1]Drug Discovery, GUSTO A Research Group, Chittagong 4000, Bangladesh
[2]Department of Microbiology, Jagannath University, Dhaka 1100, Bangladesh
Full list of author information is available at the end of the article

of Piper species has been successfully reported against several conditions such as antitumor, antimetastatic, cytotoxic, antidepressant, antibacterial, antifungal and antidiabetic [5]. These plant species have good reputation to be used as medicinal agents for a long time in Jamaica for stomach ache and insect repellents. Additionally, roots and fruits of the *Piper chaba* have been beneficial for asthma, bronchitis, pain, and fever [4]. One of the most important and less investigated Piper Species, Mountain Long Pepper (*Piper sylvaticum* Roxb.), is a terrestrial, perennial angiosperm widely distributed across South China, India, Bangladesh, and Myanmar. In the Indian subcontinent, the leaves of this plant are used as vegetables and roots as a cure for snake poison [5]. The other research indicates the possible use of *P. sylvaticum* as laxative, anthelmintic, and treatment of bronchitis, and cure remedy for the disease of spleen and liver. The photochemistry of *P. sylvaticum* has been investigated and several physiologically active compounds have been identified such as piperine, piperlonguminine, β-sitosterol and N-isobutyldeca-trans-2-trans-4-dienamide which maybe possibly responsible for anticancer effects. Pharmacological activities such as antioxidant and hepatoprotective activities have been reported [5–8].

Even though, so far, there is no report demonstrating the anthelmintic activity of the stems of *P. sylvaticum*. Therefore, the present study aims to evaluate the anthelmintic activity of the stems of *P. sylvaticum* in experimental and computer aided models.

## Methods

### Plant material

The stems of *Piper sylvaticum* (Roxb.) were collected from Kaptai, SitaPahar, Chittagong district, (22°22′N 91° 48′E), Bangladesh in October 2014 and identified by Dr. Shaikh Bokhtear Uddin, a botanist at the Department of Botany, University of Chittagong (CU), Chittagong 4331, Bangladesh and a voucher specimen with the reference (SUB 3217) has been deposited for future reference in the university herbarium.

### Extraction procedure

The collected stems were washed, cut into small parts, dried in the shade and finally ground into coarse powder. The powdered plant material (about 220 g) was taken in a clean, flat-bottomed glass container and soaked in 700 ml of methanol. The particularglass container with the contents was retained for 14 days along with frequent shaking, and the mixture solution was filtered by white sterilized cotton materials accompanied by filter paper (Whatman No.1). Then, the filtrate solution was evaporated in order to yield the methanol

extract of *P. Sylvaticum* (MEPSS: 10 g) which was then stored in a refrigerator at 4 °C until further use.

### Drugs and chemicals

Methanol, hydrochloric acid, and vanillin were purchased from Merck (Darmstadt, Germany). On the other hand, Levamisole collected from ACI Limited, Sonargaon, Bangladesh and catechin from BDH Chemicals Ltd. Poole, UK. All the chemical reagents used in this study were of analytical grade.

### Phytochemical screening

Qualitative phytochemical screening of the MEPSS was carried out to determine the presence of alkaloids, flavonoids, tannins, carbohydrates, and saponins as described previously [9].

### Determination of total condensed tannins content

Total condensed tannins content of MEPSS was estimated by Sun et al. [10, 11]. Briefly, 0.5 ml of extract (1 mg/mL) was added to 3 ml of 4% vanillin-methanol solution (v/v) and 1.5 ml of hydrochloric acid and then slightly vortexed. The final mixture was allowed to stand at room temperature for 15 min, and the measurement of the absorbance was taken at 500 nm. The experiment was carried in triple time, and total condensed tannin or proanthocyanidin content was expressed as catechin (mg/g) by using the equation of the calibration curve y = 0.5825x, $R^2$ = 0.9277, where x indicates the absorbance and y refer the catechin equivalent.

### In vitro anthelmintic activity

The Anthelmintic activity of MEPSS was determined according to the previously reported method [12, 13]. In this study, an aquarium worm (*Tubifex tubifex*) was used for the test due to its physiological and anatomical similarity with an intestinal worm, i.e., Annelida. The worms were collected from an aquarium shop (Chittagong, Bangladesh) and the average size of worms was used for the experiment from 2 to 2.5 cm in length. Here, the test was carried in triplicates and randomly divided into five groups:

Group I: used only distil water served as a negative control
Group II: used standard drug levamisole (1 mg/mL) served as positive control
Groups III, IV, and V: served as test groups at three different concentrations (5, 8 and 10 mg/mL) of MEPSS respectively.

In the present investigation, around 10 to 12 worms were taken in each petri dish in five groups, and 3 mL of extract solution (MEPSS) of different concentrations were added. Then, the starting time, time of paralysis and time of the death of the worms were observed and noted carefully. The anthelmintic activity was evaluated at two different stage 'time of paralysis' and 'time of death' of the worms.The paralysing time was counted when movement of worms could not be observed after shaking vigorously. The time of death was recorded after confirming that the worms moved neither when vigorously shaken nor when dipped in slightly warm water. The best concentration of MEPSS for anthelmintic activity on *T. tubifex* compare with Standard Levamisole (1 mg/mL) was measured by linear regression.

## In silico molecular docking study
For molecular docking study, Glide of Schrödinger-Maestro (Version 10.1) is used to predict the potent active compound *Piper sylvaticum* against the active site of TUBULIN-COLCHICINE enzymes where compounds are collected from the literature review [7].

## Ligand and protein preparation
The chemical structures of three major compounds isolated from *Piper sylvaticum* namely Piperine (PubChem CID: 638024), Piperlonguminine (PubChem CID: 5320621), N-iso butyl deca-trans-2-trans-4-dienamide (PubChem CID: 5318 516) and standard Levamisole (PubChem CID: 26879) were obtained from the PubChem Project database and were structurally plotted in 3 dimensions (3D) using Ligprep 2.5 in Schrödinger Suite, 2015 and their ionization states were generated at pH $7.0 \pm 2.0$ using Epik 2.2 in Schrödinger Suite. In case of the protein preparation, the 3D structure of TUBULIN-COLCHICINE receptor was obtained from the Protein Data Bank (PDB: 1SAO) [14]. Afterward, the structure was prepared and refined using the protein preparation wizard (Schrödinger-Maestro v 10.1) where charges and bond orders were assigned, hydrogens were added to the heavy atoms, selenomethionines were converted to methionine, and all waters portion were removed. On the othe hand, certain thiol and hydroxyl groups were reoriented, and amide groups of asparagines, glutamine, and imidazole ring of histidines, protonation states of histidines, glutamic acidand aspartic acids were optimized at neutral pH. By using force field OPLS_2005, minimization was carried out setting maximum heavy atom RMSD to 0.30 Å [15].

## Receptor grid generation
In Glide, grids were generated keeping the default parameters of van der Waals scaling factor 1.00 and charge cut-off 0.25 subjected to OPLS 2001 force field. A cubic box of specific dimensions centred around the centroid of the active site residues was generated for the receptor. The bounding box was set to 16 Å × 16 Å × 16 Å and it's essential to identify the active binding site in the target protein.

## Glide standard precision (SP) ligand docking
Flexible ligand docking was performed with Glide of Schrödinger-Maestro (version 10.1) [16, 17] within which penalties were applied to non-cis/trans amide bonds. Glide standard precision docking was performed with these molecules, and hits above 4 kcal/mol based on docking score with TUBULIN-COLCHICINE enzyme in XP mode, keeping all docking parameters as default. No bonding constraints were given during docking calculations. Using Monte Carlo random search algorithm, ligand poses were generated for each input molecule, and binding affinity of these molecules to the TUBULIN-COLCHICINE enzyme was predicted regarding Glide docking score. Potential energies of the docked molecules were also predicted with empirical E model scoring function. Post-docking minimization was performed with OPLS 2005 force field, and one pose per ligand was saved. Strain energies of ligands (bound and free forms) were calculated, and hits with more than 4 kcal/mol energy difference between the two forms (bound and free forms) received a penalty equal to the quarter of their strain energy difference, which is added to the docking score.

## ADME & toxicity analysis
As we know molecules of the desired compound must be biologically active in a high amount at the same time, it should be lower in showing toxic activities. It should be easily accessible to the concentration for better therapeutic activity in the human body. To evaluate this pharmacokinetics (i.e. the effect of a remedial compound in the body) of compounds the best way is to separate the different impacts that effect the binding of compounds into the specific active target side. For this purpose, we used Swiss ADME Analysis (http://www.swissadme.ch/) and Moleinspiration Chemoinformatics software (http://www.molinspiration.com/) to estimate the absorption, distributions metabolism, and excretion of the compounds piperine, piperlonguminine, N-isobutyl deca-trans-2-trans-4-dienamide.

## Statistical analysis
Data were analyzed by SPSS software (statistical package for social science, version 20, IBM Corporation, Armonk, NY, USA) and presented as mean ± SEM (standard error mean). Here, *P*-values less than 0.05, 0.01 and 0.001 were considered as statistically significant.

## Results
### Phytochemical screening
Phytochemical screening of MEPSS revealed the presence of alkaloids, carbohydrates, flavonoids, tannins, and saponins.

## Total condensed tannins content

The total condensed tannins content of MEPSS was expressed in catechin equivalent (CE), and the content was $55.82 \pm 0.25$ mg CE/g dried plant extract.

## In vitro anthelmintic activity

The anthelmintic activity of MEPSS was determined on *Tubifex tubifex* worms. From the result, it can be concluded that the degree of anthelmintic activity was found to be directly proportional to the concentration of the extract ranging from the lowest to highest concentration (5 to 10 mg/mL). At the concentrations of 5, 8 and 10 mg/mL, the MEPSS showed significant paralysis time of 12.86, 7.89, 4.53 min and significant death time of 43.95, 27.81 and 21.21 min respectively (Table 1) where the standard drug, Levamisole showed a paralysis time of 3.22 min and death time of 6.06 min. Besides, the best concentration of MEPSS for anthelmintic activity on *Tubifex tubifex* worms compare with the Standard drug, Levamisole (1 mg/ml) is 11.90 mg/ml, which is presented in Table 2.

## In silico study: Molecular docking for anthelmintic activity

In this study, three compounds isolated from *Piper sylvaticum* stem were selected for molecular docking study and the results shown in Table 3. Molecular docking study showed that Piperine has the best docking score against TUBULIN-COLCHICINE which is –6.22 kcal/mol. The results were compared to that of the standard drug of Levamisole which gives docking score –6.527 kcal/mol. Interactions between ligands and TUBULIN-COLCHICINE enzyme have been presented in Fig. 1.

## ADME & Toxicity Analysis

Drug-likeliness activity of the ligand molecule was classified using ADME properties Swiss ADME Analysis and Moleinspiration Chemoinformatics software. The ADME properties (absorption, distribution, metabolism, and elimination) of the piperine, piperlonguminine, and N-isobutyl deca-*trans*-2-*trans*-4-dienamide were shown

**Table 2** Determinations of the best concentration of methanol extract of *Piper sylvaticum* stem for anthelmintic activity on *Tubifex tubifex* worms equivalent with standard drug Levamisole (1 mg/ml)

| Parameter | MEPSS (mg/ml) |
|---|---|
| Equivalent concentration for time taken for paralysis (A) | 10.73 |
| Equivalent concentration for time taken for death (B) | 13.07 |
| Best concentration of MEPSS = (A + B)/2 | 11.90 |

MEPSS denote for methanol extract of *Piper sylvaticum* stem

in Table 4. The selected properties are well-known to influence cell permeation, bioavailability and metabolism. Here, predicted properties of all compounds were in the range to satisfy the Lipinski's rule of five to be recognized as drug like potential.

## Discussion

Plant-derived natural products have gained attention as a potential source of new therapeutic agents. The medicinal properties of plants have been investigated due to their potent pharmacological activities, low toxicity, and economic viability. Moreover, most of the clinically active drugs are from natural products which indicate the importance of drugs having natural sources in drug discovery process. So, it is essential to study the medicinal plants so that the discovery of active natural products ingredient can be identified for healing diseases and then the identified active ingredients could be synthesized in the laboratory [18, 19]. With this view, the plant, *P. sylvaticum* has been investigated for the evaluation of anthelmintic activity using aquarium worm followed by in silico molecular docking study and ADME/T analysis.

Helminths infection is considered to be a significant problem in human and animals that leads to a chronic and devastating disease which ultimately leads to death and also causes drug resistance to other diseases. To prevent infection of helminths, there is a need for studies focusing on natural products such as medicinal plants which give new bioactive compounds having no or fewer side effects, easily available to the peoples of developing countries and more importantly, they have the best compatibility with human physiology than conventional drugs [20–22]. In the present investigation,

**Table 1** Anthelmintic activity of methanol extract of *Piper sylvaticum* stem

| Treatment/Dose | Time is taken for paralysis (min) | Time is taken for death (min) |
|---|---|---|
| Control (Water) | 0.00 | 0.00 |
| Levamisole(1 mg/ml) | 3.32 ± 0.17 | 6.06 ± 0.45 |
| MEPSS (5 mg/ml) | 12.86 ± 0.78*** | 43.95 ± 1.85*** |
| MEPSS (8 mg/ml) | 7.89 ± 0.11*** | 27.81 ± 0.64*** |
| MEPSS (10 mg/ml) | 4.53 ± 0.34 | 21.21 ± 0.54*** |

MEPSS denote for methanol extract of *Piper sylvaticum* stem. Each value in the table is represented as mean ± SEM ($n = 3$). ***$P < 0.001$ compared with standard drug Levamisole (Dunnett's test)

**Table 3** Docking results of Levamisole (standard drug), piperine, piperlonguminine, and N-isobutyl deca-*trans*-2-*trans*-4-dienamide with TUBULIN-COLCHICINE enzyme (PDB: 1SAO) for anthelmintic activity

| Compound name | Docking Score kcal/mol | Glide e model kcal/mol | Glide Energy kcal/mol |
|---|---|---|---|
| Levamisole | −6.527 | −39.285 | −28.885 |
| Piperine | −6.22 | −49.492 | −38.113 |
| Piperlonguminine | −5.328 | −43.743 | −32.599 |
| N-isobutyl deca-*trans*-2-*trans*-4-dienamide | −0.337 | −20.961 | −20.594 |

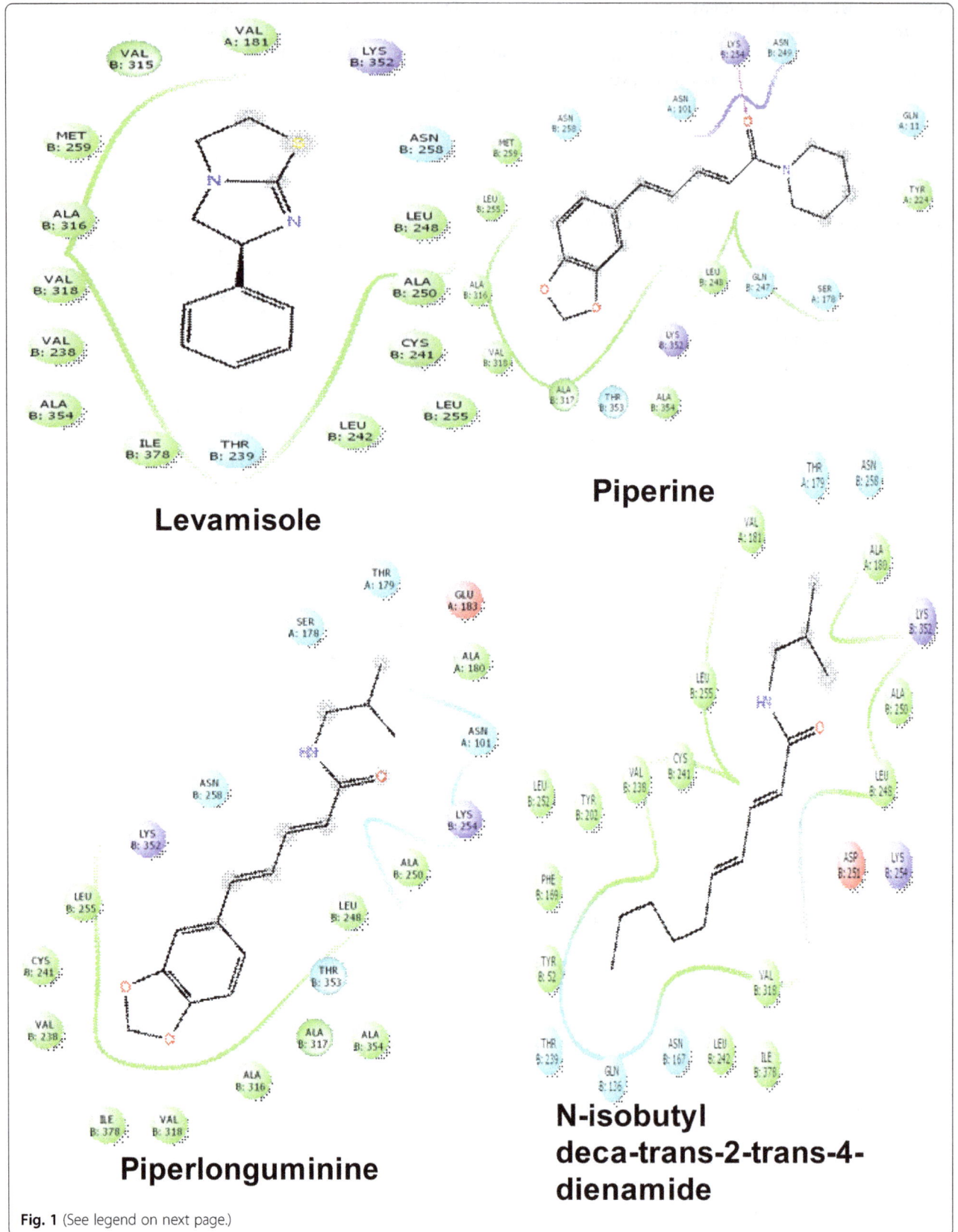

**Levamisole**

**Piperine**

**Piperlonguminine**

**N-isobutyl deca-trans-2-trans-4-dienamide**

**Fig. 1** (See legend on next page.)

(See figure on previous page.)
**Fig. 1** Docking results of Levamisole (standard drug), piperine, piperlonguminine, and N-isobutyl deca-*trans*-2-*trans*-4-dienamide with TUBULIN-COLCHICINE enzyme (PDB: 1SAO) for anthelmintic activity. The colors indicate the residue (or species) type: Red-acidic (Asp, Glu), Green-hydrophobic (Ala, Val,Ile, Leu, Tyr, Phe, Trp, Met, Cys, Pro), Purple-basic (Hip, Lys, Arg), Blue-polar (Ser, Thr, Gln, Asn, His, Hie, Hid), Light gray-other (Gly, water), Darker gray-metal atoms. Interactions with the protein are marked with lines between ligand atoms and protein residues: Solid pink—H-bonds to the protein backbone, Dotted pink-H-bonds to protein side chains, Green—pi-pi stacking interactions, Orange-pi-cation interactions. Ligand atoms that are exposed to solvent are marked with gray spheres. The protein "pocket" is displayed with a line around the ligand, colored with the color of the nearest protein residue. The gap in the line shows the opening of the pocket

observations were made for the time is taken for paralysis and time is taken for the death of individual worms against the methanol extract and the standard drug, levamisole. The standard drug, levamisole acts as a nicotinic acetylcholine receptor agonist, and it causes persistent stimulation of the parasitic worm muscles, leading to paralysis and ultimately leads to death. Several bioactive phytoconstituents such as alkaloids, tannins, saponins, and flavonoids were found predominantly during preliminary phytochemical analysis of the methanol extract of *P. sylvaticum* which have been associated with anthelmintic properties [19, 22]. Besides, the plant, *P. sylvaticum* has been already found to be rich in various plant secondary metabolites such as piperine, piperlonguminine, β-sitosterol, and N-isobutyldeca-trans-2-trans-4-dienamide [7].

Our current study concludes that MEPSS has been found to possess significant anthelmintic potential in a dose-dependent manner. This activity may be due to the presence of bioactive phytoconstituents such as alkaloids, tannins, flavonoids and saponins and also a considerable amount of condensed tannins (55.82 ± 0.25 mg CE/g). Some of these phytoconstituents such as alkaloids, tannins, phenols etc. may be responsible for the significant anthelmintic activity [23]. Here, alkaloids can produce paralysis by acting on the central nervous system (CNS) whereas tannins and polyphenols selectively bind to free proteins present in the GI tract (gastrointestinal tract) and eventually cause mortality. On the other hand, the anthelmintic efficacy of saponins is due to its membrane permeabilising property [19, 22]. The anthelmintic activity of the MEPSS may be due to a single compound or combined effect of these phytochemicals.

We have also evaluated the molecular docking of some compounds to demonstrate the collaboration between compounds and protein at the molecular level, which enables us to portray the conduct of molecule of those compounds in the coupling site of targeted proteins and to illustrate the biochemical process of the anthelminthic activity. From the result (as shown in Table 3), it is concluded that piperine (− 6.22 kcal/mol) and piperlonguminine (− 5.32 kcal/mol) showed the significant docking scores which were comparable to those of the reference drug, Levamisole (− 6.52 kcal/mol). The docking score of Piperine is relatively near about the docking score of standard drugs, Levamisole. From the result of docking study, it is clear that these compounds especially piperine can be a good candidate for new anthelmintic agent.

During the ADME analysis of compounds, we have noticed in Table 4 that three compounds show molecular weight less than 500 g/mol, Hydrogen bond donor activity is less than 5, Hydrogen bond acceptor accepting activity is less than 10, high lipophilicity (logP) is less than 5, molar refractivity are between 40 and 130. From the results of ADME and Toxicity analysis, it can be concluded that all compounds were in the range to satisfy the Lipinski's rule of five to be recognized as drug like potential in terms of better pharmacokinetics properties with less toxic effects.

## Conclusion

From above discussion we can assume that this plant can play a prominent role for anthelmintic activity. As it has been accepted in following three experiments, we can suggest *Piper sylvaticum* for further research to amend the activity of anthelmintic for better effect.

**Table 4** Toxicity and ADME analysis of the phytoconstitiuents isolated from *Piper sylvaticum* by Swiss ADME Analysis and Molinspiration Cheminformatics software

| Compound name | Molecular weight[a] (g/mol) | H-donor[b] | H-acceptor[c] | LogP value[d] | Molar refractivity[e] |
|---|---|---|---|---|---|
| Piperine | 285.34 | 0 | 3 | 3.33 | 85.47 |
| Piperlonguminine | 273.33 | 1 | 3 | 3.30 | 78.77 |
| N-isobutyl deca-*trans*-2-*trans*-4-dienamide | 223.35 | 1 | 1 | 4.26 | 71.47 |

[a]Molecular weight accepted range < 500
[b]Hydrogen bond donor acceptable range ≤ 5
[c]Hydrogen bond acceptor acceptable range ≤ 10
[d]High lipophilicity (expressed as LogP, Acceptable range < 5)
[e]Molar refractivity should be between 40 and 130

**Abbreviations**
MEPSS: Methanol extract of *Piper sylvaticum* stem; mg: milligram; ml: millilitre; RMSD: Root-mean-square deviation; SEM: Standard error mean

**Acknowledgments**
We are greatly thankful to the managing committee of the Department of Pharmacy, International Islamic University Chittagong, Bangladesh for providing all the laboratory facilities and support to complete the research work. Special thanks to A.T.M. Mostafa Kamal, Assistant Professor, Department of Pharmacy, International Islamic University Chittagong for his kind help to complete the study.

## Authors' contributions

MA and MNUC collected, dried and prepared the extract. MNUC, AP, MM[1, 6] and MSHK conceived and designed the study; MA, MM[4], MSR, and NK performed the anthelmintic experiment; MNUC, AP, MM[1, 6], and AKR, have analyzed the data and wrote the manuscript. Best concentration calculation for anthelmintic effect was given by MSHK. AP, NR, and MNUC did the molecular docking study and ADME/T analysis. All authors read and approved the final manuscript.

## Competing interests

The authors declare that they have no competing interests.

## Author details

[1]Drug Discovery, GUSTO A Research Group, Chittagong 4000, Bangladesh. [2]Department of Microbiology, Jagannath University, Dhaka 1100, Bangladesh. [3]Department of Pharmacy, International Islamic University Chittagong, Chittagong 4318, Bangladesh. [4]Department of Pharmacy, East West University, Dhaka 1212, Bangladesh. [5]Department of Pharmacy, University of Science and Technology Chittagong, Chittagong 4202, Bangladesh. [6]Department of Pharmacy, BGC Trust University Bangladesh, Chittagong 4000, Bangladesh. [7]Department of information technology, MDP Bioinformatics, University of Turku, 20500 Turku, Finland.

## References

1. Taylor CM, Wang Q, Rosa BA, Huang SC-C, Powell K, Schedl T, et al. Discovery of anthelmintic drug targets and drugs using chokepoints in nematode metabolic pathways. McKerrow J, editor. PLoS Pathog. Public Library of Science; 2013;9:e1003505.
2. Shalaby HA. Anthelmintics resistance; how to overcome it? Iran J Parasitol. Tehran University of Medical Sciences. 2013;8:18–32.
3. Geerts S, Gryseels B. Drug resistance in human helminths: current situation and lessons from livestock. Clin Microbiol Rev American Society for Microbiology (ASM). 2000;13:207–22.
4. Virinder S. Parmar, Subhash C. Jain, Kirpal S. Bisht, Rajni Jain, Poonam Taneja, Amitabh Jha, Om D. Tyagi, Ashok K. Prasad, Jesper Wengel, C.E. Olsen, Per M. Boll. Phytochemistry of the genus Piper. Phytochemistry. 1997;46 (4):597–673
5. Bezerra DP, Pessoa C, De Moraes MO, Saker-Neto N, Silveira ER, Costa-Lotufo LV. Overview of the therapeutic potential of piplartine (piperlongumine). Eur J Pharm Sci. 2013;48:453–63.
6. Wang Y-H, Morris-Natschke SL, Yang J, Niu H-M, Long C-L, Lee K-H. Anticancer principles from medicinal Piper (胡椒 Hú Jiāo) plants. J Tradit Complement Med. 2014;4(1):8–16.
7. Mahanta PK, Ghanim A, Gopinath KW. Chemical Constituents of Piper sylvaticum (Roxb.) and Piper boehmerifolium (Wall). Journal of Pharmaceutical Sciences. 1974;63(7):1160–1161
8. Ved A, Rawat AKS. and Gupta A. Antioxidant and hepatoprotective potential of phenol-rich fraction from piper sylvaticum roxb. roots. Current Topics in Nutraceuticals Research. 2016;14(3): p.207
9. Tiwari P, Kumar B, Kaur M, Kaur G, Kaur H. Phytochemical screening and extraction: A review. Int. Pharm. Sci. 2011;1:98–106
10. Sun JS, Tsuang YH, Chen IJ, Huang WC, Hang YS, Lu FJ. An ultra-weak chemiluminescence study on oxidative stress in rabbits following acute thermal injury. Burns 1998;24:225–231
11. Virinder S. Parmar, Subhash C. Jain, Kirpal S. Bisht, Rajni Jain, Poonam Taneja, Amitabh Jha, Om D. Tyagi, Ashok K. Prasad, Jesper Wengel, C.E. Olsen, Per M. Boll. Phytochemistry of the genus Piper. Phytochemistry. 1997;46(4):597–673
12. Ajaiyeoba EO, Onocha PA, Olarenwaju OT. In vitro anthelmintic properties of Buchholzia coriaceae and Gynandropsis gynandra extracts. Pharm Biol Taylor & Francis. 2001;39:217–20.
13. Shoibe M, Chy MNU, Alam M, Adnan M, Islam MZ, Nihar SW, Rahman N, Suez E. In Vitro and In Vivo Biological Activities of Cissus adnata (Roxb.). Biomedicines. 2017; 5(4):63. https://doi.org/10.3390/biomedicines5040063.
14. Berman HM, Westbrook J, Feng Z, Gilliland G, Bhat TN, Weissig H, et al. The protein data Bank, 1999–. Int Tables Crystallogr Vol F Crystallogr Biol Macromol Springer; 2006. p. 675–684.
15. Hasanat A, Chowdhury TA, Kabir MSH, Chowdhury MS, Chy MNU, Barua J, Chakrabarty N, Paul A. Antinociceptive Activity of Macaranga denticulata Muell. Arg. (Family: Euphorbiaceae): In Vivo and In Silico Studies. Medicines. 2017; 4(4):88. https://doi.org/10.3390/medicines4040088.
16. Friesner RA, Banks JL, Murphy RB, Halgren TA, Klicic JJ, Mainz DT, et al. Glide: a new approach for rapid, accurate docking and scoring. 1. Method and assessment of docking accuracy. J Med Chem ACS Publications. 2004;47: 1739–49.
17. Halgren TA, Murphy RB, Friesner RA, Beard HS, Frye LL, Pollard WT, et al. Glide: a new approach for rapid, accurate docking and scoring. 2. Enrichment factors in database screening. J Med Chem. ACS Publications. 2004;47:1750–9.
18. Saleh-e-In MM, Sultana N, Hossain MN, Hasan S, Islam MR. Pharmacological effects of the phytochemicals of Anethum sowa L. root extracts. BMC Complement Altern Med. 2016;16:464. https://doi.org/10.1186/s12906-016-1438-9.
19. Jamkhande PG, Barde SR. Evaluation of anthelmintic activity and in silico PASS assisted prediction of Cordia dichotoma (Forst.) root extract. Anc Sci Life Medknow Publications. 2014;34:39–43.
20. Sreejith M, Kannappan N, Santhiagu A, Mathew AP. Phytochemical, anti-oxidant and anthelmintic activities of various leaf extracts of Flacourtia sepiaria Roxb. Asian Pac J Trop Biomed Elsevier. 2013;3:947–53.
21. Beech RN, Skuce P, Bartley DJ, Martin RJ, Prichard RK, Gilleard JS. Anthelmintic resistance: markers for resistance, or susceptibility? Parasitology Cambridge University Press. 2011;138:160–74.
22. Maisale AB, Attimarad SL, Haradagatti DS, Karigar A. Anthelmintic activity of fruit pulp of Cordia dichotoma. Int J Res Ayurveda Pharm International Journal of Research in Ayurveda and Pharmacy. 2010;1:597–600.
23. Bate-Smith EC. The phenolic constituents of plants and their taxonomic significance. I. Dicotyledons. Bot J Linn Soc Oxford University Press. 1962;58:95–173.

# 19

# Phytochemical and pharmacological evaluation of methanolic extract of *Lathyrus sativus* L. seeds

Shovon Bhattacharjee[1], Azhar Waqar[1], Kishan Barua[1], Abhijit Das[2]* , Shukanta Bhowmik[1] and Sumitra Rani Debi[3]

**Abstract**

**Background:** *Lathyrus sativus* L. (Fabaceae) has long been used as a traditional medicine for the treatment of several ailments such as Scabies, eczema, and allergy. The aim of the study was to evaluate the phytochemical nature with Central Nervous System (CNS) depressant, analgesic, antipyretic activities of the methanolic plant extract of *Lathyrus sativus* L. seeds in different experimental models.

**Methods:** Preliminary phytochemical screening and proximate analysis was carried out using different standard methods. CNS depressant activity was evaluated observing the effects of plant extract on Swiss albino mice using open field and hole-cross method. Acetic acid induced writhing and formalin induced paw licking methods were used for the appraisal of analgesic activity while 2,4-dinitrophenol (DNP) induced pyrexia model was used to investigate the antipyretic activity. The data were analyzed by one way ANOVA followed by Dunnett's test using SPSS (version 20).

**Results:** The phytochemical analysis revealed the presence of wide range of phytoconstituents in the plant extract. Our investigation demonstrated that the methanolic plant extract significantly ($p < 0.001$) decreased the locomotor activity of mice in open field and hole-cross method at both the tested doses (200 and 300 mg/kg) which were comparable to the standard drug diazepam (1 mg/kg). The plant extracts significantly ($p < 0.001$) inhibited the writhing induced by acetic acid in mice to 87.09% and 80.65% (200 and 300 mg/kg respectively) compared to the standard indomethacin (70.97%). The extracts (200 and 300 mg/kg respectively) also significantly ($p < 0.001$) reduced the writhing to 43.39%, 64.15% in early and 46.15%, 97.44% in late phase of formalin-induced licking and biting. In 2,4-DNP induced pyrexia the extracts exhibited protection at 200 and 400 mg/kg, similar to standard drug aspirin at 150 mg/kg.

**Conclusion:** The results demonstrated that the plant extract has potential CNS depressant, analgesic and antipyretic activity.

**Keywords:** CNS depressant, Analgesic, Antipyretic, Proximate analysis, *Lathyrus sativus* L

## Background

Several herbal plants have been listed in the ancient literatures for their different medicinal values and their formulation has been found to be effective for the treatment of various diseases [1]. Medicinal plants have provided us lots of bioactive natural compounds like alkaloids, carbohydrates, glycosides, saponins, flavonoids, phenolic compounds, steroids, tannins, gum, amino acids and volatile oils having a wide range of therapeutic and pharmacological potentials which are being used as raw materials for new drug discovery and development for different ailment [2, 3].

Depression of central nervous system (CNS) can be considered as a major affective brain disorder which is very prevalent now-a-days as about 5% of the general population is found to be suffering from it [4]. For the treatment of this disorder several antipsychotic drugs are available in the local medicine stores. But these

* Correspondence: abhijitdas@nstu.edu.bd; abhi.nstu@gmail.com
[2]Department of Pharmacy, Noakhali Science and Technology University, Noakhali 3814, Bangladesh
Full list of author information is available at the end of the article

drugs are reported to be hazardous to human health as they exhibit side effects like damage of autonomic, endocrine, haematopoietic systems, neurological impairment and allergic reactions [5]. Analgesics can be described as those substances which reduces the sensation of pain by alleviating pain threshold to external stimuli [6]. Contemporary analgesics like opiates and non-steroidal anti-inflammatory medications might not continually be appropriate for all patients, significantly for those with chronic pain, because of the limitations of efficacy, facet effects and intolerability. Pyrexia or fever occurs as a result of secondary implication of inflammation while enhanced production of prostaglandins is the key factor for the induction of pain, inflammation and fever [7]. Thus, most anti-inflammatory agents are also expected to possess analgesic and antipyretic activities as they inhibit or prevent excess production of prostaglandins [8]. Based on the above adverse effects of various commercial drugs there is a high demand for these arches of new drugs with lesser or no side effects. Therefore, researchers are focusing towards traditional complementary and alternative medicines to discover new drugs for the treatment of psychiatric disorders, alleviating pain and fever [9–11].

*Lathyrus sativus* L. (grass pea), belonging to Fabaceae family and locally known as "Khesari" in Bangladesh, is widely cultivated for human consumption and livestock feed in Asia and East Africa [12]. The seeds of *L. sativus* L. contain 28 to 32% of proteins and essential amino acids [13]. Oil extracted from the seeds of *L. sativus* L. are used locally as homeopathic medicine [14]. It is also used as traditional medicine in Bangladesh to cure Scabies, eczema, and allergy [15]. It was reported by several studies that the seeds of *L. sativus* L. possess antioxidant [16] and hypoglycemic activities [17] yet no research has been conducted regarding CNS depressant, analgesic and antipyretic activities of the plant extract. Therefore, in pursuit of searching plants possessing significant medicinal and pharmacological activities in Bangladesh and for finding out new sources of CNS depressor, analgesics and anti-inflammatory agents, here we have analyzed the crude methanolic extract of *L. sativus* L. seeds for its CNS depressant, analgesic and antipyretic activities and reported the results in our preliminary investigation.

## Methods
### Drugs and chemicals
All the chemicals used in this study were of analytical grade, and purchased from Sigma Chemical Co. (St. Louis, MO, USA), and Merck (Darmstadt, Germany). Diazepam (Incepta Pharmaceuticals Ltd.), Indomethacin (Opsonin Pharma Ltd.), Aspirin (Square Pharmaceuticals Ltd.) was used for conducting the tests.

### Collection and extraction of plant material
The *L. sativus* L. seeds were collected from the Noakhali region, Bangladesh. The plant samples were identified by a taxonomist and a taxonomical sample specimen (DACB: 36575) was preserved in the National Herbarium of Bangladesh for future reference. The plant seeds were grounded into powder and 500 g of the sample was soaked in 99% methanol. The mixture was then filtrated and the extraction was concentrated using a rotary evaporator (RE200, Bibby Sterling, Ltd., UK) under reduced pressure at 4 rpm and 65 °C temperature. The gummy concentrate obtained was designated as crude methanolic extract. The crude methanolic extract was further freeze dried and preserved at + 4 °C for further analysis.

### Test animals
Healthy Swiss albino mice, six weeks of age and weighing about 25–30 g, of both sexes were obtained from the central animal house of the Department of Pharmacy, Jahangirnagar University, Savar, Dhaka-1342, Bangladesh. The mice were housed five per cage and acclimatized in standard laboratory conditions (room temperature 24 ± 2 °C, relative humidity 55–60%, and 12 h light and dark cycles) for 7 days and were fed formulated rodent food and water prior to the research work. The study was conducted following all the rules governing the use of laboratory animals. The experimental protocol was approved by the Animal Ethics Committee of Noakhali Science and Technology University, Bangladesh.

### Proximate analysis and phytochemical screening
The parameters determined for proximate analyses include moisture, ash content, crude protein and fat. The analysis was carried out using the modified method described by [18] based on method of Association of Official Analytical Chemists (AOAC, 1990). The preliminary phytochemical evaluation of the plant extract for alkaloids, carbohydrates, reducing sugar, cardiac glycosides, flavonoids, saponins, phytosterols, terpenes, phenols, proteins and amino acids, tannins and steroids were determined by using the standard procedures [19–21].

### Experimental design
The experimental animals were divided into control, standard and two test groups containing five mice each. For all test, Group-1 served as controls, Group-2 for standard and Group-3, Group-4 received experimental plant extract. Group 1 received the vehicle 1% Tween 80 in water (at the dose of 10 ml/kg body weight), group 2 received various standard drugs like Diazepam, Indomethacin, Aspirin at different doses [22–24], and group 3 and 4 received 200–400 mg/kg dose of plant extract on the basis of toxicity study of the plant extract.

## CNS depressant activity test

### Open field test

This experiment was carried out in accordance with a modified method of Adebesin et al. [25].. The mice in the control group received the vehicle 1% Tween 80 in water (at the dose of 10 ml/kg body weight) while the test groups received the crude methanolic extract of *L. sativus* L. seeds (at the doses of 200 and 300 mg/kg body weight respectively) and standard group received diazepam at the dose of 10 mg/kg body weight (b.w.) orally. The animals were placed on the floor of an open field (100 cm × 100 cm × 40 cm h) divided into a series of squares with alternative color (black and white). The number of squares visited by each animal was counted for 3 min duration started at 0, 30, 60, 90 and 120 min after the administration of test drugs.

### Hole-cross test

The method described by Hussain et al. was followed to conduct this test using a cage (30 cm × 20 cm × 14 cm) with a steel partition fixed in the middle [26]. A hole of 3 cm diameter was made at a height of 7.5 cm in the middle of the cage. The mice were divided into control (received vehicle 1% Tween 80 in water at 10 mL/kg body weight), standard (diazepam at a dose of 1 mg/kg body weight) and two test groups (received methanolic extract of seeds of *L. sativus* L. at the doses of 200 and 300 mg/kg body weight respectively) each having five mice. The number of passage of a mouse from one chamber to another through the hole was recorded for a period of 3 min at the 0, 30, 60, 90 and 120 min of the oral administration of test drugs.

## In vivo analgesic activity test

### Acetic acid induced writhing test

To evaluate the analgesic activity of the plant extract acetic acid writhing model in mice was conducted accordingly the procedure described by Koster et al. [27]. The test samples (methanolic extract of *L. sativus* L., 200 and 400 mg/kg body weight respectively), standard (indomethacin, 10 mg/kg body weight per orally) and control (1% Tween 80 in distilled water at the dose of 10 ml/kg body weight) were given and after 30 min 0.7% acetic acid was injected intra-peritoneally (i.p.). The writhing (constriction of abdomen, turning of trunk and extension of hind legs) was observed randomly after 15 min of interval and its frequency was counted for up to 25 min in each group of animals. The percent inhibition (% analgesic activity) was calculated by:

$$\%\text{Inhibition} = [(A–B)/A] \times 100$$

Where, A = Average number of writhing of the control group; B = Average number of writhing of the test or standard groups.

### Formalin induced writhing test

This test was performed according to the procedure described by Viana et al. [28]. The experimental animals were separated in four groups each having 5 mice and received 1% Tween 80 in water at 10 ml/kg body weight dose per orally (p.o.) (control group), indomethacin at 10 mg/kg body weight subcutaneously (s.c.) (standard) and methanolic extract of *L. sativus* L. seeds at the dose of 200 and 400 mg/kg body weight p.o. (test groups). At 30 min interval the test animals were injected 50 μL of freshly prepared 0.6% solution of formalin subcutaneously, under the plantar surface of the left hind paw of each mouse. The mice were placed individually in an observation chamber and monitored for one hour. The time (in second) spent in licking and biting responses of the injected paw was taken as an indicator of pain response. Anti-nociceptive effect was determined in two phases. The early phase (Neurogenic phase) was recorded during the first 5 min, while the late phase (Inflammatory phase) was recorded during the last 15–20 min after formalin injection.

## Antipyretic activity test

### 2,4-Dinitrophenol (DNP) induced pyrexia

Adult albino mice of both sexes fasted for 24 h but allowed water ad libitum were used for the experiment. They were randomized into groups of five mice each. DNP (10 mg/kg, i.p.) was administered to the mice after obtaining the basal rectal temperatures. Hyperthermia developed within 30 min of DNP administration. Different doses of extract (200 and 400 mg/kg body weight i.p.), aspirin (150 mg/kg), and distilled water (10 ml/kg, p.o.) were administered to the treatment and control groups of animals. The rectal temperature of each animal was recorded by inserting a thermometer 2 cm into the rectum at 1, 2, 3 and 4 h after administration of the test drugs [29].

## Statistical analysis

One way ANOVA with Dunnett's post Hoc test for this experiment was carried out with SPSS 18.0 for Windows® software and the results obtained were compared with the control group. Differences between groups were considered significant at a level of $p < 0.001$, $p < 0.01$ and $p < 0.05$.

## Results

### Proximate analysis

Results of proximate analysis of dried seeds of *L. sativus* L. are demonstrated in Table 1. The results revealed that the plant extract has low moisture content (10.77%) and a high ash value (6.68%). It also contains moderate concentration of protein (4.27%) and low concentration of fat (1.11%).

**Table 1** Proximate composition of dried *L. sativus* L. seeds

| Proximate Analysis | Value (%) |
| --- | --- |
| Moisture Content | 10.77 |
| Total Ash Value | 6.68 |
| Proteins | 4.27 |
| Fat | 1.11 |

## Phytochemical screening

Table 2 reveals the quantitative phytochemical analysis of *L. sativus* L. seeds. The preliminary phytochemical evaluation of the plant extract confirmed the presence of alkaloids, carbohydrates, reducing sugar, flavonoids, terpenes, phenols, proteins and amino acids, and tannins.

## CNS depressant activity

### Open field test

After statistical analysis of the experimental data (Dunnett's test), it was observed that in open field test, the number of squares traveled by the mice was suppressed significantly in the test group throughout the study period (Table 3). The CNS depressant activity observed for the extract was dose dependent and a noticeable result was found at 120 min of test sample administration. Test animals showed significant ($p < 0.001$) decrease in number of movement at the dosages of 300 mg/kg ($2.67 \pm 0.33$) and 200 mg/kg ($9.33 \pm 0.33$), as compared to $34.67 \pm 2.60$ for the control group and $24.00 \pm 1.53$ for the standard group after 120 min of administration of the extract.

### Hole-cross test

Results of the hole-cross test of *L. sativus* L. seeds are shown in Table 4. The locomotors activity reducing effect was manifested at the 2nd observation (30 min)

**Table 2** Phytochemical compositions of methanolic extract of *L. sativus* L. seeds

| Phytochemical groups | Methanolic extract |
| --- | --- |
| Alkaloids | + |
| Carbohydrates | + |
| Reducing Sugar | + |
| Cardiac Glycosides | − |
| Flavonoids | + |
| Saponins | − |
| Phytosterols | − |
| Terpenes | + |
| Phenols | + |
| Proteins and Amino acids | + |
| Tannins | + |
| Steroids | − |

(+) = Present of Phytochemicals and (−) = Absence of Phytochemicals

period and was sustained up to the 5th observation period (120 min) for the plant extract. The extract diminished the movement of the tested animals in a dose dependent manner which was comparable with standard diazepam. After 120 min of administration the extract, at the dose of 200 and 300 mg/kg, showed significant ($p < 0.001$) depressant activity by reducing the locomotion of the mice to $2.50 \pm 0.64$ ($p < 0.001$) and $1.25 \pm 0.25$ ($p < 0.001$) respectively. In comparison the standard drug diazepam reduced the movement of the tested animal to $2.50 \pm 0.29$ ($p < 0.001$) at the dose of 1 mg/kg.

## Analgesic activity

### Acetic acid induced writhing method

The results showed that the pain relief was achieved in a significant ($P < 0.01$, $P < 0.001$) dose dependent manner, at all test doses (200 and 400 mg/kg body weight) as shown in figs. 1 and 2 ensured by Dunnett's test. Maximum writhing inhibition (87.09%) was observed at 400 mg/kg dose of methanolic extract of *L. sativus* L. seeds while at 300 mg/kg dose it exhibited 80.65% inhibition. The inhibitory effect of indomethacin (10 mg/kg body weight) was lower (70.97%) than that of the highest dose of the plant extract.

### Formalin induced paw licking method

The results of the antinociceptive effects of *L. sativus* L. seeds on formalin-induced paw pain response in mice are presented in Table 5. It can be seen that the highest dose (400 mg/kg b.w.) caused a significant ($p < 0.001$) inhibitory effect, once again in a dose dependent manner, on both phases of formalin induced pain as compared to control. The percentage of inhibition was 43.39 and 46.15% for the dose of 200 mg/kg; and 64.15 and 97.44% for 450 mg/kg b.w. in the first and second phase respectively. This potency was comparable to that of indomethacin (10 mg/kg b.w.) which produced an inhibition of 54.72% during the first phase and 71.79% during the second phase of the formalin-induced pain in mice.

## Antipyretic activity

### 2, 4-Dinitrophenol (DNP) induced pyrexia test

From the results (Table 6), it was observed that, experimental mice showed a marked increase in rectal temperature, 18th h after DNP injection. The extract (200 and 400 mg/kg) significantly ($p < 0.05$–0.01) reduced the rectal temperature of the animals in the second, third and fourth hour after administration, reaching the peak of antipyretic effect with the highest dose (400 mg/kg) in the 4th h ($35.26 \pm 0.52$ °C, $p < 0.001$), in relation to control ($36.95 \pm 0.49$ °C). Standard drug (aspiring) treatment (150 mg/kg body weight) caused significant ($p < 0.05$) antipyretic effect at all time periods,

**Table 3** Effect of methanolic extract of the L. sativus L. seeds on open field test in mice

| Group | Number of Movements(Mean ± SEM) | | | | |
|---|---|---|---|---|---|
| | 0 min | 30 min | 60 min | 90 min | 120 min |
| Group-I | 57.50 ± 2.50 | 50.50 ± 2.50 | 46.67 ± 1.76 | 45.33 ± 5.33 | 34.67 ± 2.60 |
| Group-II | 45.00 ± 2.00 | 33.00 ± 2.00[*] | 31.33 ± 2.03[**] | 15.33 ± 0.88[**] | 24.00 ± 1.53[**] |
| Group-III | 38.50 ± 1.50[**] | 32.50 ± 2.50[*] | 32.00 ± 2.00[**] | 23.33 ± 1.45[*] | 9.33 ± 0.33[***] |
| Group-IV | 36.50 ± 0.50 | 29.50 ± 0.50[*] | 20.67 ± 3.04[**] | 4.33 ± 0.33[**] | 2.67 ± 0.33[***] |

Values are represented as mean ± SEM, ($n = 5$). Group I (control) animals received vehicle (1% Tween 80 in water), Group II (standard) received diazepam 1 mg/kg body weight, Group III and Group IV were treated with 200 and 300 mg/kg body weight (p.o.) of the methanolic extract of L. sativus L. seeds, respectively. ***indicates $P < 0.001$, **indicates $P < 0.01$ and *indicates $P < 0.05$; one-way ANOVA followed by Dunnett's test as compared to control

reaching the peak in the 4th h ($35.00 ± 0.49$ °C) in comparison to control.

## Discussion

In our research work we tried to explicate diverse pharmacological potency of the methanolic extract of L. sativus L. in mice along with the proximate and phytochemical analysis. The proximate analysis of the plant extract was carried out to evaluate its moisture, total ash, protein and fat content. It is a very important technique for the product development and quality control or regulatory purposes in the food industry and also for the purity and quality test of crude drugs in pharmaceutical industry [30]. Our study results demonstrated that the methanolic plant extract had a low moisture content which indicates that the preservation period of the extract will be high as it is evident that moisture content in the range of 5–15% are good for formulating and also hinder the microbial growth [31]. The moderate amount of ash content in the plant extract suggests that it is comparatively rich in different types of minerals. Ash content estimation is necessary because the inorganic elements or minerals may be the cause of a pharmacological impact [32]. Proximate analysis also revealed that the plant possess moderate amount of protein and lower amount of fat. Protein plays a major role in various body functions like body development, fluid balance, hormone and enzyme formation and also sustaining strong immune function. While low content of fat (below the range 8.3–27.0%) is reported to be poor sources of lipids and thus increase in the consumption of the vegetables would naturally lower fat intake [32].

The secondary metabolites (phytochemicals) of a plant extract are responsible for the pharmacological actions of that plant or plant parts and thus estimation of those bioactive compounds may be used to treat chronic as well as infectious diseases [30]. Our study was an evidential approach to ascertain the mentioned pharmacological functions of L. sativus L. seeds and found to have the presence of alkaloids, carbohydrates, reducing sugar, flavonoids, terpenes, phenols, proteins and amino acids, and tannins in the plant extract. Several studies reported that alkaloids possess various pharmacological activities like antihypertensive, antiarrhythmic, antimalarial and anticancer activity [33]. Pure alkaloids and their synthetic compounds have also been reported to be used as analgesic, antispasmodic and antibacterial agents [32]. Carbohydrates and reducing sugar are essential nutrient for the body as they produce energy required and supplies energy to brain, muscle and blood [34]. Terpenes possess medicinal properties such as anticarcinogenic, antimalarial, antiulcer, antimicrobial and diuretic activity [32]. Phenols, flavonoids and tannins are the major groups responsible for antioxidant activity [31]. Previous studies showed that saponins demonstrated antibacterial, antiinflammatory, anticancer, and antidiabetic activities [35].

Two different neuropharmacological models, namely open field and hole-cross test, were used to study the CNS depressant activity of L. sativus L. seed extract. The results of the study provided evidence that the plant extract significantly ($p < 0.001$) induced sedative-hyponotic activity in test animals confirming their CNS depressant

**Table 4** Effect of methanolic extract of the L. sativus L. seeds on hole cross test in mice

| Group | Number of Movements (Mean ± SEM) | | | | |
|---|---|---|---|---|---|
| | 0 min | 30 min | 60 min | 90 min | 120 min |
| Group-I | 11.75 ± 1.11 | 27.00 ± 2.45 | 19.50 ± 2.22 | 18.50 ± 1.19 | 20.00 ± 2.39 |
| Group-II | 6.50 ± 1.32[*] | 11.00 ± 1.58[**] | 5.25 ± 1.37[**] | 9.00 ± 0.58[***] | 2.50 ± 0.29[***] |
| Group-III | 2.25 ± 0.48[***] | 9.50 ± 1.08[**] | 6.25 ± 1.03[**] | 4.00 ± 0.41[***] | 2.50 ± 0.64[***] |
| Group-IV | 4.00 ± 0.91[**] | 6.50 ± 0.87[***] | 4.00 ± 0.71[***] | 2.25 ± 0.29[***] | 1.25 ± 0.25[***] |

Values are represented as mean ± SEM, ($n = 5$). Group I (control) animals received vehicle (1% Tween 80 in water), Group II (standard) received diazepam 1 mg/kg body weight, Group III and Group IV were treated with 200 and 300 mg/kg body weight (p.o.) of the methanolic extract of L. sativus L. seeds, respectively. ***indicates $P < 0.001$, **indicates $P < 0.01$ and *indicates $P < 0.05$; one-way ANOVA followed by Dunnett's test as compared to control

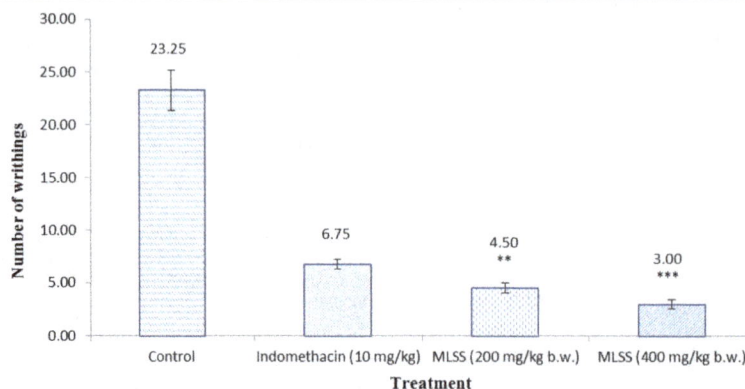

**Fig. 1** Effect of *L. sativus* L. seeds on acetic acid induced writhing in mice. Results are given as mean ± SEM of five animals in each group. ***indicates *P* < 0.001, **indicates *P* < 0.01 when compared to control. One-way ANOVA followed by Dunnett's test as compared to control. MLSS = Methanolic extract of *L. sativus* L. seeds

activity. Gamma-aminobutyric acid (GABA) is evidenced to be the major inhibitory neurotransmitter of CNS and several anxiolytic, muscle relaxant and sedative-hypnotic drugs exhibit their action via GABA [36]. Thus it can be pretended that the methanolic seed extract may act by commencing the GABAergic inhibition of the CNS through membrane hyperpolarization that lead to a reduction in the firing rate of critical neurons in the brain or the extract may simply activate the GABA receptors directly [37]. Again, research has shown that plants containing alkaloids, flavonoids and tannins are useful for the treatment of many CNS disorders as they reduce the locomotor activity of the CNS [38] which led to the postulation that these compounds may act as benzodiazepine like molecules [39]. Earlier investigation of the phytoconstituents of *L. sativus* L. proved the presence of these phytochemicals [40]. Thus it may be predicted that these compounds may also be responsible for the CNS depressant activity of the plant extracts though the key compound for producing such effect is yet to be discovered.

Among various available test to evaluate the analgesic activity of different compounds, Acetic acid-induced writhing is a well recommended protocol in evaluating the peripheral analgesic property of medicinal agents due to its sensitivity and response to the compounds at a dose which is not effective in other methods [41]. In our study, assessment of analgesic activity using the acetic acid induced writhing test revealed that oral administration of *L. sativus* L. seeds produced a statistically significant inhibition of writhes compared to the control. This is an indication of the peripheral analgesic activity of the active principle(s) of the plant extract, since any agent that lowers the writhing number, demonstrates analgesia by inhibiting prostaglandin synthesis which is a peripheral mechanism of pain inhibition [42]. Here the pain induction is caused by liberating endogenous substances as well as some other pain mediators such as arachidonic acid via cyclooxygenase, and prostaglandin biosynthesis (specifically lipoxygenase, PGE2 and PGF2α) [43]. These products enhance capillary permeability affecting local pain receptor that results in inflammation and pain [41].

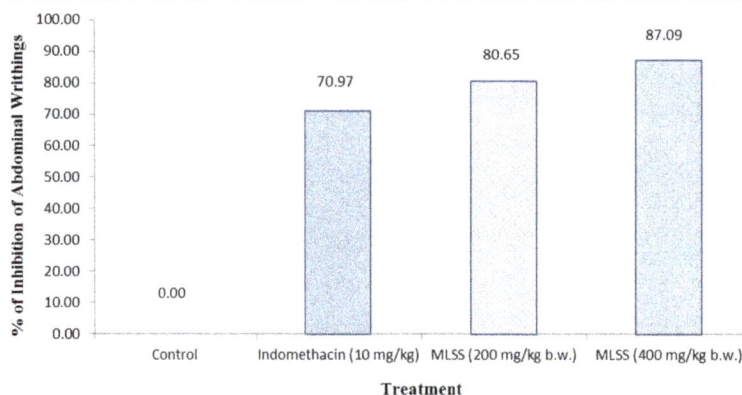

**Fig. 2** Percentage of inhibition of abdominal contractions in acetic acid induced writhing method by *L. sativus* L. seeds and standard indomethacin. MLSS = Methanolic extract of *L. sativus* L. seeds

**Table 5** Effect of methanolic extract of the *L. sativus* L. seeds on formalin induced writhing in mice

| Groups | Licking number (Mean ± SEM) | | % Inhibition | |
|---|---|---|---|---|
| | Early phase (0–5 min) | Late phase (10–15 min) | Early phase (0–5 min) | Late phase (10–15 min) |
| Group-I | 13.25 ± 0.63 | 9.75 ± 0.85 | – | – |
| Group-II | 6.00 ± 0.41 | 2.75 ± 0.25 | 54.72 | 71.79 |
| Group-III | 7.50 ± 0.65** | 5.25 ± 0.63** | 43.39 | 46.15 |
| Group-IV | 4.75 ± 0.48** | 0.25 ± 0.25*** | 64.15 | 97.44 |

Values are expressed as mean ± SEM (*n* = 5). Group I (control) animals received vehicle (1% Tween 80 in water), Group II (standard) received indomethacin 10 mg/kg body weight, Group III and Group IV were treated with 200 and 400 mg/kg body weight (p.o.) of the methanolic extract of *L. sativus* L. seeds, respectively. ***indicates *P* < 0.001, and **indicates *P* < 0.01; one-way ANOVA followed by Dunnett's t-test as compared to control. MLSS = Methanolic extract of *L. sativus* L. seeds

In order to obtain more specific evidence on the possible mechanism of analgesic activity of *L. sativus* L. seeds, the effect of different doses of the plant extract on formalin test was examined. This test model is considered as a method of persistent pain produced by the intra-plantar injection of formalin that induces a biphasic nociceptive behavior. The early phase (0–5 min) is characterized by neurogenic pain caused by C-fibre activation due to the stimulation of peripheral nociceptors caused by formalin [44]. A second burst of licking behavior occurs after 15 to 30 min and seems to be characterized by the inflammatory response elicited by formalin which is triggered by a combination of stimuli, including inflammation of the peripheral tissues and mechanisms of central sensitization [45, 46]. Again it is assumed that manifestation in the late phase is due to inflammation causing a release of serotonin, histamine, bradykinin and prostaglandins, which at least to some degree can cause the sensitization of the central nociceptive neurons [47]. It is reported that substance P is involved in the first phase whereas histamine, serotonin, prostaglandins and bradykinin are responsible for the second phase of inflammation [45]. In our research, the extract demonstrated antinociceptive activity in blocking both phases of the formalin response although the effect of the extract was more pronounced in the late phase of test. As oral pretreatment with *L. sativus* L. inhibited the first (neurogenic pain) and second (inflammatory nociception) phases of formalin-induced licking in mice therefore it may be postulated that the plant extract may possess both peripheral and central effect.

On antipyretic activity the plant extract significantly inhibited DNP induced pyrexia at both the concentrations. In generally, non-steroidal anti-inflammatory drugs (NSAIDs) exhibit their antipyretic effect through inhibiting the production of prostaglandins specifically prostaglandin E2 (PGE2) in the hypothalamus [48]. Thus it may be assumed that the plant extract may have functioned as a cyclooxygenase-2 (COX-2) antagonist through the inhibition of PGE2 production in the hypothalamus or by the enhancement of body's own antipyretic substances such as vasopressin and arginine production [29, 48]. Furthermore, the extract could have also been mediated its hypothermic activity by vasodilatation of superficial blood vessels resulting in increased dissipation of heat following resetting of hypothalamic temperature control center [49]. However, all these actions may be due to presence of certain phytochemical compounds in this plant as several studies have reported that steroids, tannins, triterpenoids, flavonoid and coumarin glycosides are responsible for antipyretic activity [50]. Our investigated plant also contains tannis, terpenoids and flavonoid which may have attributed to its potent antipyretic activity.

## Conclusion

On the basis of the findings of the present study it can be easily stated that the methanolic extract of *Lathyrus sativus* L. seeds possesses remarkable pharmacological potentialities. The results of our research work also supplicate its traditional uses for various medical purposes. Therefore, the experimental evidence obtained in the

**Table 6** Effect of methanol extract of *L. sativus* L. seeds on 2, 4-Dinitrophenol (DNP) induced pyrexia in mice

| Treatment | Temperature in °C | | | | | |
|---|---|---|---|---|---|---|
| | Initial | Pyretic | 1 h | 2 h | 3 h | 4 h |
| Group-I | 36.23 ± 0.69 | 37.23 ± 0.55 | 37.22 ± 0.54 | 37.01 ± 0.5 | 37.01 ± 0.50 | 36.95 ± 0.49 |
| Group-II | 34.95 ± 0.28 | 36.09 ± 0.22 | 35.79 ± 0.30* | 35.24 ± 0.29* | 35.08 ± 0.27* | 35.00 ± 0.28* |
| Group-III | 35.97 ± 0.73 | 36.93 ± 0.78 | 36.79 ± 0.76 | 36.41 ± 0.82 | 36.29 ± 0.77 | 36.22 ± 0.82 |
| Group-IV | 34.86 ± 0.13 | 36.09 ± 0.19 | 35.87 ± 0.13 | 35.25 ± 0.16* | 35.08 ± 0.14* | 34.87 ± 0.13** |

Values are expressed as mean ± SEM (*n* = 5). Group I (control) animals received distilled water (10 ml/kg), Group II (standard) received aspirin 150 mg/kg body weight, Group III and Group IV were treated with 200 and 400 mg/kg body weight (p.o.) of the methanolic extract of *L. sativus* L. seeds, respectively. ***indicates *P* < 0.001, and **indicates *P* < 0.01; one-way ANOVA followed by Dunnett's t-test as compared to control. MLSS = Methanolic extract of *L. sativus* L. seeds

laboratory test model could justify for the traditional use of this plant as a CNS depressant, analgesic, and antipyretic agent.

## Abbreviations

AOAC: Association of Official Analytical Chemists; b.w.: Body Weight; CNS: Central Nervous System; COX-2: Cyclooxygenase-2; DNP: Dinitrophenol; GABA: Gamma-aminobutyric acid; i.p.: Intra-Peritoneally; NSAID: Non-Steroidal Anti-Inflammatory Drug; p.o.: Per Orally; PGE2: Prostaglandin E2; s.o.: Subcutaneously

## Acknowledgements

The authors are also thankful to all the teachers and staffs of the Department of Pharmacy, Noakhali Science and Technology University for their cordial co-operation by providing laboratory support to carry out the research work.

## Funding

This research work was carried out by the author in the partial fulfillment of the requirements for the degree of Bachelor of Science (Hons) in Applied Chemistry and Chemical Engineering. Authors did not receive any funding for conducting the research work.

## Authors' contributions

MAW and KB carried out the collection of plant, extraction process and conducted the research work. AD wrote the manuscript. SB and AD* carried out conception and design of the study, statistical analysis and interpretation of data. SB and SRD helped in the plant collection procedure, revised the manuscript and guided to improve the quality of final manuscript. All authors read and approved the final manuscript.

## Competing interests

The author reports no conflict of interests in this work.

## Author details

[1]Department of Applied Chemistry and Chemical Engineering, Noakhali Science and Technology University, Noakhali 3814, Bangladesh. [2]Department of Pharmacy, Noakhali Science and Technology University, Noakhali 3814, Bangladesh. [3]Department of Environmental Science and Disaster Management, Noakhali Science and Technology University, Noakhali 3814, Bangladesh.

## References

1. Senthilkumar R, Ahmedjohn S, Archunan G, Manoharan N. Antioxidant activity of Wedelia chinensis in alloxan induced diabetic rats. Pharmacologyonline. 2008;2:640–51.
2. Hasan MM, Hossain A, Shamim A, Rahman MM. Phytochemical and pharmacological evaluation of ethanolic extract of Lepisanthes rubiginosa L leaves. BMC Complement Altern Med. 2017;17(1):496.
3. Akinmoladun AC, Ibukun EO, Afor E, Obuotor EM, Farombi EO. Phytochemical constituent and antioxidant activity of extract from the leaves of Ocimum gratissimum. Sci Res Essays. 2007;2(5):163–6.
4. Hoskeri JH, Venkatarangaiah K, Hanumanthappa SK, Vootla SK, Gadwala M. CNS depressant activity of extracts from Flaveria trinervia spring C. Mohr Phytopharmacol. 2011;1:101–8.
5. Zhang ZJ. Therapeutic effect of herbal extract and constituents in animal models of psychiatric disorders. Life Sci. 2004;75:1659–99.
6. Kumar JP, Shankar NB. Analgesic activity of Mollugo pentaphylla Linn by tail immersion method. Asian J Pharm Clin Res. 2009;2:61–3.
7. Khan MA, Baki A, Al-Bari MA, Hasan S, Mosaddik MA, Rahman MM, et al. Antipyretic activity of roots of Laportea crenulata gaud in rabbit. Res J Med Med Sci. 2007;2(2):58–61.
8. Dewanjee S, Maiti A, Sahu R, Dua TK, Mandal SC. Study of anti-inflammatory and antinociceptive activity of hydroalcoholic extract of Schima wallichii bark. Pharm Biol. 2009;47(5):402–7.
9. Selvi PT, Kumar MS, Yaswanth T, Adiyaman E, Anusha PT. Central nervous system depressant activity of aqueous extract of leaves of Azadirachta indica Linn in mice. Asian J Pharm Res. 2012;2:97–9.
10. Sulaiman MR, Zakaria ZA, Chiong HS, Lai SK, Israf DA, Tg TM, et al. Antinociceptive and anti-inflammatory effects of Stachytarpheta jamaicensis (L.) Vahl (Verbenaceae) in experimental animal models. Med Princ Pract. 2009;18:272–9.
11. Ibrahim B, Sowemimo A, van Rooyen A, Van de Venter M. Antiinflammatory, analgesic and antioxidant activities of Cyathula prostrata (Linn.) Blume (Amaranthaceae). J Ethnopharmacol. 2012;141(1):282–9.
12. Ramakrishna V, Rajasekhar S, Reddy LS. Identification and purification of metalloprotease from dry grass pea (Lathyrus sativus L.) seeds. Appl Biochem Biotechnol. 2010;160(1):63.
13. Urga K, Fufa H, Biratu E, Husain A. Evaluation of Lathyrus sativus cultivated in Ethiopia for proximate composition, minerals, β-ODAP and anti-nutritional components. African J food, Agricul Nutr. Dev. 2005;5(1):1–15.
14. Duke J. Handbook of legumes of world economic importance. Springer Science & Business Media. 2012;
15. Ahsan S, Jahan R, Ahmad I, Chowdhury H, Rahmatullah M. A survey of medicinal plants used by Kavirajes of Barisal town in Barisal district. Bangladesh American-Eurasian J Sust Agric. 2010;4(2):237–46.
16. Sarmento A, Barros L, Fernandes Â, Carvalho AM, Ferreira IC. Valorization of traditional foods: nutritional and bioactive properties of Cicer arietinum L. and Lathyrus sativus L. pulses. J Sci Food Agric. 2015;95(1):179–85.
17. Sultana A, Rahmatullah M. Antihyperglycemic activity of methanolic extract of non-boiled and boiled Lathyrus sativus L. seeds. J Chem Pharm Res. 2016; 8(8):874–6.
18. Oluduro AO. Evaluation of antimicrobial properties and nutritional potentials of Moringa oleifera lam. Leaf in South_Western Nigeria, Malaysian. J Microbiol. 2012;2(8):59–67.
19. Harborne JB. Phytochemical methods. A guide to modern techniques of plant analysis, vol. 13. London, New York: Chapman and Hall Ltd; 1973. p. 49–188.
20. Roopashree TS, Dang R, Rani SRH, Narendra C. Antibacterial activity of antipsoriatic herbs: Cassiatora, Momordica charantia and Calendula officinalis. Int J Appl Res Nat Prod. 2005;1(3):20–8.
21. Sofowora AE. Recent trends in research into African medicinal plants. J Ethnopharmacol. 1993;389:209–14.
22. Nahar L, Zahan R, Morshed MTI, Haque A, Alamand Z, Mosaddik A. Antioxidant, analgesic and CNS depressant effects of Synedrella Nodiflora. PHOG J. 2012;4(31):29–36.
23. Murugesan T, Ghosh L, Das J, Pal M, Saha BP. CNS activity of Jussiaea suffruticosa Linn. Extract in rats and mice. Pharm Pharmacol Commun. 1999;5:663–6.
24. Essien AD, Essiet GA, Akuodor GC, Akpan JL, Chilaka KC, Bassey AL, Ezeokpo BC, Nwobodo NN. Pharmacological evaluation of the aqueous stem bark extract of Bombax buonopozense in the relief of pain and fever. Afr J Pharm Pharmacol. 2016;10(5):59–65.
25. Adebesin IF, Akindele AJ, Adeyemi OO. Evaluation of neuropharmacological effects of aqueous leaf extract of Albizia glaberrima (Leguminosae) in mice. J Ethnopharmacol. 2015;160:101–8.
26. Hussain J, Ur Rehman N, Hussain H, Al-Harrasi A, Ali L, Rizvi TS. Analgesic, anti-inflammatory, and CNS depressant activities of new constituents of Nepeta clarkei. Fitoterapia. 2012;83(3):593–8.
27. Koster R, Anderson M, DeBeer EJ. Acetic acid analgesic screening. Fed Proc. 1959;18:418–20.
28. Viana GS, Do Vale TG, Rao VSN, Matos FJA. Analgesic and antiinflammatory effects of two chemotypes of Lippia alba: a comparative study. Pharm Biol. 1998;36(5):347–51.
29. Okokon J, Davis KA, Azare BA. Antipyretic and antimalarial activities of Solenostemon monostachyus. Pharm Biol. 2016;54(4):648–53.
30. Shukla A, Vats S, Shukla RK. Phytochemical screening, proximate analysis and antioxidant activity of Dracaena reflexa lam. Leaves. Indian J Pharm Sci. 2015;77(5):640.

31. Islam MZ, Hossain MT, Hossen F, Mukharjee SK, Sultana N, Paul SC. Evaluation of antioxidant and antibacterial activities of *Crotalaria pallida* stem extract. Clinical Phytosci. 2018;4(1):8.

32. Achi NK, Onyeabo C, Ekeleme-Egedigwe CA, Onyeanula JC. Phytochemical, proximate analysis, vitamin and mineral composition of aqueous extract of *Ficus capensis* leaves in south eastern Nigeria. J Appl Pharm Sci. 2017;7(3):117–22.

33. Saxena M, Saxena J, Nema R, Singh D, Gupta A. Phytochemistry of medicinal plants. J Pharmacog Phytochem. 2013;1(1):168–82.

34. Ejelonu BC, Lasisi AA, Olaremu AG, Ejelonu OC. The chemical constituents of calabash (*Crescentia cujete*). African J Biotechnol. 2011;10(84):19631–6.

35. Urzúa A, Rezende MC, Mascayano C, Vásquez L. A structure-activity study of antibacterial diterpenoids. Molecules. 2008;13:882–91.

36. Wong CG, Bottiglieri T, Snead OC. Gaba, γ-hydroxybutyric acid, and neurological disease. Annals Neurol. 2003;54(S6):S3-12.

37. Kolawole OT, Makinde JM, Olajide OA. Central nervous system depressant activity of *Russelia equisetiformis*. Niger J Physiol Sci. 2007;22:59–63.

38. Hossain MS, Akter S, Das A, Sarwar MS. CNS depressant, antidiarrheal and antipyretic activities of ethanolic leaf extract of *Phyllanthus acidus* L. on Swiss albino mice. British J Pharm Res. 2016;10(5):1.

39. Verma A, Jana GK, Sen S, Chakraborty R, Sachan S, Mishra A. Pharmacological evaluation of *Saraca indica* leaves for central nervous system depressant activity in mice. J Pharm Sci Res. 2010;2(6):338–43.

40. Campbell CG. Grass pea, *Lathyrus sativus* L. In: Bioversity International; 1997.

41. Muhammad N, Saeed M, Khan H. Antipyretic, analgesic and anti-inflammatory activity of *Viola betonicifolia* whole plant. BMC Complement Altern Med. 2012;12:59.

42. Loganayaki N, Siddhuraju P, Manian S. Antioxidant, anti-inflammatory and anti-nociceptive effects of *Ammannia baccifera* L. (Lythracceae), a folklore medicinal plant. J Ethnopharmacol. 2012;140:230–3.

43. Khan H, Saeed M, Gilani AUH, Khan MA, Dar A, Khan I. The antinociceptive activity of *Polygonatum verticillatum* rhizomes in pain models. J Ethnopharmacol. 2010;127(2):521–7.

44. Alam MA, Subhan N, Awal MA, Alam MS, Sarder M, Nahar L, et al. Antinociceptive and anti-inflammatory properties of *Ruellia tuberosa*. Pharm Biol. 2009;47:209–14.

45. Abdala S, Dévora S, Martín-Herrera D, Pérez-Paz P. Antinociceptive and anti-inflammatory activity of *Sambucus palmensis* link, an endemic Canary Island species. J Ethnopharmacol. 2014;155:626–32.

46. Milano J, Oliveira SM, Rossato MF, Sauzem PD, Machado P, Beck P, Zanatta N, et al. Antinociceptive effect of novel trihalomethyl-substituted pyrazoline methyl esters in formalin and hot-plate tests in mice. Eur J Pharmacol. 2008; 581:86–96.

47. Verma PR, Joharapurkar AA, Chatpalliwar VA, Asnani A. Antinociceptive activity of alcoholic extract of *Hemidesmus indicus* r.Br. In mice. J Ethnopharmacol. 2005;102:298–301.

48. Binny K, Kumar SG, Dennis T. Anti-inflammatory and antipyretic properties of the rhizome of *Costus speciosus* (koen.) sm. J Basic Clinical Pharm. 2010; 1(3):177.

49. Rang HP, Dale MM, Ritter JM, Moore PK. Pharmacology. 6th ed. Edinburgh: Churchill Livingstone; 2007.

50. Hossain E, Mandal SC, Gupta JK. Phytochemical screening and in-vivo antipyretic activity of the methanol leaf-extract of *Bombax malabaricum* DC (Bombacaceae). Tropical J Pharma Res. 2011;10(1)

# 20

# Hepatoprotective potentials of methanol extract of *T. conophorum* seeds of carbon tetrachloride induced liver damage in Wistar rats

Kelly Oriakhi[1*], Patrick O. Uadia[2] and Ikechi G. Eze[3]

## Abstract

**Background:** *Tetracarpidium conophorum* (TC) is a tropical plant used in ethno medicine for treating various diseases including hepatic ailments. The present study investigated the effect of methanol extract of *T. conophorum* seeds in rats intoxicated with $CCl_4$ 24 h and 48 h after intoxication respectively.

**Methods:** Thirty-five male Wistar rats were distributed equally into seven groups. Group IA (control) received distilled water and olive oil (i.p), group IIA rats were intoxicated with $CCl_4$ in olive oil (600 mg/kg, i.p.) only on the 8th day, while groups IIIA, IVA and VA were given 100 mg/kg of sylimarin, 250 mg/kg and 500 mg/kg of methanol extract respectively for 7 days, thereafter they were intoxicated with $CCl_4$ on the 8th day. Groups VIA and VIIA were intoxicated with $CCl_4$ on the 8th day and administered 250 mg/kg and 500 mg/kg of methanol extract of *T. conophorum* seeds at 1 h, 6 h, 12 h, 18 h and 24 h and the animals were sacrificed 24 h after intoxication with $CCl_4$. This procedure was repeated for a different set of thirty-five (groups IB-VIIB) male rats but the animals were sacrificed 48 h after intoxication with $CCl_4$. Fasting blood sample was collected by cardiac puncture for biochemical analyses.

**Results:** There were significant increases ($p < 0.05$) in serum hepatic enzyme markers (ALT, AST, ALP, and γ-GT) activities, as well as bilirubin and significant reduction in antioxidant enzymes ($P < 0.05$) in rats intoxicated with $CCl_4$ when compared to control group, but administration (pre-treatment and post-treatment) of methanol extract of *T. conophorum* seeds at doses of 250 and 500 mg/kg body weight and standard sylimarin drug attenuated the toxic insult of $CCl_4$ in a dose-dependent manner at 24 h and 48 h after intoxication respectively.

**Conclusions:** Our findings confirm that methanol extract of TC exhibited hepatoprotective activity against $CCl_4$ induced liver damage.

**Keywords:** African walnut, Liver damage, Hepatoprotection and carbon tetrachloride, Antioxidant

## Background

Liver disease is a main cause of death in many developing countries. It is an organ of prime importance and plays a significant role not only in metabolism and detoxification of exogenous toxins and therapeutic agents but also in the bio-regulation of fats, carbohydrates, amino acids, proteins, blood coagulation and immuno-modulation [1]. However, impairment of the liver generally occurs from excessive exposure to toxicants, alcohol, chemotherapeutic agents, viruses and protozoan infections [1]. An experimental model to induce liver damage by carbon tetrachloride ($CCl_4$) has been established. $CCl_4$ is activated by cytochrome (CYP) 2E1, CYP2B1 or CYP2B2, and possibly CYP3A, to form the trichloromethyl radical, $CCl_3^-$ [2]. This radical can bind to cellular molecules (nucleic acid, protein, lipid), impairing crucial cellular processes such as lipid metabolism, which

---

* Correspondence: kelly.oriakhi@uniben.edu
[1]Department of Medical Biochemistry, School of Basic Medical Sciences, University of Benin, Benin City, Nigeria
Full list of author information is available at the end of the article

results in fatty degeneration (steatosis) [3]. $CCl_3^-$ forms adducts with DNA, which initiate the onset of hepatocellular carcinoma. This radical can also react with oxygen to form the trichloromethylperoxy radical $CCl_3OO^-$, a highly reactive species. $CCl_3OO^-$ reacts with polyunsaturated fatty acids and phospholipids to initiates the chain reaction of lipid peroxidation. This affects the permeabilities of mitochondrial, endoplasmic reticulum, and plasma membranes, resulting in the loss of cellular calcium sequestration and homeostasis, which can contribute heavily to subsequent cell damage [4, 5]. Among the degradation products of fatty acids are reactive aldehydes, especially 4–hydroxynonenal, which bind easily to functional groups of proteins and inhibit important enzyme activities (loss of glucose-6-phosphatase activation) [6] thereby leading to liver injury [7]. $CCl_4$ intoxication is mediated by two types of nonparenchymal liver cells, viz.; Kupffer cells and stellate cells. The activation of Kupffer cells by $CCl_4$ mediate inflammatory processes via the nuclear factor kappa B (NF-kB) signal transduction pathway with production of pro-inflammatory cytokines such as tumor necrosis factor-$\alpha$ (TNF-$\alpha$), interleukin-1$\beta$ (IL-1$\beta$), interleukin-6(IL-6) and other inflammatory mediators; inducible nitric oxide synthase (iNOS), and cyclooxygenase-2 (Cox-2) [8, 9], which in turn causes full activation of the mitogen activated protein kinase (MAPK)/extracellular signal-related kinase (ERK) and the Janus kinase (Jak)-signal transducer and activator of transcription protein (STAT) pathway. These pathways are involved in the regulation of cell proliferation and apoptosis [10]. Stellate cells, are normally quiescent and fat-storing cells, but after activation by agents such as $CCl_4$, it display a typical acute-phase response [11], take on a fibroblast like appearance, release nitric oxide, begin to overproduce type-I collagen, and thus promote hepatic fibrosis [12].

However, there are current orthodox drugs for managing/treating hepatic diseases, but these drugs have adverse side effects, and resistance to many of them can develop after variable time periods [13]. To circumvent this challenge, our present study is designed to use alternative medicine (phytotherapy) in the treatment of liver disease. Medicinal plants have always been rich sources of biologically active compounds vital to human health [14]. Thus a search for a new molecule with hepatoprotective properties from plants could be a useful strategy [15]. One of such plants is *T. conophorum* (African walnut) which belongs to the family of Euphorbiaceae and it is commonly known in Southern Nigeria as ukpa (Igbo), in Western Nigeria as awusa or asala (Yoruba) and okhue in Bini [16]. Isolation and structural elucidation of phytochemicals such as steroidal terpenoids, flavonoids, and phenols from *T. conophorum* seed have been reported by our research group (data not provided). This plant possesses multiple medicinal properties such as antioxidant and immunostimulatory properties [17], improve fertility, antimicrobial [18] and anticancer activities [19]. It is against this background that this research seeks to evaluate the hepatoprotective effect of the methanol extract of *T. conophorum* seeds.

## Methods
### Collection of plant materials
The seeds of *T. conophorum* used in this study were collected from an open forest at Ovia North East Local government Area of Edo state, Nigeria. The fresh walnut seeds were identified by Professor M.E. Osawaru and authenticated by Professor MacDonald Idu both of the Department of Plant Biology and Biotechnology of the University of Benin, Benin City, Nigeria. Herbarium specimen (voucher number UBHe0153) was deposited at the Herbarium of the University of Benin.

### Extract preparation
Air-dried and powdered seeds of *T. conophorum* (1 kg) were extracted with absolute methanol (5 L) at room temperature for 72 h. The samples were filtered with Whatman No. 50 filter paper and the filtrate evaporated to dryness with a rotary evaporator (RE 300, Bibby Scientific, UK) to give 320 g. The resultant yield was stored in an air-tight container and kept in the refrigerator maintained at 4 °C.

### Chemicals
Carbon tetrachloride ($CCl_4$), 1-chloro-2,4-dinitrobenzene (CDNB), 5′,5′-dithiobis-2-nitrobenzoic acid (DTNB), reduced glutathione (GSH), epinephrine, hydrogen peroxide ($H_2O_2$), trichloroacetic acid (TCA), and thiobarbituric acid (TBA) were purchased from Sigma (St. Louis, MO, USA). Alanine aminotransferase (ALT) kit, aspartate aminotransferase kit, g-glutamyl transferase (g-GT) kit, total bilirubin, total protein and alkaline phosphatase kit were obtained from Randox laboratories Ltd. (Admore, Crumlin, Co-Antrim, UK). All other reagents were of analytical grade and were obtained from BDH (Poole, Dorset, UK).

### Animals
Albino rats (Wistar strain) (150–170 g), bred in the Department of Biochemistry, Faculty of Life Science, University of Benin, Benin City, Nigeria, were used for the study. They were kept in clean cages in a 12 h light/dark cycle with litter changed daily. The animals were housed in galvanized rat cages and acclimatized for two weeks before the commencement of the experiment. They were fed with guinea growers' mash and had access to water ad libitum. Experiments were performed according to guidelines for the care and use of laboratory animals. Weights of the rats were monitored throughout the period of the experiment. The handling of the animals

was in accordance with the principles of laboratory animal care [20].

## Experimental design

Effect of methanol extract of *T. conophorum* seeds on rats intoxicated with carbon tetrachloride after 24 h of intoxication. Thirty-five (35) albino rats (Wistar strain) of average weight $150 \pm 10$ g were used in this study, with 5 rats per group.

**Group IA (control):** Rats were administered olive oil (i.p) on the 8th day and distilled water only (orally).

**Group IIA:** Rats were administered carbon tetrachloride ($CCl_4$) in olive oil (600 mg/kg, i.p) on the 8th day.

**Group IIIA:** Rats were given silymarin (100 mg/kg body weight) daily for 1 week orally, then on the 8th day, the rats were intoxicated with $CCl_4$ in olive oil (600 mg/kg, i.p), fasted overnight, thereafter fasting blood samples were collected after 24 h of intoxication of $CCl_4$.

**Groups IVA&VA:** Rats were given methanol extract of *T. conophorum* seed (250 and 500 mg/kg body weight, respectively) daily for 1 week orally, then on the 8th day, the rats were intoxicated with $CCl_4$ in olive oil (600 mg/kg, i.p), fasted over night, thereafter blood samples were collected after 24 h of intoxication with $CCl_4$.

**Groups VIA&VIIA:** Rats were administered carbon tetrachloride ($CCl_4$) in olive oil(600 mg/kg, i.p), and then given methanol extract of *T. conophorum* seed (250 and 500 mg/kg body weight respectively, orally) at 1 h, 6 h, 12 h, 18 h and 24 h. Fasting blood samples were collected after the last administration of the extract at 24 h.

Effect of methanol extract of *T. conophorum* seeds intoxicated with carbon tetrachloride after 48 h of intoxication. Thirty (35) albino rats (Wistar strain) of average weight $150 \pm 10$ g were used in this study, with 5 rats per group.

**Group IB (control):** Rats were administered olive oil (i.p) on the 8th day and distilled water only (orally).

**Group IIB:** Rats were administered CCl4 in olive oil 600 mg/kg (i.p) on the 8th day.

**Group IIIB:** Rats were given silymarin (100 mg/kg body weight) daily for 1 week orally, then on the 8th day, the rats were intoxicated with $CCl_4$ in olive oil (600 mg/kg, i.p), thereafter fasting blood samples were collected after 48 h of intoxication with $CCl_4$.

**Groups IVB&VB:** Rats were given methanol extract of *T. conophorum* seed (250 and 500 mg/kg body weight, respectively) daily for 1 week orally, then on the 8th day, the rats were intoxicated with CCl4 in olive oil (600 mg/kg, i.p), thereafter fasting blood samples were collected after 48 h of intoxication with $CCl_4$.

**Groups VIB&VIIB:** Rats were administered $CCl_4$ in olive oil (600 mg/kg, i.p), and then given methanol extract of *T. conophorum* seed (250 and 500 mg/kg body weight respectively, orally) at 1 h, 6 h, 12 h, 18 h and 24 h. Fasting blood samples were collected after the last administration of the extract at 48 h of intoxication with $CCl_4$.

## Blood sample collection

Twenty-four and 48 h after the last treatment of groups A and B respectively, rats were killed by cervical dislocation and dissected. The livers were quickly removed and rinsed in ice-cold 1.15% KCl, dried and weighed. The livers were then minced with scissors in 4 volumes of ice-cold 0.1 M phosphate buffer, pH 7.4 and homogenized in a Potter–Elvehjem homogenizer. The homogenates were later centrifuged at 12,000 g for 15 min at 4 °C to obtain post-mitochondrial fraction (PMF). Blood was collected from the heart by the heart puncture technique into sample tubes. The blood samples were centrifuged at 3000 g for 10 min in a bench centrifuge to obtain serum, which was later used for the estimation of biochemical parameters.

## Determination of hepatic enzymes

Alanine aminotransferase and aspartate aminotransferase (AST) were determined using the method of Reitman and Frankel [21]. For determination of ALT activity, the serum sample was added to the buffered solution containing DL-alanine and $\alpha$-ketoglutarate (pH 7.4) and incubated for 30 min at 37 °C. After incubation 1.0 mM, DNPH was added, followed by the addition of 0.4 M NaOH. The absorbance was read at 500 nm and the ALT activity deduced, while in AST activity; the serum sample was added to the buffered solution containing L-aspartic and $\alpha$-ketoglutarate (pH 7.4) and incubated for 1 h at room temperature. After incubation 1.0 mM, DNPH was added, followed by the addition of 0.4 M NaOH and absorbance read at 500 nm. For determination of $\gamma$-GT activity [22] the serum sample was added to a substrate solution containing glycylglycine, MgCl2, and $\gamma$-glutamyl-p-nitroanilide in 0.05 M Tris (free base) pH 8.2. The mixture was incubated at 37 °C for 1 min and absorbance read at 405 nm at 1 min interval for 5 min. The activity of $\gamma$-GT was calculated from the absorbance value using the formula.

ALP activity was determined using Teco kit and method described by Kochmar and Moss, [23], precisely 0.5 ml of alkaline phosphatase substrate was placed into test tubes and equilibrated for 3 min at 37 °C. At the timed interval, 0.05 ml for each standard, control, and the sample was added to their respective test tubes, mix gently and incubate for 10 mins at 37 °C. Alkaline phosphatase color developer (2.5 ml) was added to the respective test tubes and absorbance read at 590 nm.

## Determination of Total protein

Total protein was determined using Radox kit and described by Tietz, [24].

## Determination of Total bilirubin

Total bilirubin was determined using Radox kit and described by Tietz Jendrassik and Grof [25].

## Determination of oxidative stress parameters

### Superoxide dismutase (SOD) activity

The level of SOD activity was determined according to the method of Misra and Fridovich, [26]. The liver fraction was reacted with epinephrine solution and the rate of inhibition of adrenochrome solution from the autooxidation of epinephrine was measured spectrophotometrically at 480 nm.

### Catalase activity

Catalase activity in the liver was determined as previously described by Asru [27]. The liver fraction was added to 0.2 M $H_2O_2$ solution and samples of this mixture were withdrawn at various intervals into a dichromate/acetic acid buffered solution. The rate of decomposition of hydrogen peroxide was determined spectrophotometrically at 480 nm.

### Reduced glutathione

The determination of reduced glutathione (GSH) level of tissue was based on the measurement of the absorbance of 2 nitro 5-thiobenzoic acid formed, at 412 nm [28], when Ellman's reagent reacted with GSH. An aliquot of the liver fraction was deproteinized in 4% sulphosalicylic acid and centrifuged at 17,000 rpm for 15 min at 4 °C. The supernatant was reacted with Ellman's reagent and the absorbance of the complex formed read at 412 nm. The amount of GSH in the liver fraction was determined from a standard GSH calibration curve.

### Glutathione-S-transferase activity

The activity of GST in the liver fraction was determined as described by Habig et al. [29]. The 1.0 mM GSH and 1.0 nM CDNB were reacted with the tissue fraction and the change in optical density at 340 nm within 30 s intervals for 3 min was taken. The activity was calculated with an extinction coefficient of 9.6 mM/cm.

### Glutathione peroxidase activity

The activity of glutathione peroxide (GPx) was determined by the method described by Rotruck et al. [30]. The mixture containing 0.5 ml of sodium phosphate buffer, 0.1 ml of 10 mM sodium azide, 0.2 ml of 4 mM reduced glutathione, 0.1 ml of 2.5 mM Hydrogen peroxide (H2O2) was performed. Precisely 0.5 ml of the sample was taken from the mixture into test tubes and was incubated at 37 °C for 3 min and the reaction was terminated using 0.5 ml TCA (10%). The mixture was centrifuged to obtain the supernatant and thereafter 1 ml of the DNTB reagent was added to developed the colour, and absorbance read at 412 nm using a spectrophotometer. The enzyme activity was expressed as Units/mg protein (one unit is the amount of enzyme that converts 1 mol GSH to GSSG in the presence of hydrogen peroxide/min).

## Determination of lipid peroxidation

Lipid peroxidation was assessed in terms of malondialdehyde (MDA) formation in the rat liver 10,000 g supernatant fraction. The measurement of thiobarbituric acid reacting substances (TBARS) was performed as described previously by Varshney and Kale, [31]. MDA was quantitated by using $\Sigma = 1.56 \times 105$ $M^{-1}$ $cm^{-1}$ [32].

## Histology

Portions of the liver were fixed in 10% neutral buffered formalin for histology. Thin sections of the liver were dissected and processed using Leica TP2010 automatic tissue processor for 18 h. The processor passed the tissues through fixation, dehydration, dealcoholisation, and paraffinization. Ultra-thin sections of 5 μm were sliced from the paraffinated sections using a Thermo scientific semi-automated rotary microtome. The tissues were then subjected to hematoxylin and eosin staining and viewed under a microscope using 10 X magnification.

## Statistical analysis

Data were expressed as the mean ± S.E.M of triplicate determinations using the statistical package for social science (SPSS) version 17.0 for windows. Statistical significance was calculated by one-way analysis of variance. Differences between means were estimated by Duncan's multiple range tests.

## Results

### Effect of methanol extract of *T. conophorum* seeds on serum aspartate aminotransferase, alanine aminotransferase and alkaline phosphatase in $CCl_4$ induced hepatotoxicity in rats after 24 h of intoxication

The effect of methanol extract of *T. conophorum* seeds on serum hepatic enzymes (AST, ALT, and ALP) in $CCl_4$ induced hepatotoxicity in rats after 24 h of intoxication is shown in Fig. 1. Administration of $CCl_4$ at a dose of 600 mg/kg body weight significantly increased ($p < 0.05$) the activities of the serum enzymes AST, ALT, ALP by 65.9%, 61.5%, 76.6% respectively when compared with the normal control (Group IA). Pre-treatment of the rats with the methanol extract of *T. conophorum* seeds at a dose of 250 and 500 mg/kg body weight for one week before administering $CCl_4$ showed a significant decrease ($p < 0.05$) in AST, ALT, ALP when compared to rats administered

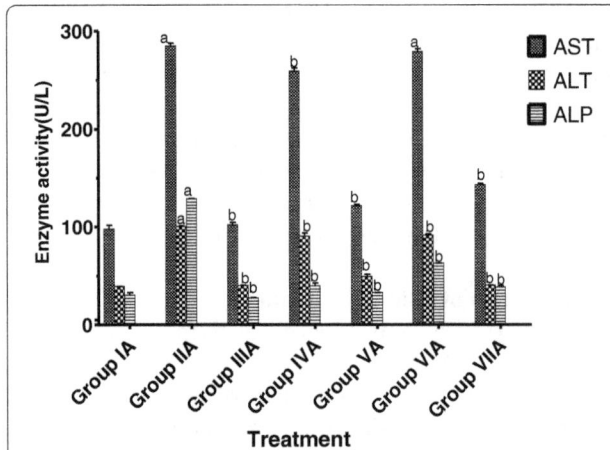

**Fig. 1** Effect of methanol extract of *T. conophorum* seeds on serum Aspartate aminotransferase, Alanine aminotransferase and Alkaline phosphatase activities in CCl$_4$ induced hepatotoxicity in rats after 24 h of intoxication. Values are Mean ± SEM, *n* = 5 rats in each group. *p* < 0.05, a as compared with the normal control group; b as compared with the CCl$_4$ only (group IIA). AST- Aspartate aminotransferase; ALT- Alanine aminotransferase; ALP- Alkaline phosphatase; CCl$_4$ - Carbon tetrachloride. Group IA (control) received distilled water and olive oil (i.p), group IIA rats were intoxicated with CCl$_4$ in olive oil (600 mg/kg, i.p.) only on the 8th day, while groups IIIA, IVA and VA were given 100 mg/kg of silymarin, 250 mg/kg and 500 mg/kg of methanol extract respectively for 7 days, thereafter intoxicated with CCl$_4$ on the 8th day. Groups VIA and VIIA were intoxicated with CCl$_4$ on the 8th day and administered 250 mg/kg and 500 mg/kg of methanol extract of *T. conophorum* seeds at 1 h, 6 h, 12 h, 18 h and 24 h. Fasting blood samples were collected after the last administration of the extract at 24 h of intoxication with CCl$_4$

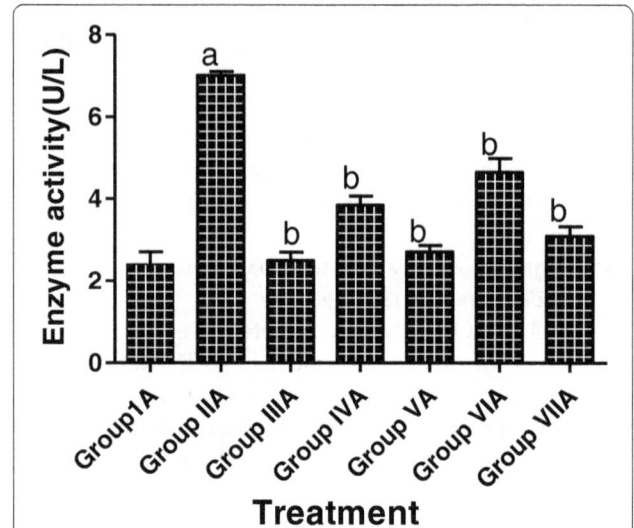

**Fig. 2** Effect of methanol extract of *T. conophorum* seeds on Gamma gtutamyl transferase activities in CCl$_4$ induced hepatotoxicity in rats after 24 h of intoxication. Values are Mean ± SEM, *n* = 5 rats in each group. *p* < 0.05, a as compared with the normal control group; b as compared with the CCl$_4$ only (group IIA) . γ-GT – Gamma gtutamyl transferase CCl$_4$, Carbon tetrachloride. Group IA (control) received distilled water and olive oil (i.p), group IIA rats were intoxicated with CCl$_4$ in olive oil (600 mg/kg, i.p.) only on the 8th day, while groups IIIA, IVA and VA were given 100 mg/kg of silymarin, 250 mg/kg and 500 mg/kg of methanol extract, respectively for 7 days, thereafter intoxicated with CCl$_4$ on the 8th day. Groups VIA and VIIA were intoxicated with CCl$_4$ on the 8th day and administered 250 mg/kg and 500 mg/kg of methanol extract of *T. conophorum* seeds at 1 h, 6 h, 12 h, 18 h and 24 h. Fasting blood samples were collected after the last administration of the extract at 24 h of intoxication with CCl$_4$

CCl$_4$ only (Group IIA). The standard drug silymarin at a dose of 100 mg/kg also significantly prevented the elevation of the serum enzymes. Pre-treatment for a week with the crude methanol extract (250 and 500 mg/kg) and silymarin exhibited a protection of 8.93%, 57.2% and 64.1% in AST levels, 9.9%, 51.02% and 60.3% in ALT levels, 66% 74.6%, and 78.9% in ALP levels respectively. Post-treatment of rats with the extract after CCl$_4$ administration at 250 and 500 mg/kg significantly restored liver damage in a dose-dependent manner.

### Effect of methanol extract of *T. conophorum* seeds on gamma gtutamyl transferase and Total bilirubin in CCl$_4$ induced hepatotoxicity in rats after 24 h of intoxication

The effect of methanol extract of *T. conophorum* seeds on serum γ-GT and total bilirubin in CCl$_4$ induced hepatotoxicity in rats after 24 h of intoxication is shown in Figs. 2 and 3 respectively. Administration of CCl$_4$ at a dose of 600 mg/kg body weight significantly increased (*p* < 0.05) the levels of the serum γ-GT and total bilirubin by 65.62% and 87.1% respectively when compared with the normal control (Group IA). Pre-treatment of the rats with the methanol extract of *T. conophorum* seeds at a dose of 250 and 500 mg/kg body weight for one week before administering CCl$_4$ showed a

significant decrease (*p* < 0.05) in γ-GT and total bilirubin levels when compared to rats administered CCl$_4$ only (Group IIA). The standard drug silymarin at a dose of 100 mg/kg also significantly prevented the elevation of the γ-GT and total bilirubin levels. Pre-treatment for a week with the crude methanol extract (250 and 500 mg/kg) and silymarin exhibited a protection of 45.1%, 61.3% and 64.3% in γ-GT activities and 46.8%, 75.8% and 88.7% in total bilirubin concentrations respectively. Post-treatment of rats with the extract after CCl$_4$ administration at 250 and 500 mg/kg significantly restored liver damage in a dose-dependent manner.

### Effect of methanol extract of *T. conophorum* seeds on antioxidant enzyme activity in CCl$_4$ induced hepatotoxicity in rats after 24 h of intoxication

The effect of methanol extract of *T. conophorum* seeds on antioxidant enzymes in CCl$_4$ induced hepatotoxicity in rats after 24 h of intoxication is shown in Table 1. There was a significant (*P* < 0.05) decrease in the hepatic enzymatic (CAT, SOD, GPx, and GST) and non-enzymatic (GSH) antioxidants recorded in rats following CCl$_4$ administration. However pre-treatment of the rats with the methanol extract of *T. conophorum* seeds at a dose of 250 and 500 mg/

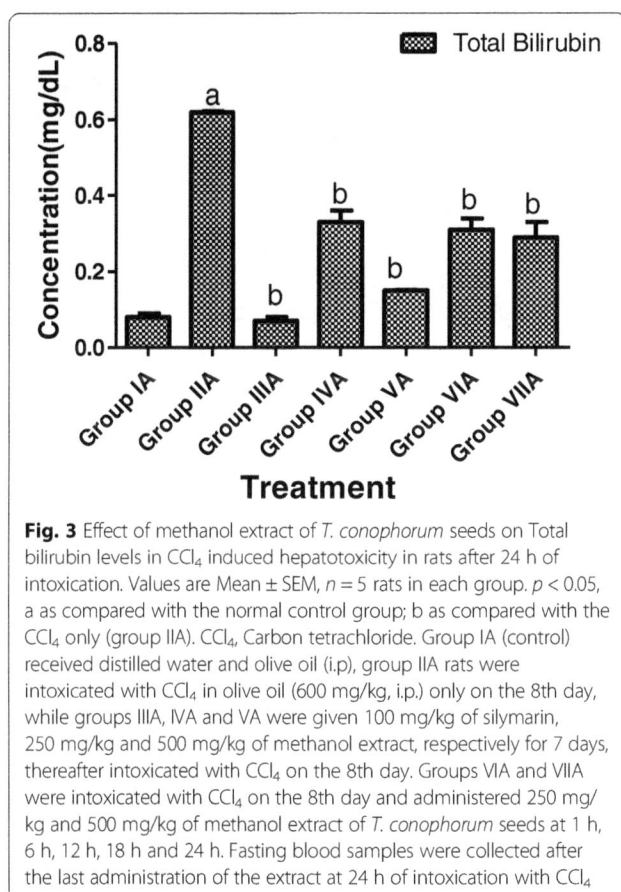

**Fig. 3** Effect of methanol extract of *T. conophorum* seeds on Total bilirubin levels in CCl$_4$ induced hepatotoxicity in rats after 24 h of intoxication. Values are Mean ± SEM, $n = 5$ rats in each group. $p < 0.05$, a as compared with the normal control group; b as compared with the CCl$_4$ only (group IIA). CCl$_4$, Carbon tetrachloride. Group IA (control) received distilled water and olive oil (i.p), group IIA rats were intoxicated with CCl$_4$ in olive oil (600 mg/kg, i.p.) only on the 8th day, while groups IIIA, IVA and VA were given 100 mg/kg of silymarin, 250 mg/kg and 500 mg/kg of methanol extract, respectively for 7 days, thereafter intoxicated with CCl$_4$ on the 8th day. Groups VIA and VIIA were intoxicated with CCl$_4$ on the 8th day and administered 250 mg/kg and 500 mg/kg of methanol extract of *T. conophorum* seeds at 1 h, 6 h, 12 h, 18 h and 24 h. Fasting blood samples were collected after the last administration of the extract at 24 h of intoxication with CCl$_4$

kg body weight for one week before administration of CCl$_4$ showed significant increases ($p < 0.001$; $p < 0.05$) in CAT, SOD, GSH and GPx, activities in a dose-dependent manner compared to rats intoxicated with CCl$_4$ only (group IIA), while non-significant increase in GST activities were observed at the two different doses when compared to group IIA. The standard drug silymarin at a dose of 100 mg/kg

also significantly increased the antioxidant status in rats in group IIIA. However, post-treatment of the rats in groups VIA and VIIA with the extract at a dose of 250 and 500 mg/kg showed significant increases in CAT and GSH activities in a dose-dependent manner. There was no significant difference in SOD and GPx activities in rats administered with 250 mg/kg of extract (group VIA) but significantly increased ($p < 0.05$) when given 500 mg/kg of the extract (group VIIA).

**Effect of methanol extract of *T. conophorum* seeds on liver lipid peroxidation in CCl$_4$ induced hepatotoxicity in rats after 24 h of intoxication**

The effect of methanol extract of *T. conophorum* seeds on lipid peroxidation levels in CCl$_4$ induced hepatotoxicity in rats after 24 h of intoxication is shown in Fig. 4. Hepatic MDA level was remarkably increased by 55.1% ($p < 0.05$) in CCl$_4$ treated group as compared to control group, 24 h after CCl$_4$ administration. Pre-treatment with the extract at different doses (250 and 500 mg/kg) significantly decreased hepatic MDA levels. MDA levels were decreased by 58.6%, 22.9% and 52.1% in groups IIIA, IVA and VA respectively, compared to CCl$_4$ treated group (group IIA), while post-treatment of the rats in groups VIA and VIIA with the extract at a dose of 250 and 500 mg/kg showed significant decrease in MDA levels in a dose-dependent manner.

**Effect of methanol extract of *T. conophorum* seeds on serum aspartate aminotransferase, alanine aminotransferase and alkaline phosphatase in CCl$_4$ induced hepatotoxicity in rats after 48 h of intoxication**

The effect of methanol extract of *T. conophorum* seeds on serum biochemical parameters (AST, ALT, ALP) in CCl$_4$ induced hepatotoxicity in rats after 48 h of intoxication is shown in Fig. 5. Administration of CCl$_4$ at a dose of 600 mg/kg body weight significantly increased ($p < 0.05$)

**Table 1** Effect of methanol extract of *T. conophorum* seeds on liver antioxidant status in CCl$_4$ induced hepatotoxicity in rats after 24 h of intoxication

| Treatment | Parameters | | | | |
|---|---|---|---|---|---|
| ($n = 5$) | CAT (Unit/mg protein) | SOD (Unit/mg protein) | GPx (Unit/mg protein) | GST (Unit/mg protein) | GSH (µg/mg protein) |
| Group1A | 32.20 ± 1.20 | 6.00 ± 0.50 | 4.20 ± 0.22 | 0.53 ± 0.03 | 14.50 ± 0.25 |
| Group IIA | ***16.42 ± 1.12[a] | ***2.55 ± 0.08[a] | ***2.69 ± 0.10[a] | **0.30 ± 0.05[a] | ***6.41 ± 0.15 |
| Group IIIA | ***30.25 ± 0.50[b] | ***5.50 ± 0.15[b] | ***4.12 ± 0.11[b] | *0.50 ± 0.05[b] | ***18.20 ± 0.45 |
| Group IVA | ***25.50 ± 0.55[b] | *3.50 ± 0.05[b] | **3.46 ± 0.05[b] | 0.35 ± 0.01[a] | ***15.20 ± 0.40 |
| Group VA | ***28.00 ± 0.40[b] | ***5.06 ± 0.20[b] | **3.43 ± 0.02[b] | *0.45 ± 0.05[b] | ***15.00 ± 0.06 |
| GroupVIA | ***23.30 ± 0.30[b] | 2.80 ± 0.08[b] | 3.13 ± 0.04[b] | 0.32 ± 0.03[b] | ***15.70 ± 0.16 |
| GroupVIIA | ***27.62 ± 0.60[b] | **4.00 ± 0.12[b] | ***3.54 ± 0.09[b] | 0.40 ± 0.01[a] | ***16.20 ± 0.20 |

Values are Mean ± SEM, n = 5 rats in each group, *P<0.05; **$p < 0.01$; ***$p < 0.001$, a as compared with the normal saline (control) group; b as compared with the CCl$_4$ only group SOD Superoxide dismutase; CAT Catalase; GPx Glutathione peroxidase; GST Glutathione-S-Transferase
Group IA (control) received distilled water and olive oil (i.p), group IIA rats were intoxicated with CCl$_4$ in olive oil (600 mg/kg, i.p.) only on the 8th day, while groups IIIA, IVA and VA were given 100 mg/kg of silymarin, 250 mg/kg and 500 mg/kg of methanol extract respectively for 7 days, thereafter intoxicated with CCl$_4$ on the 8th day. Groups VIA and VIIA were intoxicated with CCl$_4$ on the 8th day and administered 250 mg/kg and 500 mg/kg of methanol extract of *T. conophorum* seeds at 1 h, 6 h, 12 h, 18 h and 24 h. Fasting blood samples were collected after the last administration of the extract at 24 h of intoxication with CCl$_4$

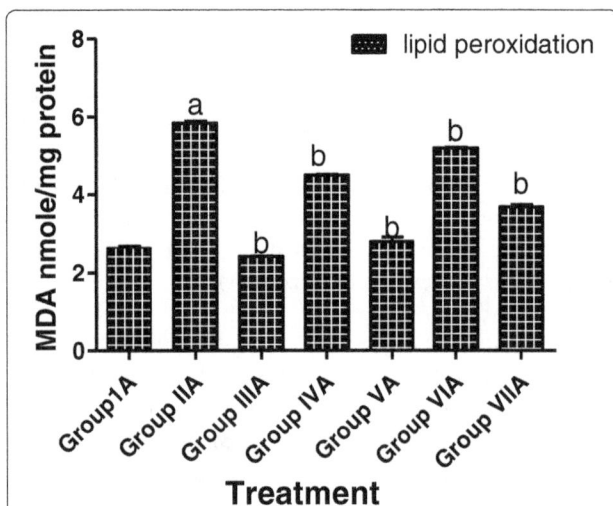

**Fig. 4** Effect of methanol extract of *T. conophorum* seeds on lipid peroxidation levels in CCl$_4$ induced hepatotoxicity in rats after 24 h of intoxication. Values are Mean ± SEM, *n* = 5 rats in each group. *p* < 0.05, a as compared with the normal control group; b as compared with the CCl$_4$ only (group IIA). CCl$_4$, Carbon tetrachloride, MDA-malondialdehyde. Group IA (control) received distilled water and olive oil (i.p), group IIA rats were intoxicated with CCl$_4$ in olive oil (600 mg/kg, i.p.) only on the 8th day, while groups IIIA, IVA and VA were given 100 mg/kg of silymarin, 250 mg/kg and 500 mg/kg of methanol extract, respectively for 7 days, thereafter intoxicated with CCl$_4$ on the 8th day. Groups VIA and VIIA were intoxicated with CCl$_4$ on the 8th day and administered 250 mg/kg and 500 mg/kg of methanol extract of *T. conophorum* seeds at 1 h, 6 h, 12 h, 18 h and 24 h. Fasting blood samples were collected after the last administration of the extract at 24 h of intoxication with CCl$_4$

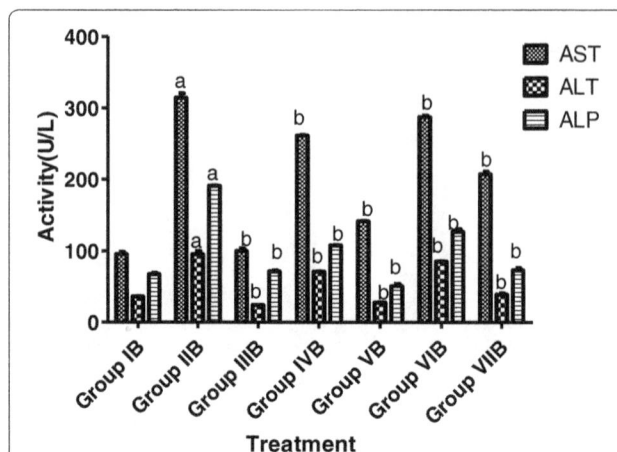

**Fig. 5** Effect of methanol extract of *T. conophorum* seeds on serum Aspartate aminotransferase, Alanine aminotransferase and Alkaline phosphatase activities in CCl$_4$ induced hepatotoxicity in rats after 48 h of intoxication. Values are Mean ± SEM, *n* = 5 rats in each group. *p* < 0.05, a as compared with the normal control group; b as compared with the CCl$_4$ only (group IIB). AST- Aspartate aminotransferase; ALT- Alanine aminotransferase; ALP - Alkaline phosphatase; CCl$_4$ - Carbon tetrachloride. Group IB (control) received distilled water and olive oil (i.p), group IIB rats were intoxicated with CCl$_4$ in olive oil (600 mg/kg, i.p.) only on the 8th day, while groups IIIB, IVB and VB were given 100 mg/kg of silymarin, 250 mg/kg and 500 mg/kg of methanol extract respectively for 7 days, thereafter intoxicated with CCl$_4$ on the 8th day. Groups VIB and VIIB were intoxicated with CCl$_4$ on the 8th day and administered 250 mg/kg and 500 mg/kg of methanol extract of *T. conophorum* seeds at 1 h, 6 h, 12 h, 18 h and 24 h. Fasting blood samples were collected after the last administration of the extract at 48 h of intoxication with CCl$_4$

the activities of the serum enzymes, AST ALT, ALP by 69.6%, 62.5%, and 64.7% respectively after 48 h of intoxication when compared with the control. Pre-treatment of the rats with the methanol extract of *T. conophorum* seeds at a dose of 250 and 500 mg/kg body weight for one week before the administration of CCl$_4$ showed a significant decrease (p < 0.05) in AST, ALT and ALP. The standard drug silymarin at a dose of 100 mg/kg also significantly prevented the elevation of serum enzymes. Pre-treatment with crude methanol extract (250 and 500 mg/kg) and silymarin exhibited a protection of 16.7%, 55% and 68.1% in AST levels, 25%, 70.8% and 75% in ALT levels, 43.3%, 73.4% and 62.4% in ALP levels respectively. Post-treatment of rats with the methanol extract after CCl$_4$ administration at 250 and 500 mg/kg significantly restored liver damage in a dose dependent manner.

**Effect of methanol extract of *T. conophorum* seeds on gamma gtutamyl transferase and Total bilirubin levels in CCl$_4$ induced hepatotoxicity in rats after 48 h of intoxication**
The effect of methanol extract of *T. conophorum* seeds on serum γ-GT and total bilirubin levels in CCl$_4$ induced hepatotoxicity in rats after 48 h of intoxication is shown in Figs. 6 and 7 respectively. Administration of CCl$_4$ at a

dose of 600 mg/kg body weight significantly increased (p < 0.05) the levels of the serum γ-GT and total bilirubin by 70.6% and 87.5% respectively when compared with the normal control (Group IB). Pre-treatment of the rats with the methanol extract of *T. conophorum* seeds at a dose of 250 and 500 mg/kg body weight for one week before administering CCl$_4$ showed a significant decrease (*p* < 0.05) in γ-GT and total bilirubin levels when compared to rats administered CCl$_4$ only (Group IIB). The standard drug silymarin at a dose of 100 mg/kg also significantly prevented the elevation of the γ-GT and total bilirubin. Pre-treatment for a week with the crude methanol extract (250 and 500 mg/kg) and silymarin exhibited a protection of 49%, 64.1% and 70.2% in γ-GT activities and 62.5%, 70.8% and 80.6% in total bilirubin concentrations respectively. Post-treatment of rats with the extract after CCl$_4$ administration at 250 and 500 mg/kg significantly restored liver damage in a dose-dependent manner.

**Effect of methanol extract of *T. conophorum* seeds on antioxidant enzyme activities in CCl$_4$ induced hepatotoxicity in rats after 48 h of intoxication**
The effect of methanol extract of *T. conophorum* seeds on antioxidant enzymes and lipid peroxidation in CCl$_4$

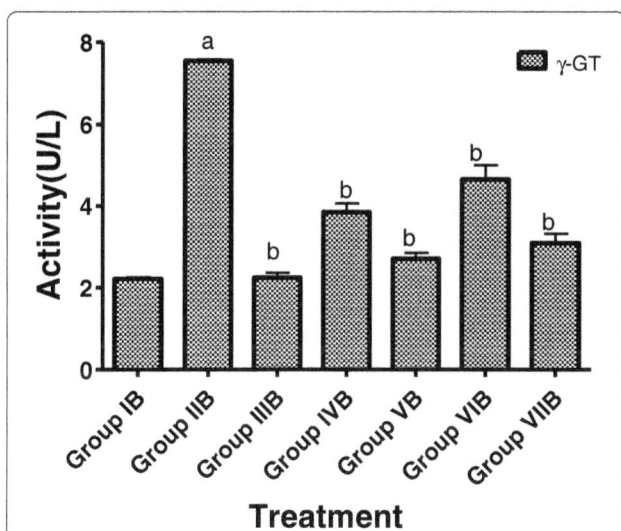

**Fig. 6** Effect of methanol extract of *T. conophorum* seeds on Gamma gtutamyl transferase activities in CCl$_4$ induced hepatotoxicity in rats after 48 h of intoxication. Values are Mean ± SEM, *n* = 5 rats in each group. *p* < 0.05, a as compared with the normal control group; b as compared with the CCl$_4$ only (group IIB). γ-GT – Gamma gtutamyl transferase CCl$_4$- Carbon tetrachloride. Group IB (control) received distilled water and olive oil (i.p), group IIB rats were intoxicated with CCl$_4$ in olive oil (600 mg/kg, i.p.) only on the 8th day, while groups IIIB, IVB and VB were given 100 mg/kg of silymarin, 250 mg/kg and 500 mg/kg of methanol extract, respectively for 7 days, thereafter intoxicated with CCl$_4$ on the 8th day. Groups VIB and VIIB were intoxicated with CCl$_4$ on the 8th day and administered 250 mg/kg and 500 mg/kg of methanol extract of *T. conophorum* seeds at 1 h, 6 h, 12 h, 18 h and 24 h. Fasting blood samples were collected after the last administration of the extract at 48 h of intoxication with CCl$_4$

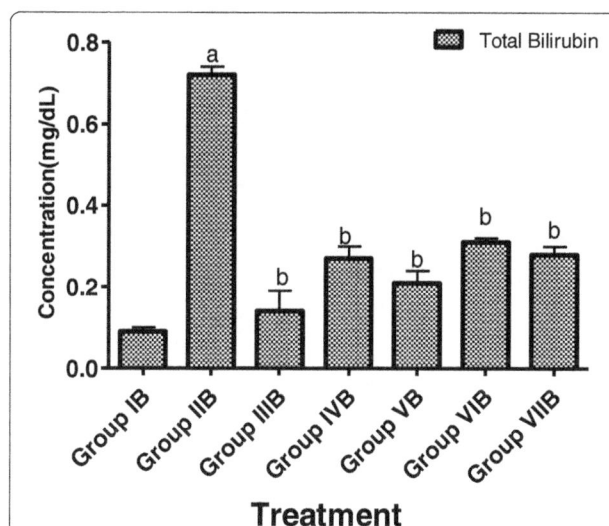

**Fig. 7** Effect of methanol extract of *T. conophorum* seeds on Total bilirubin in CCl$_4$ induced hepatotoxicity in rats after 48 h of intoxication. Values are Mean ± SEM, n = 5 rats in each group. p < 0.05, a as compared with the normal control group; b as compared with the CCl$_4$ only(group IIB), CCl$_4$, Carbon tetrachloride. Group IB (control) received distilled water and olive oil (i.p), group IIB rats were intoxicated with CCl$_4$ in olive oil (600 mg/kg, i.p.) only on the 8th day, while groups IIIB, IVB and VB were given 100 mg/kg of silymarin, 250 mg/kg and 500 mg/kg of methanol extract, respectively for 7 days, thereafter intoxicated with CCl$_4$ on the 8th day. Groups VIB and VIIB were intoxicated with CCl$_4$ on the 8th day and administered 250 mg/kg and 500 mg/kg of methanol extract of *T. conophorum* seeds at 1 h, 6 h, 12 h, 18 h and 24 h. Fasting blood samples were collected after the last administration of the extract at 48 h of intoxication with CCl$_4$

induced hepatotoxicity in rats after 48 h of intoxication is shown in Table 2. There was a significant (*p* ‹ 0.05) decrease in the hepatic enzymatic (CAT, SOD, GPx, and GST) and non-enzymatic (GSH) antioxidants recorded in rats following CCl$_4$ administration. However pre-treatment of the rats with the methanol extract of *T. conophorum* seeds at doses of 250 and 500 mg/kg body weight for 7 days before the administration of CCl$_4$ showed significant increases (*p* ‹ 0.001; *P* ‹ 0.05) in CAT, SOD, GSH and GPx, activities in a dose-dependent manner compared to rats intoxicated with CCl$_4$ only (group IIB), while non-significant increase in GST activities was observed at 250 mg/kg extract dose (group IVB) when compared to group IIB, but there was a significant increase (*p* ‹ 0.05) when given 500 mg/kg dose of the extract to group VB. Standard drug silymarin at a dose of 100 mg/kg also attenuated the toxic effect of CCl$_4$ in group IIIB rats. However, post-treatment of the rats in groups VIB and VIIB with the extract at a dose of 500 mg/kg showed significant increases in CAT, SOD, GPx, GST activities and GSH levels in a dose-dependent manner. There was no significant difference in CAT, SOD and GPx activities in rats administered with 250 mg/kg of the extract (group VIB).

## Effect of methanol extract of *T. conophorum* seeds on liver lipid peroxidation in CCl$_4$ induced hepatotoxicity in rats after 48 h of intoxication

The effect of methanol extract of *T. conophorum* seeds on lipid peroxidation levels in CCl$_4$ induced hepatotoxicity in rats after 48 h of intoxication is shown in Fig. 8. Hepatic MDA level was remarkably increased by 79.5% (*p* ‹ 0.05) in CCl$_4$ treated group only compared to control group, after 48 h of intoxication. Pre-treatment with the extract before administration of CCl$_4$ at different doses (250 and 500 mg/kg) significantly decreased hepatic MDA levels. MDA levels were decreased by 80.8%, 46.2% and 71.8% in groups IIIB, IVB and VB respectively, compared to CCl$_4$ treated group (group IIB), while post-treatment of the rats in groups VIB and VIIB with the extract at a dose of 250 and 500 mg/kg showed significant decrease in MDA levels in a dose-dependent manner.

### Histopathological examination of the liver

Histopathological examination of the liver of normal control rats and rats intoxicated with CCl$_4$ after 24 h and 48 h intoxication is shown in Figs. 9 and 10 respectively. Figures 9 and 10 are sections of the liver from a

**Table 2** Effect of methanol extract of *T. conophorum* seeds on Liver Antioxidant Status in CCl$_4$ induced hepatotoxicity in rats after 48 h of intoxication

| Treatment | Parameters | | | | |
|---|---|---|---|---|---|
| (n = 5) | Catalase (Unit/mg protein) | SOD (Unit/mg protein) | GPx (Unit/mg protein) | GST (Unit/mg protein | GSH (µg/mg protein) |
| Group1B:Normal control | 70.20 ± 3.50 | 6.70 ± 0.53 | 3.80 ± 0.16 | 0.62 ± 0.02 | 16.80 ± 0.53 |
| Group IIB | ***44.50 ± 1.20[a] | ***2.50 ± 0.50[a] | ***1.50 ± 0.06[a] | ***0.29 ± 0.001[a] | ***7.01 ± 0.50[a] |
| Group IIIB | ***70.50 ± 2.50[b] | ***6.50 ± 0.25[b] | ***4.40 ± 0.15[b] | ***0.51 ± 0.06[b] | ***17.02 ± 0.25[b] |
| Group IVB | 50.00 ± 1.17[b] | *4.20 ± 0.20[b] | ***3.46 ± 0.10[b] | 0.26 ± 0.01[a] | ***10.20 ± 0.15[b] |
| Group VB | ***66.90 ± 2.00[b] | ***6.05 ± 0.15[b] | ***3.43 ± 0.21[b] | **0.43 ± 0.001[b] | ***15.20 ± 0.40[b] |
| Group VIB | 48.50 ± 3.80[b] | 2.62 ± 0.60[b] | ***2.69 ± 0.07[b] | 0.30 ± 0.003[b] | ***11.80 ± 0.30[b] |
| Group VIIB | ***68.00 ± 2.55[b] | ***5.50 ± 0.11[b] | **3.12 ± 0.20 | **0.45 ± 0.02[b] | ***14.00 ± 0.28[b] |

Values are Mean ± SD, n = 4 rats in each group. *P$^<$0.05; **$p < 0.01$; ***$p < 0.001$, a as compared with the normal saline (control) group; b as compared with the CCl$_4$ only group *SOD* Superoxide dismutase; *CAT* Catalase; *GSH* Reduced glutathione; *GPx* Glutathione peroxidase; *GST* Glutathione-S-Transferase,*CCl$_4$* Carbon tetrachloride

Group IB (control) received distilled water and olive oil (i.p), group IIB rats were intoxicated with CCl$_4$ in olive oil (600 mg/kg, i.p.) only on the 8th day, while groups IIIB, IVB and VB were given 100 mg/kg of silymarin, 250 mg/kg and 500 mg/kg of methanol extract respectively for 7 days, thereafter intoxicated with CCl$_4$ on the 8th day. Groups VIB and VIIB were intoxicated with CCl$_4$ on the 8th day and administered 250 mg/kg and 500 mg/kg of methanol extract of *T. conophorum* seeds at 1 h, 6 h, 12 h, 18 h and 24 h.Fasting blood samples were collected after the last administration of the extract at 48 h of intoxication with CCl$_4$

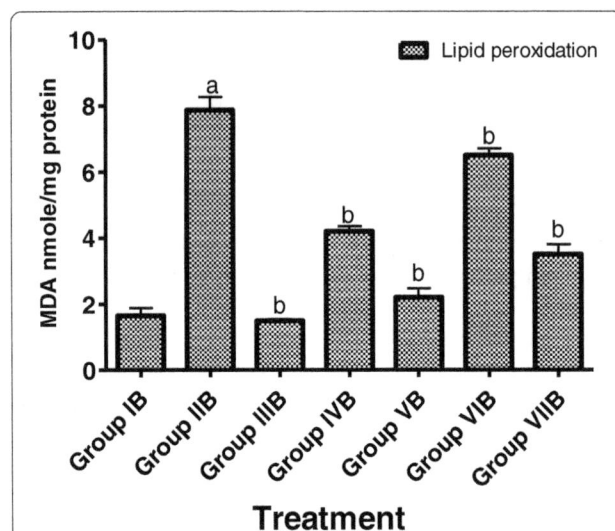

**Fig. 8** Effect of methanol extract of *T. conophorum* seeds on lipid peroxidation levels in CCl$_4$ induced hepatotoxicity in rats after 48 h of intoxication. Values are Mean ± SEM, n = 5 rats in each group. p < 0.05, a as compared with the normal control group; b as compared with the CCl$_4$ only (group IIB), CCl$_4$, Carbon tetrachloride, MDA-malondialdehyde. Group IB (control) received distilled water and olive oil (i.p), group IIB rats were intoxicated with CCl$_4$ in olive oil (600 mg/kg, i.p.) only on the 8th day, while groups IIIB, IVB and VB were given 100 mg/kg of silymarin, 250 mg/kg and 500 mg/kg of methanol extract, respectively for 7 days, thereafter intoxicated with CCl$_4$ on the 8th day. Groups VIB and VIIB were intoxicated with CCl$_4$ on the 8th day and administered 250 mg/kg and 500 mg/kg of methanol extract of *T. conophorum* seeds at 1 h, 6 h, 12 h, 18 h and 24 h. Fasting blood samples were collected after the last administration of the extract at 48 h of intoxication with CCl$_4$

representative rat in each of the five groups. Figures 9 and 10, show that under the conditions of this experiment, carbon tetrachloride caused damage to the liver mainly by inducing macrovesicular steatosis, congestion of the centriole and extensive hemorrhagic necrosis. The plant extract was able to ameliorate the harmful effects of carbon tetrachloride to varying degrees; with the highest dose seeming most effective. The results observed in this study supported the biochemical results.

## Discussion

Carbon tetrachloride induced hepatotoxicity in rats is a well characterized experimental model for evaluating the hepatoprotective potential of various herbal extract/natural compounds [33, 34]. Hepatic cytochrome P450 metabolizes CCl$_4$ and forms the trichloromethyl free radical (CCl$_3^-$). This CCl$_3^-$ radical forms a more toxic trichloromethyl peroxyl radical (CCl$_3$O$_2$) in the presence of oxygen. It is capable of abstracting hydrogen from polyunsaturated fatty acids of the cell membrane to initiate lipid peroxidation and formation of oxidation products such as malondialdehyde and 4-hydroxynonenal [35]. As a result, plasma membrane becomes more permeable to Ca$^{2+}$ leading to perturbations in calcium homeostasis that culminates in necrotic cell death [36].

The current study showed that treatment with CCl$_4$ at a dose of 600 mg/kg after 24 and 48 h of intoxication respectively led to the development of hepatic injury in rats. Serum activities of AST, ALT, ALP, γ-GT and total bilirubin level were significantly increased (P$^<$ 0.05) in the rats treated with CCl4 only when compared with the rats in the control groups (Figs. 1, 2 and 3). These serum enzymes according to Zimmerman [37] have been identified to be increased in cytotoxic and cholestatic hepatic injuries. Elevation of AST has been reported to be an

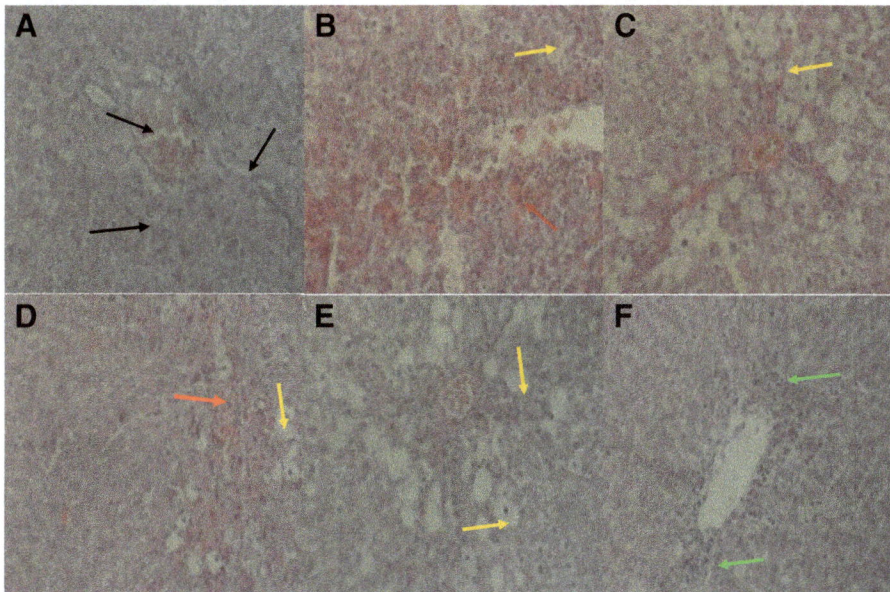

**Fig. 9** Photomicrographs of liver sectionsfrom **a** Control rats showing normal liver histology: Black arrow heads indicatenormal portal vein and hepatocytes with well fenestrated sinusoidal space, **b** rats intoxicated with $CCl_4$on the 8th day **c** rats treated with 250 mg/kg bw.TC seed for 7 days,thereafter intoxicated with $CCl_4$ on the 8th day **d** rats treated with 500 mg/kg bw.TC seed for 7 days,thereafter intoxicated with $CCl_4$ on the 8th day **e** rats intoxicated with $CCl_4$and then given methanol extract of TCseed (250 mg/kg body weight orally) at 1 h, 6 h, 12 h, 18 h and 24 h **f** rats intoxicated with $CCl_4$and then given methanol extract of TCseed (500 mg/kg body weight orally) at 1 h, 6 h, 12 h, 18 h and 24 h. The liver sections were stained with H/E and observed with a 10X objective. Arrow heads (Orange): Vesicular steatosis/fatty accumulation; (Dark Red): Extensive hemorrhagic necrosis; (Light Red): Mild hemorrhagic necrosis; (Green): Mild portal hepatitis. TC: *Tetracarpidium conophorum*

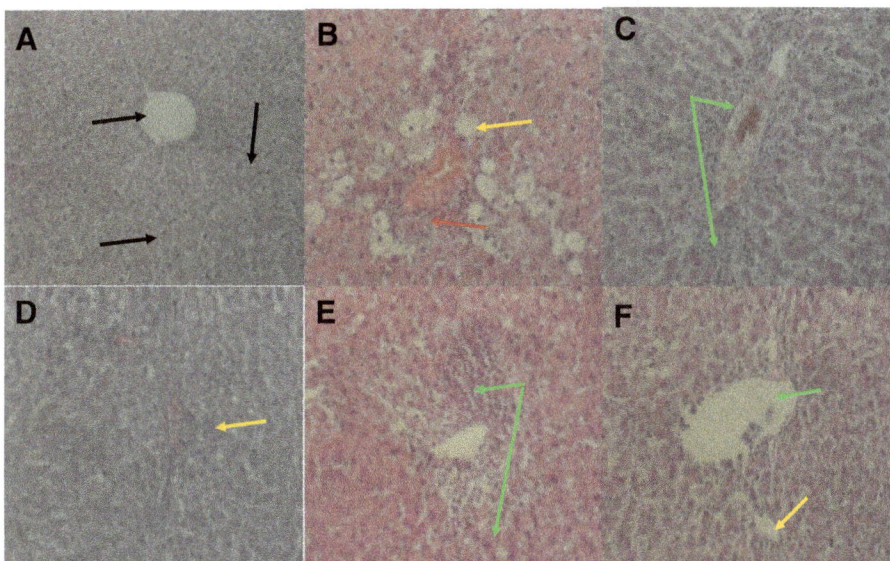

**Fig. 10** Photomicrographs of liver sections from **a** Control rats showing normal liver histology: Black arrow heads indicate normal central vein, hepatocytes, sinusoids **b** rats intoxicated with $CCl_4$on the 8th day **c** rats treated with 250 mg/kg bw.TC for 7 days, thereafter intoxicated with $CCl_4$ on the 8th day **d** rats treated with 500 mg/kg bw.TC seed for 7 days,thereafter intoxicated with $CCl_4$ on the 8th day **e** rats intoxicated with $CCl_4$and then given methanol extract of TC seed (250 mg/kg body weight orally) at 1 h, 6 h, 12 h, 18 h and 24 h **f** rats intoxicated with $CCl_4$and then given methanol extract of TC seed (500 mg/kg body weight orally) at 1 h, 6 h, 12 h, 18 h and 24 h. The liver sections were stained with H/E and observed with a 10 X objective. Arrow heads (Orange): Vesicular steatosis/fatty accumulation; (Dark Red): Extensive hemorrhagic necrosis; (Green): Mild/patchyportal hepatitis. TC: *Tetracarpidium conophorum*

index of hepatocellular injury in rats, while ALT elevation is more associated with the necrotic state [38]. Serum ALP and γ-GT, are important enzymes in assessing obstructive liver injury [39, 40], and were found to be significantly elevated in CCl₄-treated rats. The administration of methanol extract of *T. conophorum* seeds, however, was able to attenuate the toxic effects of CCl₄ by reducing the increased activities of the serum enzymes (AST, ALT, ALP, γ-GT) and total bilirubin at both 250 mg/kg and 500 mg/kg in a dose-dependent manner. This is in agreement with Eidi et al. [41], who stated that administration of walnut leaf extract (ranging from 0.2 to 0.4 g/kg body weight) significantly lowered serum ALT, AST and ALP levels in the CCl₄-treated rat. Post-treatment of rats with the extract at 250 and 500 mg/kg respectively after CCl₄ administration significantly restored liver damage in a dose-dependent manner. Similarly pre/post-administration of standard silymarin also reduced the toxic effect of CCl₄ induced liver damage.

Oxidative stress induced by CCl₄ in rats in this study show a significant decrease in the antioxidant enzymes. Oral administration of the methanol extract of *T. conophorum* seeds gave rise to increase in the antioxidant parameters investigated in this study. The increases were observed significantly at both 250 and 500 mg/kg extract for catalase, superoxide dismutase, reduced glutathione and glutathione peroxidase, except glutathione S- transferase when compared with CCl₄ treated rats. Antioxidants have been observed to exert their action in vivo by inhibiting the generation of reactive oxygen species by suppressing the CytP450 bioactivation of chemicals and drugs to reactive metabolites [42]. Antioxidants also carry out their mechanism of action by directly scavenging free radicals, a process known as mopping up, by up-regulating the expression of the genes coding for SOD, CAT, glutathione peroxidase and glutathione reductase [43, 44]. This may be achieved by activating nuclear transcription factor erythroid-derived 2-like 2 (Nrf2), a transcriptional regulator that controls the expression of genes involved in oxidative defense. Mechanistically, Nrf2 is inactive in the cytoplasm due to the formation of a complex with its inhibitor Keap-1 [45]. Following the release of Keap-1 from complex induced by oxidative stress, Nrf2 is translocated to the nucleus, where it binds to promoters containing antioxidant response elements (AREs), resulting in the transactivation of the respective genes for antioxidant enzymes [45]. The methanol extract of *T. conophorum* seeds, known for its antioxidant activity, may increase the levels of phosphorylated AKT and extracellular signal-regulated protein kinase (ERK) in hepatocytes, increasing Nrf2 phosphorylation at serine or tyrosine residues, which help in the dissociation of the Nrf2/Keap1 complex that

maintains Nrf2 in the cytosol. This increases the translocation of Nrf2 to the nucleus where it binds to the antioxidant responsive element (ARE) to increase the expression and activity of GPx, GST, and GR, resulting in a decrease of the oxidative stress status [46]. Carbon tetrachloride administration significantly induced lipid peroxidation, a marker of oxidative stress. However, administration of the methanol extract of *T. conophorum* seeds led to significant reduction of lipid peroxidation. This was in agreement with Theophile et al. [47], who posited that plants with antioxidant activities could be protected from oxidative damage.

## Conclusion
The methanol extract of *T. conophorum* seeds at doses up to 500 mg/kg was able to ameliorate the biochemical changes and injuries associated with the effect of CCl₄ poisoning which could be attributed to the presence of phytochemicals and antioxidant activities. It could therefore be suggested based on these findings that methanol extract of *T. conophorum* seeds possesses protective effect against CCl₄-induced hepatotoxicity through its antioxidant mechanism of action.

**Abbreviations**
*AKT: Protein kinase B*; ALP: Alkaline phosphatase; ALT: Alanine aminotransferase; AST: Aspartate aminotransferase; CAT: Catalase; CCl₄: Carbon tetrachloride; GSH: Glutathione; GSH-Px: Glutathione peroxidase; GST: Glutathione-S-transferase; Keap-1: Kelch-like ECH-associated protein 1; MDA: Malondialdehyde; SOD: Superoxide dismutase; TC: *Tetracarpidium conophorum*; γ-GT: Gamma glutamyl transferase

**Acknowledgements**
I appreciate Mr. Keke Collins Obinna, Miss Blessing Titus and Osazee Imasuen for providing technical services.

**Funding**
The work was supported by Tertiary Trust Fund, University of Benin to Oriakhi Kelly, Department of Medical Biochemistry, School of Basic Medical Sciences.

**Authors' contributions**
Professor Patrick.O. Uadia designed the experiments, Dr. Ikechi.G. Eze prepared and interpreted the liver histology slides and Dr. Kelly Oriakhi carried out the experimental bench work, analysed, wrote the manuscript and interpreted the data. All authors read and approved the final manuscript.

**Competing interests**
The authors declare that they have no competing interests.

**Author details**
[1]Department of Medical Biochemistry, School of Basic Medical Sciences, University of Benin, Benin City, Nigeria. [2]Department of Biochemistry, Faculty of Life Sciences, University of Benin, Benin City, Nigeria. [3]Department of Anatomy, School of Basic Medical Sciences, University of Benin, Benin City, Nigeria.

**References**
1. Juza RM, Pauli EM. Clinical and surgical anatomy of the liver: a review for clinicians. Clin Anat. 2014;27:764–9.
2. Slater TF. Free radical mechanisms in tissue injury. Biochem J. 1984;222:1–15.
3. Raucy JL, Kramer JC, Lasker JM. Bioactivation of halogenated hydrocarbons by cytochrome P450 2E1. CRC Crit Rev Toxicol. 1993;23:1–20.
4. Weber LW, Boll M, Stamp FA. Hepatotoxicity and mechan- ism of action of haloalkanes: carbon tetrachloride as a toxicological model. Crit Rev Toxicol. 2003;33(3):105–36.
5. Mehendale HM, Roth RA, Gandolfi RA, Klaunig JE, Lemasters JJ, Curtis LR. Novel mechanisms in chemically induced hepatotoxicity. FASEB J. 1994;8: 1285–95.
6. Boll M, Weber LW, Becker E, Stampfl A. Mechanism of carbon tetrachloride induced hepatotoxicity. Hepatocellu- Lar damage by reactive carbon tetrachloride metabolites. Z Naturforsch. 2001;56(7–8):649–59.
7. Sevanian A, Ursini G. Lipid peroxidation in membrane and low-density lipoproteins: similarities and differences. Free Rad Biol Med. 2000;29:306–11.
8. Gallucci RM, Simeonova PP, Toriumi W, Luster MI. TNF-α regulates transforming growth factor-α expression in regenerating murine liver and isolated hepatocytes. J Immunol. 2000;164:872–8.
9. Gruebele A, Zawaski K, Kaplan D, Novak RF. Cytochrome P450 2E1– and cytochrome P450 2B1/2B2–catalyzed carbon tetrachloride metabolism: effects on signal transduction as demonstrated by altered immediate-early (c-Fos and c-Jun) gene expression and nuclear AP-1 and NF-κB transcription factor levels. Drug Metabol Disp. 1996;24:15–22.
10. Bak J, Je NK, Chung HY, Yokozawa T, Yoon S, Moon JO. Oligonol ameliorates CCl₄-induced liver injury in rats via the NF-Kappa B and MAPK signaling pathways. Oxid Med Cell Longev. 2016;1:1–12.
11. Nieto N, Dominguez-Rosales JA, Fontana L, Salazar A, Armendariz-Borunda J, Greenwel P, Rojkind M. Rat hepatic stellate cells contribute to the acute-phase response with increased expression of alpha1(I) and alpha1(IV) collagens, tissue inhibitor of metallo-proteinase-1, and matrix-metalloproteinase-2 messenger RNAs. Hepatol. 2000;33:597–607.
12. Lee KS, Buck M, Houglum K, Chojkier M. Activation of hepatic stellate cells by TGF alpha and collagen type I is mediated by oxidative stress through c-myb expression. J Clin Invest. 1995;96:2461–8.
13. Karou D, Dicko MH, Simpore J, Traore AS. Antioxidant and antibacterial activities of polyphenols from ethnomedicinal plants of Burkina Faso. Afri J Biotechnol. 2005;4:823–8.
14. Wolf AT, Maurer R, Glickman J, Grace ND. Hepatic venous pressure gradient supplements liver biopsy in the diagnosis of cirrhosis. J Clin Gastroenterol. 2008;42:199–203.
15. Abbas KS, Xiaoqin T, Ridhwi M, Huaping Z, Barbara NT, Mark SC. Withaferin a, a cytotoxic steroid from Vassobia breviflora, induces apoptosis in human head and neck squamous cell carcinoma. J Nat Prod. 2010;73:1476–81.
16. Oke OL. Leaf protein research in Ibadan, Nigeria. University of Ibadan Press; 1995.
17. Uadia PO, Oriakhi K, Osemwenkae PO, Emokpae MA. Effect of methanolic extract of Tetracarpidium conophorum seed on haematological parameters in carbon tetrachloride administered albino rats. Nig J Biochem Mol Bio. 2012b;27(1):63–5.
18. Ajaiyeoba EO, Fadare DA. Antimicrobial potential of extracts and fractions of the African walnut-Tetracarpidium conophorum. Afr J Biotechnol. 2006;5(22):2322–5.
19. Herbert JR, Hurley TG, Olendzki BC, Teas J, Ma Y, Ha JS. Nutritional and socioeconomic factors in reaction to prostate cancer mortality: a cross-national study. J Nat Cancer Inst. 1998;90:1637–47.
20. NIH. Guidelines for the care and use of laboratory animals. NIH publication No. 85–23, Revised 1985. 1985
21. Reitman S, Frankel S. A colorimetric method for the determination of serum glutamate-oxaloacetate and pyruvate transaminass. Am J Clin Pathol. 1957;28:56–63.
22. Teitz NN. Determination of Gamma glutamyl Transferase. In: Fundamentals of clinical chemistry ed 3 Philadelphia, W. B Saunders Co: 1987; pg 391.
23. Kochmar JF, Moss DW. Determination of alkaline phosphatase. In: Tietz NW, editor. Fundamentals of clinical chemistry. Philadelphia: W.B. Saunders and company; 1976. p. 604.
24. Tietz NW, editor. Clinical Guide to Laboratory Tests. 3rd ed. Philadelphia: W. B. Saunders; 1995.
25. Jendrassik L, Grof P. Determination of direct and indirect bilirubin. Biochem Z. 1938;297:81.
26. Misra HP, Fridovich I. The role of superoxide anion in the autooxidation of epinephrine and a simple assay for Superoxide dismustase. J Biol Chem. 1972;247:3170–5.
27. Asru KS. Colorimetric assay of catalase. Anal Biochem. 1972;47:389–94.
28. Beutler E, Duron O, Kelly BM. Improved method for the determination of blood glutathione. J Lab Clin Med. 1963;61:882–8.
29. Habig WH, Pabst MJ, Jacoby WB. Glutathione-S-transferase, the first enzymatic step in mercaptroic acid formation. J Biol Chem. 1974;249:7130–9.
30. Rostruck JT, Pope AL, Ganther HE, Swanson AB, Hafeman DG, Hoekstra WG. Selenium: biochemical role as a component of glutathione peroxidase. Sci. 1973;179:588–90.
31. Varshney R, Kale RK. Effect of calmodulin antagonists on radiation induced lipid peroxidation in microsomes. Int J Rad Biol. 1990;58:733–43.
32. Buege JA, Aust SD. Microsomal lipid peroxidation. Methods Enzymol. 1978; 52:302–10.
33. Akindele AJ, Ezenwanebe KO, Anunobi CC, Adeyemi OO. Hepatoprotective and in vivo antioxidant effects of Byrsocarpus coccineus Schum and Thonn. (Connaraceae). J. Ethnopharmacol. 2010;129(1):46–52.
34. Jaishree V, Badami S. Antioxidant and hepatoprotective effect of swertiamarin from Enicostemma axillare against D-galactosamine induced acute liver damage in rats. J Ethnopharmacol. 2010;130:103–6.
35. Karakus E, Karadeniz A, Simsek N. Protective effect of Panax ginseng against serum biochemical changes and apoptosis in liver of rats treated with carbon tetrachloride (CCl₄). J Hazard Mater. 2011;195:208–13.
36. Waller RL, Glende EA, Recknagel RO. CCl₄ and bromotrichloromethane toxicity. Dual role of covalent binding of metabolic cleavage products and lipid peroxidation in depression of microsomal calcium sequestration. Biochem Pharmacol. 1983;32:1613–7.
37. Zimmerman DJ. Drug –induced liver disease. Drugs. 1978;16(1):25–45.
38. Navarro VJ, Senior JR. Drug related hepatotoxicity. New England J Med. 2006;354:731–9.
39. Kaplan MM. Serum alkaline phosphatase-another piece is added to the puzzle. Hepatol. 1986;6:526–8.
40. Bulle F, Mavier P, Zafrani ES. Mechanism of gammaglutamyl transpeptidase release in serum during intrahepatic and extrahepatic cholestasis in the rat: a histochemical, biochemical and molecular approach. Hepatol. 1990;11: 545–50.
41. Eidi A, Mortazavi P, Moghadam JZ, Mousar P. Hepatoprotective effects of Portulaca oleracea extract against CCl₄-induced damage in rats. Pharm Bio. 2014;1:1–10.
42. Uadia PO, Oriakhi K, Osemwenkae PO, Emokpae MA. Phytochemical screening and antioxidant capacity of methanolic extract of Tetracarpidium conophorum seeds. Nig J Biochem and Mol Bio. 2012a;27(1):16–26.
43. Aruoma OI. Free radical, antioxidants and international nutrition. Asia Pasific J Clin Nutr. 1999;8(1):53–63.
44. Kamalakkannan N, Rukkumani R, Aruna K, Varma PS, Viswanathan P, Menon VP. Protective effect of N-acetyl cysteine in carbon tetrachloride-induced liver damage. Iranian J Pharm and ther. 2005;42:118–23.
45. Martín MA, Ramos S, Granado-Serrano AB, RodríguezRamiro I, Trujillo M, Bravo L, Goya L. Hydroxytyrosol induces antioxidant/detoxificant enzymes and Nrf2 translocation via extracelular regulated kinases and phosphatidylinositol-3kinase/protein kinase B pathways in HepG2 cells. Mol Nutr Food Res. 2010;54:956–66.
46. Echeverria F, Ortiz M, Valenzuela R, Videla LA. Hydroxytyrosol and cytoprotection: a projection for clinical interventions. Int J Mol Sci. 2017;18:930.
47. Theophile D, Emery TD, Desire DDP, Veronique PB, Njikam N. Effects of Alafia multiflora staff on lipid peroxidation and antioxidant enzyme status in carbon tetrachloride-treated rats. Pharmacol Online. 2006;2:76–8.

# 21

# Hepatoprotective, antihyperglycemic and antidiabetic effects of *Dendrophthoe pentandra* leaf extract in rats

Mahadi Hasan[1†], Mohammad Tuhin Ali[2*†] ⓘ, Rifat Khan[3], Parag Palit[2], Aminul Islam[3], Veronique Seidel[4], Rabeya Akter[1] and Laizuman Nahar[1]

## Abstract

**Background:** *Dendrophthoe pentandra* (L.) Miq. is a mistletoe species used in traditional medicine. Juice of leaves is used in wound healing, skin infection and cancer; whereas the whole plant is used to treat hypertension and cough. *D. pentandra* leaf extract has attracted interest due to its pharmacological properties including antioxidant, cytotoxicity and anti-inflammatory effects. In this study, we have investigated the hepatopotective, antihyperglycemic and antidiabetic potential of *D. pentandra* leaf extracts in rats.

**Methods:** *D. pentandra* leaf methanolic extract (DPLME) at a fixed dose of 400 mg/kg body weight was evaluated for its effects on fasting glucose levels of rats. DPLME at the same dose was also used to determine the antidiabetic potential in alloxan-induced diabetic rats and the hepatopotective effects on Paracetamol (PCM) intoxicated rats.

**Results:** Oral administration of DPLME exhibited a significantly notable oral glucose tolerance in rats. Single doses of the DPLME displayed very significant antidiabetic activity which was comparable to the activity of the standard antihyperglycemic agent Metformin (MET). DPLME also offered significant hepatoprotection to PCM-intoxicated rats at levels commensurable to the standard hepatoprotective drug Silymarin (SIL).

**Conclusions:** The results of the present study showed that the DPLME possesses hepatopotective, antihyperglycemic and antidiabetic activity. All these results could be due to the presence of the bioactive components in the extract and this warrant further investigation on the nature of the phytochemical(s) responsible for the observed effects.

**Keywords:** *Dendrophthoe pentandra*, Oral glucose tolerance test, Antidiabetic activity, Hepatoprotective activity

## Background

*Dendrophthoe pentandra* is a hemiparasitic woody shrub that belongs to the Loranthaceae family of mistletoes and is commonly found on tropical trees [1]. This plant has been extensively used in folklore medicine despite being commonly considered as an unwanted plant due to its parasitic nature. It is widely distributed in China, Cambodia, India, Indonesia, Laos, Malaysia, Myanmar, Philippines, Thailand, and Vietnam [2]. In Indonesia, the leaves of *D. pentandra* has been reported used in the traditional medicine to treat wounds and skin infection; while whole part of the plant is used to cure hypertension and cough [3]. It is also used for its antidiuretic activity in Indonesian traditional medicine [1]. In Sulawesi Island, this plant has been used as medicine to cure cancer [3]. Previous investigations on this species have demonstrated that the *D. pentandra* leaf extract stimulated the proliferation of mice splenocytes and thymocytes in a time- and dose-dependent manner [4]. Artanti et al. reported the antioxidant activity of this plant on the basis of DPPH free radical scavenging ability and later confirmed the exact chemical identity of the active antioxidant to be quercetin-3-O-rhamnoside, a flavonol glycoside on the basis of isolation and multiple spectrophotometric techniques [2]. Consequent phytochemical analysis revealed that flavonoids are the main active fraction of the leaf extracts of *D. pentandra*. The existence of other plant

---

* Correspondence: m.tuhinali@gmail.com

†Mahadi Hasan and Mohammad Tuhin Ali contributed equally to this work.
²Department of Biochemistry and Molecular Biology, Faculty of Biological Sciences, University of Dhaka, Dhaka 1000, Bangladesh
Full list of author information is available at the end of the article

secondary metabolites including: saponins and tannins being present in extracts of solvents of varying polarity [1, 2].

There has been a worldwide upsurge in the incidence of diabetes mellitus. It is projected to rise from 171 million in 2000 to 366 million in 2030 [5]. Diabetes mellitus is a metabolic disorder of multiple etiologies in which chronic hyperglycemia results from absent or inadequate pancreatic insulin secretion, with or without concurrent impairment of insulin action [6]. Long-term complications associated with hyperglycemia, such as retinopathy, neuropathy and angiopathy, result in significant disability and mortality [7]. Standard treatments to tackle diabetes include recombinant insulin and oral antidiabetic drugs, but these are faced with challenges such as ensuring adequate production of insulin to meet the soaring demands and difficult patient compliance due to the recurrent side effects of antidiabetic drugs [8, 9]. Hepatic diseases refer to aberrations of the structure or changes in the biochemical activity of liver cells. They occur in almost every age group and account for a global mortality of one million in 2010 [10]. Despite the immense advancements in the field of modern medicine, the absence of potent and effective hepatoprotective agents has remained a constant issue [11].

A large number of medicinal preparations based on plants are recommended for the treatment of hyperglycemia and for their hepatoprotective effect [12, 13]. The World Health Organization (WHO) expert committee on diabetes has listed as one of its recommendations that traditional methods of treatment for diabetes should be further investigated [14]. On the other hand, natural products are also an invaluable pool of molecular scaffolds to discover new drug leads and most currently marketed drugs derive directly or indirectly from plant constituents [15]. As a part of our ongoing research of pharmacological screening of the Bangladeshi medicinal plants, the methanolic extract of *D. pentandra* had been chosen for the present study. In this study, we have investigated the hepatopotective, antihyperglycemic and antidiabetic potential of *D. pentandra* leaf extracts in rats for the first time. We concluded for further study for the identification of key active compounds responsible for the observed effects.

## Methods

### Plant material

Fresh leaves of *D. pentandra* (L.) Miq were collected from the Gazipur district, Bangladesh. Subsequent botanical identification and verification was completed at the Bangladesh National Herbarium, Mirpur-1, Dhaka, Bangladesh (DACB Accession no. 45823).

### Preparation of the plant extracts

Leaves were thoroughly washed with water, chopped into small pieces and air-dried for 4 days. The dried material was ground to a fine powder and stored in an air-tight container for further use. Extracts were prepared as described previously [16]. Briefly, dried powdered *D. pentandra* leaves (300 g) were extracted at room temperature with methanol at a ratio of 1:4 (powder/solvent) in a flat-bottom glass container with occasional shaking for 4 days. The extracts were subsequently filtered through a cotton plug and then through Whatman's no.1 filter paper. The resulting filtrate was concentrated to dryness under reduced pressure.

### Animals

Swiss albino rats (80–115 g) of either sex, aged 7–8 weeks, were purchased from the animal research branch of the International Centre for Diarrhoeal Disease and Research, Bangladesh (ICDDR'B). The animals were kept under standard conditions of $25 \pm 3$ °C, relative humidity 35–60% and on a 12 h dark/light cycle for 1 week before and during the experiments. A standard rodent diet (Lipton, India) was provided with ad libitum administration of water. Food intake was withdrawn 18–24 h prior to the start of the experiments. All experiments were performed in accordance with the Ethical Principles and Guidelines for Scientific Experiments on Animals (1995) formulated by The Swiss Academy of Medical Sciences and the Swiss Academy of Sciences. The experimental period lasted for eight weeks.

### Oral glucose tolerance test (OGTT)

Tests were carried out according to a previously described protocol with some minor modifications [17]. Swiss albino rats that had fasted for 16 h prior to the experiment were randomly divided into three groups each containing four rats. Group III was orally administered with DPLME 400 mg/kg body weight followed by oral administration of 1 g/kg glucose solution. The standard group (Group II) was treated with the antihyperglycemic drug MET (Square Pharmaceuticals Ltd., Kaliakoir, Bangladesh) at a dose of 50 mg/kg body weight, followed by 1 g/kg oral glucose administration while the control group (Group I) received no glucose solution. Blood samples were subsequently collected from tail veins at 0, 30, 60, and 120 min following oral glucose administration and glucose levels were measured using a glucometer test strip [18].

### Antidiabetic activity

The antidiabetic activity of DPLME was evaluated according to a previously published method [19]. Non-diabetic and alloxan-induced diabetic rats were used in the experiment and were divided into four groups consisting of six rats in each group. Group I was the non-diabetic control group, Group II was the alloxan-induced diabetic control group. Diabetic rats in

Group III were treated with MET 50 mg/kg body weight. Diabetic rats in Group IV were orally administered with DPLME at a concentration of 400 mg/kg body weight. Following a period of 2 h, all rats were orally administered of 1 g/kg glucose solution. All treatments were carried out for seven consecutive days. At the end of the experimental period, all surviving animals were fasted overnight. Blood samples were collected from the tail veins at 0, 30, 60, and 120 min following glucose administration for five successive days and glucose levels were measured using a standard glucose oxidase test [20].

### PCM-induced hepatotoxicity and analysis of liver function parameters

The hepatoprotective activity of *D. pentandra* leaf extract was evaluated according to a previously published method [21]. Rats were divided into four groups with four rats in each group. Group I received no treatment and served as the control group. Group II was administered PCM (Beximco Pharmaceuticals Ltd., Tongi, Bangladesh) in normal saline at a dose of 20 mg/kg body weight. Group IV was orally administered with DPLME at the dose of 400 mg/kg body weight. Group III was treated with the hepatoprotective drug SIL (Radiant Nutraceuticals Ltd., Dhaka, Bangladesh) at a dose of 40 mg/kg body weight. All treatments lasted for seven consecutive days. On the fifth day of the respective treatments, PCM at a dose of 20 mg/kg body weight was administered and the animals were sacrificed 48 h later. Blood samples were collected, allowed to clot and then centrifuged to obtain serum samples. The levels of key liver function parameters including aspartate aminotransferase (AST), serum alanine aminotransferase (ALT), total cholesterol and total protein were measured using commercial assay kits (Span Diagnostic, Surat) [22].

### Statistical analyses

In all cases the experimental values are expressed as mean ± SEM (Standard error of the mean). One-way analysis of variance (ANOVA) followed by the Dunnett Multiple Comparison t-test was used for statistical comparison. Here, p ($p$-value) ≤ 0.05 was considered as statistically significant difference when any group of rats compared with the control group rats. All statistical analysis was done using GraphPad Prism software (version 5.01) from GraphPad Software, Inc., San Diego California, USA.

## Results

### Oral glucose tolerance test (OGTT)

The results of the OGTT performed in rats are summarised in Table 1 and illustrated in Fig. 1. We observed that at the ultimate 120 min interval following oral glucose intake, the rats that had received the DPLME 400 mg/kg was able to metabolise glucose more efficiently than those in the standard group that had received the antihyperglycemic drug MET 50 mg/kg. The blood glucose levels of rats from group III decreased significantly in compared to the control group I ($p < 0.05$). The rats from group III, in particular, that had received the DPLME showed a greater ability to metabolise glucose as depicted by the sharp reduction in their blood glucose levels at different intervals throughout the entire time span of 120 min.

### Antihyperglycemic activity

The data obtained are summarized in Table 2 and illustrated in Fig. 2. We observed that the rats from Group IV treated with DPLME showed distinctly reduced blood glucose levels compared with the diabetic control group ($p < 0.001$). Animals in Group IV treated with the DPLME 400 mg/kg had the lowest blood glucose levels throughout the entire five-day period. The progression rate in the decrease of blood glucose levels in rats of Group IV was found to parallel that observed in the rats of Group III that had received the standard antihyperglycemic drug MET. From the third day of administration onwards, we found that the DPLME 400 mg/kg (Group IV) could lower blood glucose in diabetic rats to a level that is comparable to the steady blood glucose level of non-diabetic rats (Group I). On the fifth day of administration, the rats in Group IV also had blood glucose levels lower than that in the corresponding control group (Group I) and the group receiving the MET (Group III). This data demonstrates an evident anti-hyperglycemic activity and a potential anti-diabetic role of DPLME.

### Effects of extracts on key liver function parameters

The results of the protective effect of *D. pentandra* extracts on PCM-induced hepatotoxicity are shown in Table 3 and illustrated in Fig. 3. The rats that had received DPLME (group IV) along with the rats treated with the hepatoprotective drug, SIL (group III) showed liver function parameters at levels similar to the untreated control group (group I). However, the rats from Group IV treated with DPLME at a concentration of 400 mg/kg displayed distinct reductions in the levels of the different liver function parameters compared with the PCM-intoxicated group (Group II) and to levels that are comparable to the levels observed for the group treated with the standard hepatoprotective drug, SIL (group III) ($p < 0.05$). Therefore, it can be suggested that DPLME offers hepatoprotection up at a concentration of 400 mg/kg at levels commensurable to that observed for SIL.

**Table 1** Effect of methanolic leaf extract of *D. pentandra* on fasting Rats after oral glucose intake

| Groups | Serum glucose level (mg/dl) | | | |
|--------|--------|--------|--------|--------|
| | 0 min | 30 min | 60 min | 120 min |
| Group I: Control group | 90.18 ± 1.32 | 261.00 ± 2.22 | 275.40 ± 2.34 | 291.60 ± 1.68 |
| Group II: MET 50 mg/kg | 91.98 ± 1.20 | 142.20 ± 0.66* | 133.20 ± 0.90* | 135.00 ± 1.14* |
| Group III: DPLME 400 mg/kg | 126.00 ± 7.44 | 111.60 ± 3.78* | 117.00 ± 4.62* | 103.50 ± 4.08* |

Data are expressed as mean ± standard error of the mean (SEM) ($n = 4$). * $p < 0.05$ denotes statistically significant result for a group when it was compared with the hyperglycemic control group (Group I)

## Discussion

Medicinal plants have remained integral components of traditional systems of medicine in many countries worldwide and are still relied upon today for various healthcare and medicinal needs [23]. Many plant-derived substances can serve as leads or precursors for the synthesis of modern drugs and have been reported to alleviate a range of ailments including diabetes and hepatic injuries [24, 25]. Hyperglycemia is the result of either insulin deficiency or insulin resistance that confers a reduced ability of liver and muscle cells to store glucose [26]. Though oral antihyperglycemic agents are widely used in practice, they present some disadvantages owing to their poor pharmacokinetic attributes and accompanying side effects [27].

Several biological activities of the extracts of *D. pentandra* have been already reported in a number of previous literatures. According to Endharti et al., the *D. pentandra* methanolic leaf extract containing quercetin has therapeutic potential to ameliorate TNBS (2,4,6-trinitrobenzene sulfonic acid) induced colitis syndrome in mice. It was also reported that

the same extract can inhibit the differentiation of Th17 cells by inhibiting IL-17 production. These findings suggest that the extract of this plant has the important role in inhibiting intestinal inflammation [1]. Extracts of *D. pentandra* have also been reported to effectively inhibit inflammation, proliferation and induce p53 expression on mice models of colitis-associated colon cancer [28].Analysis of cytotoxicity revealed that the extracts of *D. pentandra* had cytotoxic effects on K562 and MCM-B2 cell lines thus suggestive of a potential anticancer activity of this plant [29]. Methanolic extracts of *D. pentandra* leaves have been also found to exert potent anti-proliferative effects on BCR/ABL-Positive and Imatinib Resistant Leukemia Cell lines [30]. On the other hand, Artanti et al. observed significant antioxidant activities for the methanolic extracts and identified an active flavonol glycoside, quercetin-3-O-rhamnoside as antioxidant where as anti-diabetic activity had been exhibited by both the methanolic and aqueous extracts [3].

In our OGTT, which measures the body's ability to metabolise glucose and clear it out of the bloodstream [17], *D. pentandra* methanolic leaf extracts showed prominent activity. Extracts also exhibited some potential for controlling diabetes via significant antihyperglycemic activity at a concentration of 400 mg/kg in comparison to the standard drug MET, an oral antihyperglycemic agent used in addition to regulation in diet and exercise for the management of type 2 (non-insulin dependent) diabetes mellitus [31]. It has been already discussed that the main active bioactive components in the *D. pentandra* leaf extract are flavonoids. Presence of flavonoids in the *D. pentandra* extract explains its different biological and pharmacological activities [1, 2]. According to Fitrilia et al., different extracts of *D. pentandra* was found out to be rich in flavonoids, tannins and saponins [32]. Most recently, Yee et al. in [33] also reported the presence various phytochemicals including alkaloids, flavonoids, saponins, and tannins in the ethyl acetate leaf extract of this plant. Other extracts of plants indigenous to the Indian sub-continent such as, *Allium cepa*, *Allium sativum*, *Cajanus cajan*, *Coccinia indica*, have been attributed some

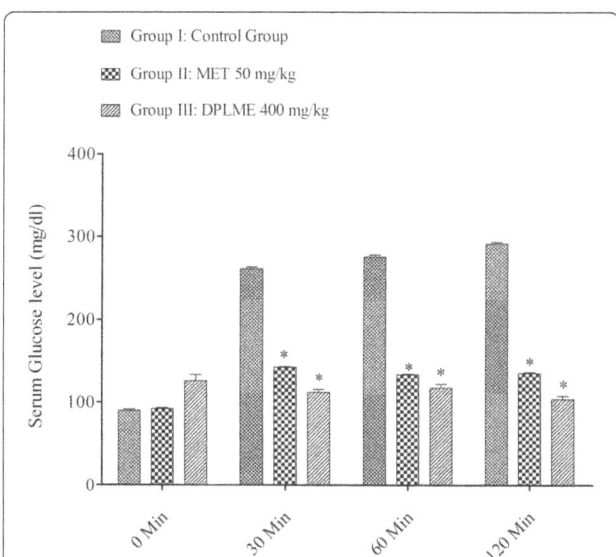

**Fig. 1** Effects of *D. pentandra* leaf methanolic extract on fasting rats after oral glucose intake. Values are expressed as mean ± SEM ($n = 4$). * $p < 0.05$ denotes statistically significant result for a group when it was compared with the hyperglycemic control group (Group I)

**Table 2** Effect of methanolic leaf extract of *D. pentandra* on Alloxan induced diabetic Rats

| Groups | Serum glucose level (mg/dl) | | | | |
|---|---|---|---|---|---|
| | Day 1 | Day 2 | Day 3 | Day 4 | Day 5 |
| Group I: Nondiabetic control | 91.80 ± 1.02*** | 102.06 ± 2.82*** | 89.64 ± 0.78*** | 99.00 ± 2.10*** | 90.00 ± 1.56*** |
| Group II: Diabetic control | 209.70 ± 2.52 | 256.14 ± 1.86 | 308.88 ± 2.94 | 261.72 ± 1.92 | 322.74 ± 3.06 |
| Group III: MET 50 mg/kg | 224.28 ± 4.02 | 157.50 ± 1.86*** | 99.54 ± 1.62*** | 80.28 ± 0.84*** | 76.68 ± 1.92*** |
| Group IV: DPLME 400 mg/kg | 125.28 ± 3.24*** | 112.68 ± 2.28*** | 104.40 ± 1.68*** | 95.04 ± 1.14*** | 77.40 ± 1.62*** |

Data are expressed as mean ± SEM values ($n = 6$). *** $p < 0.001$ denotes statistically very significant result for a group when it was compared with the control group (Group II)

anti-hyperglycemic activity and it has been suggested that the presence of phytochemicals such as flavonoids, alkaloids and other phenolics may contribute to the activity [34]. Indeed, the role of flavonoids has already been reported in the stimulation of peripheral glucose uptake, enhancement of lipogenesis and facilitation of insulin release and conversion from pro-insulin to insulin [35]. Considering all these studies, it can be concluded that the antidiabetic and anti-hyperglycemic activities of the methanolic leaf extract of *D. pentandra* is mostly associated with its flavonoids content. These studies also suggest that *D. pentandra* methanolic leaf extracts could either stimulate the pancreatic insulin secreting cells or improve the receptor responsiveness of tissues to insulin for an increased glucose uptake. Alloxan is a chemical that confers its toxicological effects by the selective necrosis of pancreatic islet cells, leading to a 3 to 4 times increase in blood glucose levels compared to the untreated animals [36, 37]. It is possible that the administration of *D. pentandra* methanolic leaf extracts to alloxan-induced diabetic animals leads to elevated

insulin secretion from regenerated or remnant beta cells or augmented stimulation of glucose uptake by peripheral tissues [38, 39].

The liver plays a vital role in the detoxification of a wide range of xenobotics [40]. Liver damage mediated by the excessive exposure to drugs (e.g. high doses of paracetamol) and environmental pollutants leads to cellular necrosis, plasma membrane damage, depletion in glutathione (GSH) levels accompanied with elevated levels of serum markers of liver damage such as ALT, AST and alkaline phosphatase (ALP) [41]. The rise in total cholesterol, total bilirubin and hypoproteinemia are also key features of liver damage in PCM-intoxicated rats [42, 43]. Several indigenous medicinal plants from the Indian sub-continent including, *Bixa orellana*, *Cajanus cajan*, *Glycosmis pentaphylla* and *Casuarina equisetifolia* are known to possess some hepatoprotective activity [44]. In our study, PCM-treated rats showed a significant rise in the levels of their liver function parameters (AST, ALT, total cholesterol, and total protein) while the levels were significantly lowered following administration of *D. pentandra* methanolic leaf extracts.

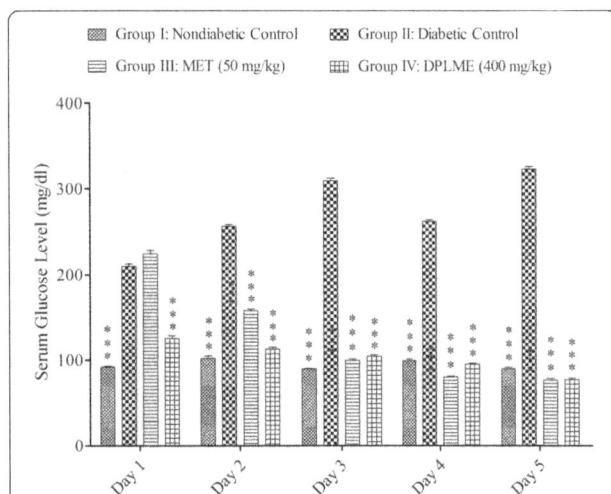

**Fig. 2** Effects of *D. pentandra* leaf methanolic extract on blood glucose levels in non-diabetic and diabetic rats. Values are expressed as mean ± SEM ($n = 6$). *** $p < 0.001$ denotes statistically very significant result for a group when it was compared with the control group (Group II)

**Table 3** Effect of methanolic leaf extract of *D. pentandra* on key liver function parameters of Rats having PCM induced hepatotoxicity

| Groups | AST (U/L) | ALT (U/L) | Total cholesterol (mg/dl) | Total protein (U/L) |
|---|---|---|---|---|
| Group I: Control | 33.75 ± 7.28* | 47.28 ± 5.26* | 114.00 ± 2.79* | 4.83 ± 1.01* |
| Group II: PCM 20 mg/kg | 127.75 ± 17.18 | 169.21 ± 16.71 | 136.50 ± 6.10 | 8.07 ± 2.09 |
| Group III: SIL 40 mg/kg | 40.88 ± 3.42* | 45.82 ± 6.59* | 116.61 ± 9.89* | 2.41 ± 0.54* |
| Group IV: DPLME 400 mg/kg | 108.39 ± 6.30* | 129.34 ± 11.06* | 112.00 ± 4.30* | 5.74 ± 0.84 |

Data are expressed as mean ± SEM ($n = 4$). * $p < 0.05$ denotes statistically significant results for a group when it was compared with the PCM group (Group II)

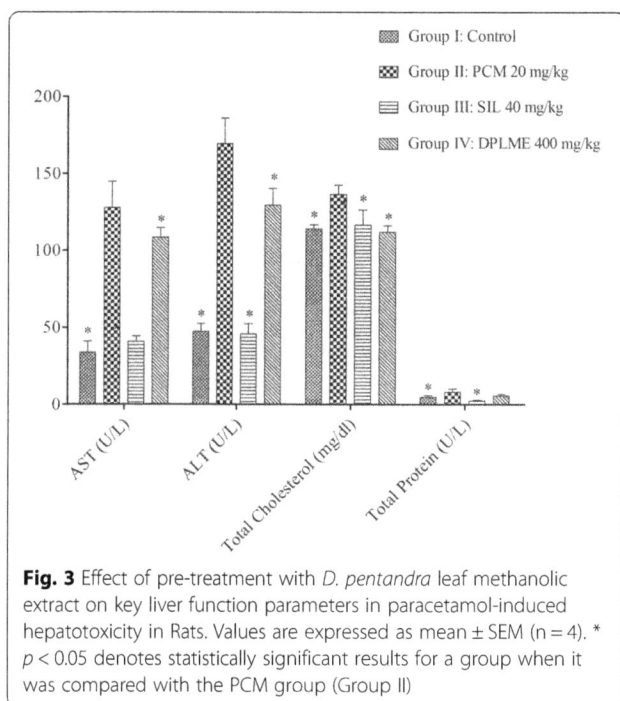

**Fig. 3** Effect of pre-treatment with *D. pentandra* leaf methanolic extract on key liver function parameters in paracetamol-induced hepatotoxicity in Rats. Values are expressed as mean ± SEM (n = 4). * $p < 0.05$ denotes statistically significant results for a group when it was compared with the PCM group (Group II)

**Abbreviations**
ALT: Alanine aminotransferase; AST: Aspartate aminotransferase; DPLME: *D. pentandra* leaf methanolic extract; MET: Metformin; OGTT: Oral glucose tolerance test; PCM: Paracetamol; SEM: Standard error of the mean; SIL: Silymarin

**Acknowledgements**
The authors acknowledge the Department of Pharmacy, School of Science and Engineering, Southeast University, Dhaka, Bangladesh for providing support and necessary research facilities to conduct this study.

**Funding**
This research work did not receive any specific funding.

**Authors' contributions**
MH and LN conceived and designed the experiments; MH and RA performed the experiments; MH and MTA analysed the data; MTA, RK, PP, AI, and VS wrote the paper. All authors read and approved the manuscript.

**Competing interests**
The authors declare that they have no competing interests.

**Author details**
[1]Department of Pharmacy, School of Science and Engineering, Southeast University, Banani, Dhaka 1213, Bangladesh. [2]Department of Biochemistry and Molecular Biology, Faculty of Biological Sciences, University of Dhaka, Dhaka 1000, Bangladesh. [3]Department of Pharmacy, Faculty of Sciences and Engineering, East West University, Dhaka 1212, Bangladesh. [4]Natural Products Drug Discovery Research Group, Strathclyde Institute of Pharmacy and Biomedical Sciences, University of Strathclyde, Glasgow, UK.

This hepatoprotective effect was comparable to the one observed for rats treated with silymarin, a popular hepatoprotective herbal remedy prepared from *Silybum marianum* (milk thistle) [45, 46]. Various secondary metabolites have been identified in the leaf extract of *D. pentandra* including flavonoids, alkaloids, saponins and tannins. Flavonol glycosides i.e., quercetin-3-O-rhamnoside was also isolated from this plant extract [2, 32, 33]. These secondary metabolites have been reported to be associated with the hepatoprotective effects of different medicinal plants [47, 48]. The observed hepatoprotective effect of *D. pentandra* extract might be associated with the presence of these flavonol as well as other secondary metabolites. It is possible that *D. pentandra* extracts help improve the functions of hepatocytes by stabilising cell membranes and/or enhancing the regeneration of parenchymal cells [11]. Overall, this suggests that *D. pentandra* methanolic leaf extracts can effectively control liver damage and restore liver functions.

## Conclusions

Our results have highlighted, for the first time, the antihyperglycemic, antidiabetic and hepatoprotective activity of the methanolic extract of *D. pentandra* leaves in vivo. Further research aimed at the elucidation of key phytochemicals responsible for the observed effects is necessary to consolidate the use of this medicinal plant as a therapeutic option for the treatment of hepatic injuries and diabetes.

**References**
1.  Endharti AT, Permana S. Extract from mango mistletoes *Dendrophthoe pentandra* ameliorates TNBS-induced colitis by regulating CD4+ T cells in mesenteric lymph nodes. BMC Complement Altern Med. 2017;17(1):468.
2.  Syazana NA, Zainuddin NASN, Sul'ain MD. Phytochemical analysis, toxicity and cytotoxicity evaluation of *Dendropthoe pentandra* leaves extracts. Int J Appl Biol Pharm. 2015;6:109–16.
3.  Artanti N, Ma'arifa Y, Hanafi M. Isolation and identification of active antioxidant compound from star fruit (*Averrhoa carambola*) mistletoe (*Dendrophthoe pentandra* L.) Miq. Ethanol extract. J Appl Sci. 2006;6:1659–63.
4.  Ang HY, Subramani T, Yeap SK, Omar AR, Ho WY, Abdullah MP, et al. Immunomodulatory effects of *Potentilla indica* and *Dendrophthoe pentandra* on mice splenocytes and thymocytes. Exp Ther Med. 2014;7(6):1733–7.
5.  Wild SH, Roglic G, Green A, Sicree R, King H. Global prevalence of diabetes: estimates for the year 2000 and projections for 2030: response to Rathman and Giani. Diabetes Care. 2004;27(10):2569.
6.  David EJ, Ohio James MF. Evaluation and prevention of diabetic neuropathy. Am Fam Physician. 2005;71(11):2123–8.
7.  Kristova V, Liskova S, Sotnikova R, Vojtko R, Kurtanský A. Sulodexide improves endothelial dysfunction in streptozotocin-induced diabetes in rats. Physiol Res. 2008;57(3):491–4.
8.  Chaudhury A, Duvoor C, Dendi VSR, Kraleti S, Chada A, Ravilla R, et al. Clinical review of antidiabetic drugs: implications for type 2 diabetes mellitus management. Front Endocrinol. 2017;8:6.
9.  Muniyappa R, Lee S, Chen H, Quon MJ. Current approaches for assessing insulin sensitivity and resistance in vivo: advantages, limitations, and appropriate usage. Am J Physiol Endocrinol Metab. 2008;294(1):E15–26.
10. Byass P. The global burden of liver disease: a challenge for methods and for public health. BMC Med. 2014;12(1):159.

11. Chattopadhyay RR. Possible mechanism of hepatoprotective activity of *Azadirachta indica* leaf extract: part II. J Ethnopharmacol. 2003;89(2):217–9.

12. Rajagopal K, Sasikala K. Antihyperglycaemic and antihyperlipidaemic effects of *Nymphaea stellata* in alloxan-induced diabetic rats. Singap Med J. 2008; 49(2):137–41.

13. Mukherjee PK, Sahoo AK, Narayanan N, Kumar NS, Ponnusankar S. Lead finding from medicinal plants with hepatoprotective potentials. Expert Opin Drug Discov. 2009;4(5):545–76.

14. Alberti KGMM, Zimmet PZ. Definition, diagnosis and classification of diabetes mellitus and its complications. Part 1: diagnosis and classification of diabetes mellitus. Provisional report of a WHO consultation. Diabet Med. 1998;15(7):539–53.

15. Newman DJ, Cragg GM. Natural products as sources of new drugs over the last 25 years. J Nat Prod. 2007;70(3):461–77.

16. Mathew S, Abraham TE. In vitro antioxidant activity and scavenging effects of *Cinnamomum verum* leaf extract assayed by different methodologies. Food Chem Toxicol. 2006;44(2):198–206.

17. Joy K, Kuttan R. Anti-diabetic activity of *Picrorhiza kurroa* extract. J Ethnopharmacol. 1999;67(2):143–8.

18. Hönes J, Müller P, Surridge N. The technology behind glucose meters: test strips. Diabetes Technol Ther. 2008;10(Suppl 1):10–26.

19. Kumar D, Kumar S, Kohli S, Arya R, Gupta J. Antidiabetic activity of methanolic bark extract of *Albizia odoratissima* Benth. In alloxan induced diabetic albino mice. Asian Pac J Trop Med. 2011;4(11):900–3.

20. Barham D, Trinder P. An improved colour reagent for the determination of blood glucose by the oxidase system. Analyst. 1972;97(151):142–5.

21. Achliya GS, Wadodkar SG, Dorle AK. Evaluation of hepatoprotective effect of Amalkadi Ghrita against carbon tetrachloride-induced hepatic damage in rats. J Ethnopharmacol. 2004;90(2–3):229–32.

22. Gowda S, Desai PB, Hull VV, Math AAK, Vernekar SN, Kulkarni SS. A review on laboratory liver function tests. Pan Afr Med J. 2009;3:17.

23. Petrovska BB. Historical review of medicinal plants' usage. Pharmacogn Rev. 2012;6(11):1–5.

24. Balunas MJ, Kinghorn AD. Drug discovery from medicinal plants. Life Sci. 2005;78(5):431–41.

25. Eddouks M, Maghrani M, Lemhadri A, Ouahidi M-L, Jouad H. Ethnopharmacological survey of medicinal plants used for the treatment of diabetes mellitus, hypertension and cardiac diseases in the south-east region of Morocco (Tafilalet). J Ethnopharmacol. 2002;82(2):97–103.

26. Klein R. Hyperglycemia and microvascular and macrovascular disease in diabetes. Diabetes Care. 1995;18(2):258–68.

27. Bolen S, Feldman L, Vassy J, Wilson L, Yeh H-C, Marinopoulos S, et al. Systematic review: comparative effectiveness and safety of oral medications for type 2 diabetes mellitus. Ann Intern Med. 2007;147(6):386–99.

28. Endharti AT, Wulandari A, Listyana A, Norahmawati E, Permana S. *Dendrophthoe pentandra* (L.) Miq. Extract effectively inhibits inflammation, proliferation and induces p53 expression on colitis-associated colon cancer. BMC Complement Altern Med. 2016;16(1):374.

29. Elsyana V, Bintang M, Priosoeryanto BP. Cytotoxicity and antiproliferative activity assay of clove mistletoe (*Dendrophthoe pentandra* (L.) Miq.) leaves extracts. Adv Pharmacol Sci. 2016;2016:3242698.

30. Zamani A, Jusoh SAM, Al-Jamal HAN. Sul'ain MD, Johan MF. Anti-proliferative effects of *Dendrophthoe pentandra* methanol extract on BCR/ABL-positive and imatinib-resistant leukemia cell lines. Asian Pac J Cancer Prev. 2016;17(11):4857–61.

31. Foretz M, Guigas B, Bertrand L, Pollak M, Viollet B. Metformin: from mechanisms of action to therapies. Cell Metab. 2014;20(6):953–66.

32. Fitrilia T, Bintang M, Safithri M. Phytochemical screening and antioxidant activity of clove mistletoe leaf extract (*Dendrophthoe pentandra* (L.) Miq.). IOSR J Pharm. 2015;5(8):13–8.

33. Yee L, Fauzi N, Najihah N, Daud N, Sulain M. Study of *Dendrophthoe pentandra* ethyl acetate extract as potential anticancer candidate on safety and toxicity aspects. J anal. Pharm Res. 2017;6(1):00167.

34. Grover J, Yadav S, Vats V. Medicinal plants of India with anti-diabetic potential. J Ethnopharmacol. 2002;81(1):81–100.

35. Cordero-Herrera I, Martín MA, Bravo L, Goya L, Ramos S. Cocoa flavonoids improve insulin signalling and modulate glucose production via AKT and AMPK in HepG2 cells. Mol Nutr Food Res. 2013;57(6):974–85.

36. Szkudelski T. The mechanism of alloxan and streptozotocin action in B cells of the rat pancreas. Physiol Res. 2001;50(6):537–46.

37. Zhang X, Liang W, Mao Y, Li H, Yang Y, Tan H. Hepatic glucokinase activity is the primary defect in alloxan-induced diabetes of mice. Biomed Pharmacother. 2009;63(3):180–6.

38. Grover J, Vats V, Rathi S. Anti-hyperglycemic effect of *Eugenia jambolana* and *Tinospora cordifolia* in experimental diabetes and their effects on key metabolic enzymes involved in carbohydrate metabolism. J Ethnopharmacol. 2000;73(3):461–70.

39. Patel D, Prasad S, Kumar R, Hemalatha S. An overview on antidiabetic medicinal plants having insulin mimetic property. Asian Pac J Trop Biomed. 2012;2(4):320–30.

40. Ekins S, Wrighton SA. The role of CYP2B6 in human xenobiotic metabolism. Drug Metab Rev. 1999;31(3):719–54.

41. Giannini EG, Testa R, Savarino V. Liver enzyme alteration: a guide for clinicians. Can Med Assoc J. 2005;172(3):367–79.

42. Wolf PL. Biochemical diagnosis of liver disease. Indian J Clin Biochem. 1999; 14(1):59–90.

43. Kumar G, Banu GS, Pappa PV, Sundararajan M, Pandian MR. Hepatoprotective activity of *Trianthema portulacastrum* L. against paracetamol and thioacetamide intoxication in albino rats. J Ethnopharmacol. 2004;92(1):37–40.

44. Ahsan MR, Islam KM, Bulbul IJ, Musaddik MA, Haque E. Hepatoprotective activity of methanol extract of some medicinal plants against carbon tetrachloride-induced hepatotoxicity in rats. Eur J Sci Res. 2009;37(2):302–10.

45. Pradhan S, Girish C. Hepatoprotective herbal drug, silymarin from experimental pharmacology to clinical medicine. Indian J Med Res. 2006; 124(5):491–504.

46. Al-Sayed E, Martiskainen O, Seif el-Din SH, Sabra A-NA, Hammam OA, El-Lakkany NM, et al. Hepatoprotective and antioxidant effect of *Bauhinia hookeri* extract against carbon tetrachloride-induced hepatotoxicity in mice and characterization of its bioactive compounds by HPLC-PDA-ESI-MS/MS. Biomed Res Int. 2014;2014:245171.

47. Nithianantham K, Shyamala M, Chen Y, Latha LY, Jothy SL, Sasidharan S. Hepatoprotective potential of *Clitoria ternatea* leaf extract against paracetamol induced damage in mice. Molecules. 2011;16(12):10134–45.

48. Atta A, Elkoly T, Mounier S, Kamel G, Alwabel N, Zaher S. Hepatoprotective effect of methanol extracts of *Zingiber officinale* and *Cichorium intybus*. Indian J Pharm Sci. 2010;72(5):564–70.

# 22

# Phytochemical, anti-inflammatory, anti-ulcerogenic and hypoglycemic activities of *Periploca angustifolia* L extracts in rats

Khaled Abo-EL-Sooud[1*] (iD), Fatma A. Ahmed[2], Sayed A. El-Toumy[3], Hanona S. Yaecob[2] and Hanan M. ELTantawy[2]

## Abstract

**Background:** In traditional North Africa, medicine decoctions of the leaves of *Periploca angustifolia* are used to treat diarrhea, inflammation, ulcers, edema and diabetes. The aim of the study was to evaluate the phytochemical, anti-inflammatory, anti-ulcerogenic, and hypoglycemic activities of an ethanolic extract of *P. angustifolia* L. in rats.

**Methods:** An extract of air-dried powdered *P. angustifolia* plant was obtained using 96% ethanol. The extract was concentrated and the total phenolic and flavonoids contents were estimated colorimetrically. The phenolic and flavonoid compounds were quantified and identified using high performance liquid chromatography (HPLC). The anti-inflammatory, anti-ulcerogenic and hypoglycemic activities of the extract were evaluated in three rat models respectively: formaldehyde-induced paw edema, ethanol induced gastric damage and alloxan induced hyperglycemia.

**Results:** The total flavonoids and total phenolics constituted 15% and 2.69% of the extract, respectively and are expressed as quercetin equivalent and µg/mg gallic acid equivalent (GAE). Coumarin, resorcinol, isorhamnetin, quercetin, and naphthalene were isolated from the ethanolic extract of *P. angustifolia*. Oral administration of the ethanolic extract at 500 mg/kg body weight (b.wt.) significantly reduced paw inflammation, gastric lesions, ulcer index scores and blood glucose levels in normal and diabetic rats.

**Conclusion:** The crude ethanolic extract of *P. angustifolia* exhibited promising anti-inflammatory, anti-ulcerogenic, and hypoglycemic activities in accordance with the plant's uses in folk medicine suggesting that *P. angustifolia* may be a safe alternative to chemical drugs.

**Keywords:** *Periploca angustifolia*, Phytochemical, Anti-inflammatory, Anti-ulcerogeni, Hypoglycemic

## Background

*Periploca* is a genus of plants from the Asclepiadaceae family in the major group of angiosperms. Several species of this family, such as *P. angustifolia* are widely used in traditional medicine as anti-diabetic, anti-mutagenic, and anti-rheumatic agents [1]. In Egypt, the leaves of *P. angustifolia* are used to treat rheumatic diseases and the roots are used for hemorrhoids, gastric ulcer and diabetes. Its resin is used as a hypotensive [2] a masticator when burning. *P. angustifolia* L was used by the Bedouins as animal food and herbal remedies [3]. Different plant extracts of the Asclepiadaceae family have shown significant anti-inflammatory [4] and

anti-ulcerogenic properties [5]. In addition, the methanolic extract of *P. angustifolia* leaves has been shown to have antioxidant effects and exert antidotal effects on cadmium-induced hepatotoxicity [6]. There is a relationship between the antioxidant capacity and anti-hyperglycemic potential of *Periploca sylvestre* and it may be due to flavonoids and phenolic contents in the plant that impart these properties [7]. *Gymnema sylvestre* (Asclepiadaceae) has been used since ancient times as a folk medicine for the treatment of diabetes, obesity, and stomach stimulation uses [8]. Aerial parts of *P. angustifolia* L. collected from southern Tunisia possess antioxidant activity against 2, 2′-azino-bis (3-ethyl-benzothiazoline-6-sulphonic acid (ABTS) and 2,2-diphenyl-1-picrylhydrazyl radical (DPPH) [9]. Samples of *Hemidesmus indicus var. indicus* and *var. pubescens* during the flowering season possess higher antiulcer and anti-

* Correspondence: kasooud@cu.edu.eg
[1]Pharmacology Department, Faculty of Veterinary Medicine, Cairo University, Giza 12211, Egypt
Full list of author information is available at the end of the article

hepato-carcinogenic effects [10, 11]. The chemical composition of the root bark of *P. angustifolia*, at the flowering stage showed the presence of C-heterosids (anthracenic derivatives), anthocyans, saponins, free quinons and proanthocyanidols [12]. In this study we determined the phytochemical composition and, in particular the phenolic and flavonoids composition of the ethanolic extract of *P. angustifolia* L., and we assessed anti-inflammatory, anti-ulcerogenic, and hypoglycemic activities.

## Methods
### Plant material
*P. angustifolia* L. was collected from the Sallum Plateau (northwestern coast of Egypt) during 2012–2013. The plants were air dried at lab-temperature until their weight plateaued, and then ground to a fine powder. The different parts of the plants were identified, confirmed and authenticated by comparing with an authentic specimen at the Plant Taxonomy Unit, Desert Research Center, Cairo, Egypt. The samples were extracted by percolation in ethanol 70%, filtered and this step was repeated several times. The ethanolic extract was concentrated under reduced pressure at temperatures not exceeding 40 °C. The obtained ethanol extract of *P. angustifolia* L. constituted 10% from the entire dried plant and was used for subsequent investigations. Scheme of separation for flavonoids and phenolics from the whole plant of *P. angustifolia* L was illustrated in Fig. 1.

### Drugs
Diclofenac sodium (Voltarin®) was obtained from Novartis Pharma Co. (Cairo, Egypt) under license from Novartis Pharma AG, (Basle, Switzerland). Ranitidine hydrochloride tablets (Zantac® Batch No. 001716C) were manufactured by Glaxo-Wellcome Egypt (Elsalam City, Cairo, Egypt, each tablet contained 150 mg ranitidine). Glibenclamide (Daonil®) was purchased from Aventis Co., under license from Aventis Pharma Co., West Germany.

### Animals
Wistar Albino rats (150–170 g) and Swiss mice (18–22 g) were obtained from the Laboratory Animal Colony, Helwan, Egypt. Animals were maintained in the Animal House of the Pharmacology Department (Faculty of Veterinary Medicine, Cairo University) under controlled conditions [temperature 23 ± 2 °C, humidity 50 ± 5% and 12-h light-dark cycles]. All animals were acclimatized for 7 days before the study. The animals were housed in sanitized polypropylene cages, containing sterile paddy husk as bedding. Animals were habituated to laboratory conditions for 48 h prior to the experimental protocol to minimize non-specific stress. All animals were fed a balanced diet of wheat bran, soybean powder, fish-meal and dietary fibers (manufactured by Cairo Agricultural Development Co.). Water was provided ad libitum. The Institutional Animal Care and Use Committee (IACUC), Cairo University approved this study.

### Estimation of Total flavonoids
The flavonoid content in extract was determined spectrophotometrically according to the method described by Djeridane et al. [13], which is based on the formation of a flavonoid–aluminum complex with a maximum absorbance at 430 nm. Total flavonoids are expressed as mg quercetin equivalent.

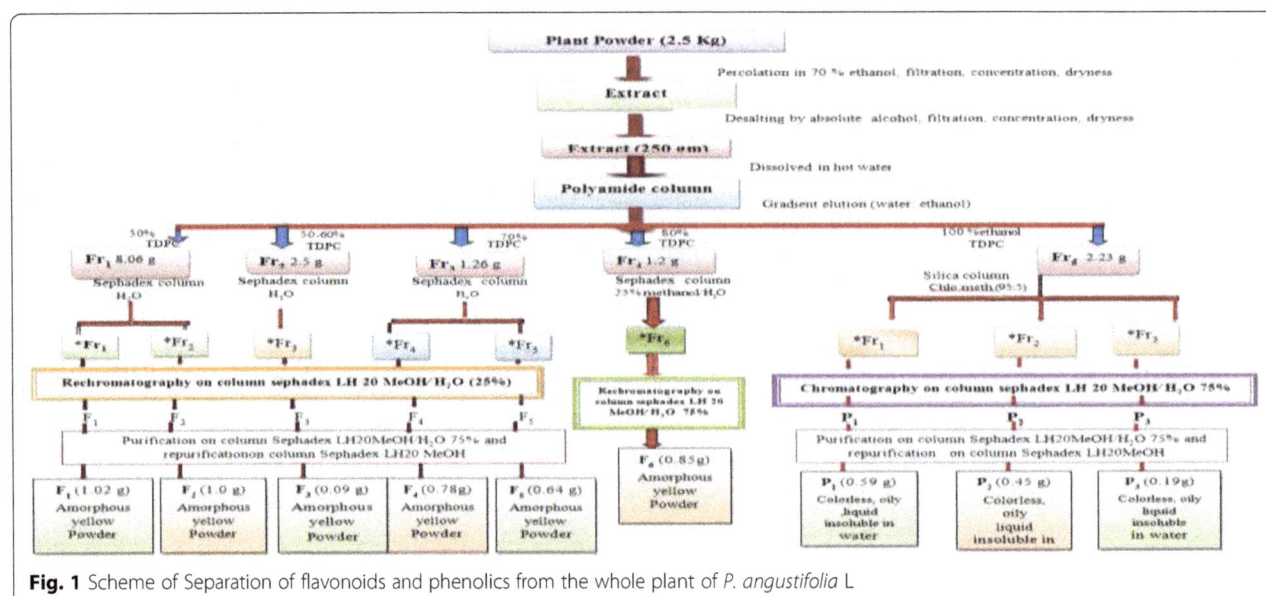

**Fig. 1** Scheme of Separation of flavonoids and phenolics from the whole plant of *P. angustifolia* L

## Estimation of Total phenolic content (TPC)

The Folin-Ciocalteu method [14] was used to determine the TPC spectrophotometrically in the different extracts using gallic acid as standard. The TPC was expressed as µg/mg gallic acid equivalent (GAE).

## Identification of phenolic and flavonoids

HPLC was used to identify phenolics and flavonoids. A known weight of air-dried plant powder was soaked in 25 ml sterilized water and agitated on a rotary shaker for 24 h at 200 rpm. Slurry was filtered through Whatmann 3MM filter paper under a vacuum, followed by centrifugation at 12.5 rpm for 30 min at 80 °C. The aqueous extract was acidified to pH 2.5 using diluted phosphoric acid. The sample was sacked three times through a separating funnel with an equal volume of diethyl ether. The combined diethyl ether layer was evaporated to dryness under reduced pressure at 30 °C. The resulting residue was re-dissolved in 3 ml of HPLC-grade methanol and filtered through a sterile membrane with a pore size of a 0.2 µm prior to HPLC analysis [15]. Identification of individual phenolic compounds of the plant sample was performed using a Dionex (Model 3000) HPLC, using a BDS Hypersil $C_{18}$ reversed-phase column (250 × 4.6 mm) with 10 µm particle size. Injection by means of Rheodyne injection valve (Model 7125) with a 50 µl fixed loop. A constant flow rate of 1 ml/min was used with two mobile phases: distilled water (A), and acetonitrile (B), using a UV detector set at wavelength 254 nm. Phenolic compounds of each sample were identified by comparing their relative retention times with those of the standard mixture chromatogram. The concentration of an individual compound was calculated on the basis of peak area measurements, and then converted to µg/g phenolic dry weight. All chemicals and solvents used were HPLC spectral grade. Standards phenolic compounds were obtained from Sigma (St. Louis, USA) and Merck (Munich, Germany).

## Acute toxicity

The acute toxicity ($LD_{50}$) of ethanolic extract of *P. angustifolia* administered orally was estimated in mice using Lorke [16] method. Three groups of five animals received 10, 100, 1000 mg/kg of the extract suspended in Tween80 (vehicle 3% v/v). The animals were observed for 72 h for signs of toxicity and death. When no deaths were recorded another four groups of five mice were administrated 2000, 3000, 4000 and 5000 mg/kg of the extract orally. The animals were observed for 72 h for signs of toxicity and the number of deaths was recorded. Control animals were received the equivalent volume of vehicle. The $LD_{50}$ values were calculated as the geometric mean of the highest non-lethal and the lowest lethal doses mathematically according to the Kerber method [17] using the following formula:

$$LD50 = LD100 - \Sigma \, (z \times d)/m$$

where z is half of the sum animals that died with the two next doses; d is the interval between two next doses and m is the number of animals/group.

## Anti-inflammatory activity

The extract was evaluated for its anti-inflammatory activity in rats using the formaldehyde-induced paw edema method [18]. Acute inflammation was produced by sub-plantar injection of 0.2 ml formaldehyde (1% w/v) into the hind paw 1 h after oral administration of ethanolic extract of *P. angustifolia* (500 mg/kg b.wt.) or diclofenac sodium (50 mg/kg b.wt.) as a standard anti-inflammatory agent. The paw volume was measured in mm by a plethysmometer (Ugo-Basile, Italy) at 1, 2, 3, and 4 h after the formaldehyde injection. Inhibition of inflammation was calculated using the following formula: % inhibition = 100 (1-Vt/Vc), where 'Vc' represents edema volume in the control group and 'Vt' represents edema volume in the test group.

## Anti-ulcerogenic activity

All rats were fasted for 48 h but were given water ad libitum till the start of the experiment. To prevent excessive dehydration during the fasting period, rats were supplied with sucrose (BDH) 8% (w/v) solution in NaCl (BDH) 0.2% (w/v), which was removed 1 h before experiments [19]. The animals were randomly separated into three groups of six rats. One group was pretreated with ethanolic extract of *P. angustifolia* orally at 500 mg/kg b.wt., another group received ranitidine (100 mg/kg orally) and the control group received equivalent volumes of saline instead of plant extract. One hour later, all groups were treated with ethanol (50%) at a dose of 10 ml/kg. One hour after ethanol administration, all rats were euthanized by an overdose of chloroform and the abdomen was opened. The stomach was removed, opened along the greater curvature, and gently rinsed under running water. The tissues were fixed with 10%

**Table 1** Phenolic and flavonoid compounds identified in the ethanolic extract of *P. angustifolia* L. using HPLC

| Compound No. | Name | % of extract |
|---|---|---|
| 1 | Coumarin | 0.16 ± 0.01 |
| 2 | Resorcinol | 56.54 ± 3.41 |
| 3 | Isorhamnetin | 40.53 ± 2.24 |
| 4 | Quercetin | 0.002 ± 0.001 |
| 5 | Naphthalene | 2.76 ± 0.78 |

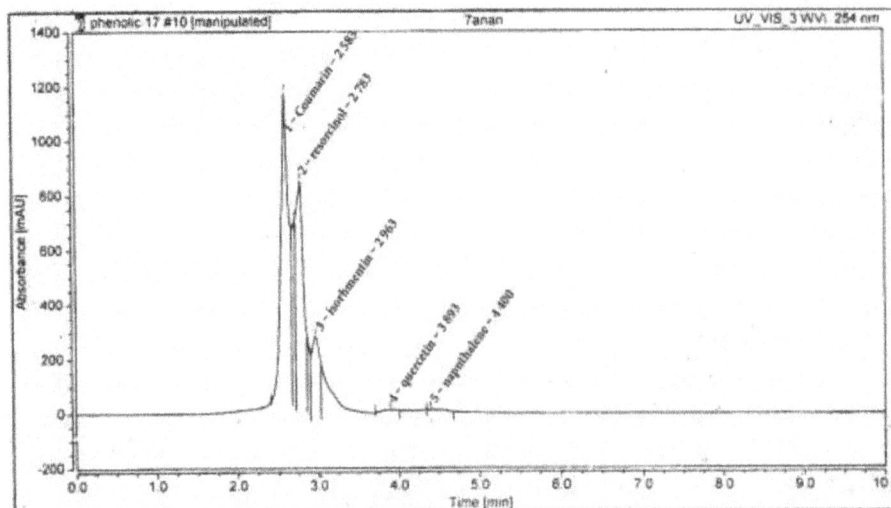

**Fig. 2** HPLC chromatogram of the phenolic and flavonoid compounds of the *P. angustifolia* L

formaldehyde in saline. Macroscopic examination was carried out under a hand lens and the presence of ulcer lesions was scored [20]. Lesions in the glandular part of the stomach were measured under an illuminated magnifying microscope (10 x). Long lesions were counted and measured along their greater length. Petechial lesions were counted with the aid of 1-mm squares grid [21]. Each five petechial lesions were considered to represent a 1-mm ulcer. The ulcer index (%) for each group was calculated as the sum of the lengths of long ulcers and petechial lesions divided by its number.

## Hypoglycemic effect of *P. angustifolia* L. extract
### Induction of diabetes
Rats were rendered diabetic by subcutaneous injection of alloxan monohydrate (Oxford) at a dose of 150 mg/kg/day for 3 days (early ketosis) and normal feeding was maintained [22]. Five days later, blood samples were drawn and the blood glucose level was measured to establish the occurrence of diabetes. The threshold for

diabetes in the present study was a glucose level of ≥225 mg/dl.

### Effect of *P. angustifolia* L. extract on hyperglycemic rats
The hypoglycemic effect of *P. angustifolia* L. extract was studied in alloxan-induced diabetic rats. The animals were fasted for 8 h but allowed free access to water. The diabetic animals were randomly divided into three groups of 10 rats and received oral *P. angustifolia* L. extract (500 mg/kg b.wt.), glibenclamide (0.2 mg/kg) or 20% *v*/v Tween 80 (5 ml/kg b.wt.).

### Effect of *P. angustifolia* L. extract on Normoglycemic rats
Non-diabetic rats were fasted overnight and then, randomly divided into three groups of 10 rats. As with the diabetic rats, the non-diabetic received oral *P. angustifolia* L. extract (500 mg/kg b.wt.), glibenclamide (0.2 mg/kg b.wt.) or 20% v/v Tween 80 (5 ml/kg b.wt.). One milliliter of blood was collected before and after two hours of treatments from each rat in all groups. Blood

**Table 2** Formaldehyde induced paw edema measured as paw thickness in rats treated with *P. angustifolia* L. extract and in control rats (n = 5)

| Group | Paw thickness (mm) | | | | |
|---|---|---|---|---|---|
| | Dose mg/kg | 1 h | 2 h | 3 h | 4 h |
| Negative Control | – | 0.30 ± 0.02 | 0.30 ± 0.01 | 0.30 ± 0.01 | 0.30 ± 0.01 |
| Control positive (formaldehyde) | solvent | 0.60 ± 0.02 | 0.68 ± 0.03 | 0.72 ± 0.05 | 0.66 ± 0.04 |
| *P. angustifolia* L. extract | 500 | 0.45 ± 0.03* | 0.49 ± 0.03* | 0.43 ± 0.01** | 0.38 ± 0.03** |
| Diclofenac sodium | 50 | 0.41 ± 0.02** | 0.44 ± 0.03** | 0.40 ± 0.03** | 0.36 ± 0.03** |

*P < 0.05 **P < 0.01 as compared to control positive

glucose was estimated by the glucose oxidase method using the Randox kit (Randox Laboratories Ltd., Ardmore, UK) according to the manufacturer's instructions.

## Statistical analysis

The results are expressed as the mean ± standard error (SE). The differences between the experimental groups were analyzed by one-way analysis of variance (ANOVA), followed by Bonferroni's test using SPSS 16.0 (SPSS Inc., Chicago, IL, USA). The results were considered statistically significant when $p$ values less than 0.05 and 0.01 were considered significant (*$p$ < 0.05, **$p$ < 0.01).

## Results

### Acute toxicity

There were no changes in the general behavior of the animals at any dose and, there were no deaths after 72 h at the highest administered dose (5000 mg/kg) of the extract. The safety of the extract was shown by the high $LD_{50}$ value of the extract (> 5 g/kg).

### Total flavonoids and phenolic contents

The total flavonoids and phenolic contents of P. angustifolia L were 3.15 ± 0.7% as quercetin equivalent and 2.69 ± 0.6% as gallic acid equivalent, respectively.

### Identification and quantification of phenolic and flavonoid compounds

Quantitative and qualitative analysis of the phenolic and flavonoid compounds in the ethanolic extract of P. angustifolia L. was performed using HPLC, where each compound was separated and identified using authentic standard. The compounds were, coumarin, resorcinol, isorhamnetin, quercetin, and naphthalene with different concentration ranges (Table 1 and Fig. 2). Resorcinol reached its maximum value of 56.54% in ethanolic extract of P. angustifolia L. followed by isorhamnetin at 40.53%, while quercetin was estimated to have a minimum value of 0.002%.

### Anti-inflammatory activity

The formaldehyde-induced paw edema model showed that sub-plantar injection of formaldehyde in rats caused a time-dependent increase in paw thickness and the maximal increase was observed 4 h after formaldehyde administration (Table 2). However, rats that received the ethanolic extract of P. angustifolia pretreatment showed significantly less ($P$ < 0.05, $P$ < 0.01) formaldehyde-induced inflammation at each time point than the animals that received formaldehyde only as did those that received the reference anti-inflammatory drug diclofenac sodium ($P$ < 0.01). Oral administration of P. angustifolia L. extract at 500 mg/kg resulted in a maximal inhibition of paw inflammation 42.42%

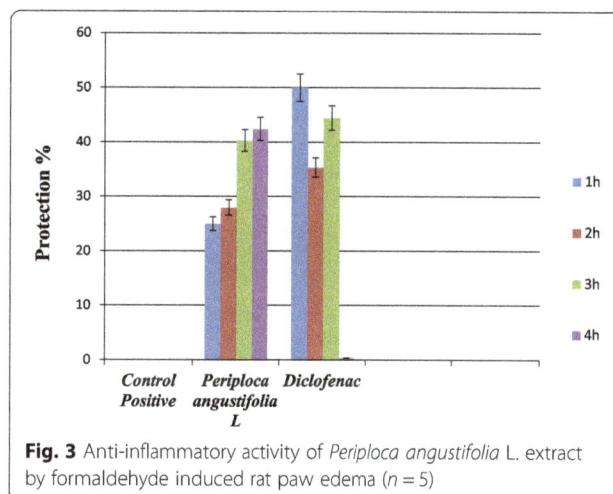

**Fig. 3** Anti-inflammatory activity of Periploca angustifolia L. extract by formaldehyde induced rat paw edema ($n = 5$)

that was close to that of diclofenac sodium 45.45% at 50 mg/kg 4 h post formaldehyde administration (Fig. 3).

### Anti-ulcer activity

Ethanol caused extensive gastric damage in the mucosa of the control animals. The lesions were characterized by multiple long hemorrhagic red bands of different sizes along the axis of the glandular stomach with petechial patches. By contrast, oral treatment with the ethanolic extract of P. angustifolia L showed significantly fewer ($p$ < 0.01) the gastric lesions and lower ulcer index than those observed in the control animals. The crude ethanolic extract of P. angustifolia L. had a protective index of 44.93%, whereas ranitidine as a reference standard (100 mg/kg) exhibited a protective index of 46.99% indicating a potent anti-ulcerogenic effect of P. angustifolia L. extract (Table 3 and Fig. 4).

### Hypoglycemic activity

Subcutaneous injection of rats with alloxan resulted in a significant increase in serum glucose levels. Administration of the crude ethanolic extract of P. angustifolia significantly reduced blood glucose levels at 2 h compared with those untreated diabetic rats. Specifically, the ethanolic extract significantly reduced the postprandial blood glucose level of diabetic rats from 211.16 to 124.33 mg/dl (Table 4 and Fig. 5). Similarly, the extract of P.

**Table 3** The effect of P. angustifolia L. extract on alcohol-induce ulcer in rats (n = 5)

| Group | Dose mg/kg | Alcohol-induce ulcers | |
|---|---|---|---|
| | | Ulcer index | Curative ratio% |
| Control | Saline | 24.15 ± 1.60 | – |
| Periploca angustifolia L. | 500 | 13.30 ± 1.20** | 44.93 |
| Ranitidine | 100 | 12.80 ± 1.10** | 46.99 |

**$P$ < 0.01; when compared with the control group

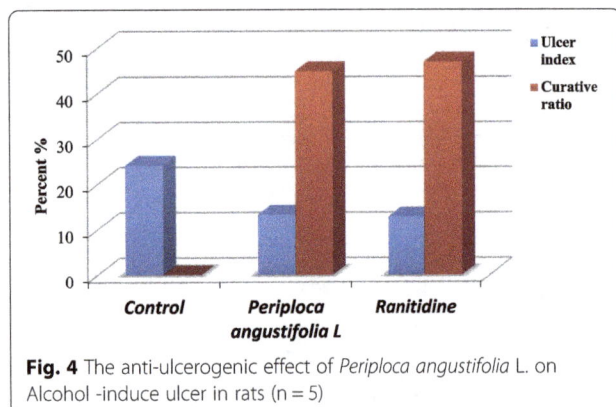

**Fig. 4** The anti-ulcerogenic effect of *Periploca angustifolia* L. on Alcohol -induce ulcer in rats (n = 5)

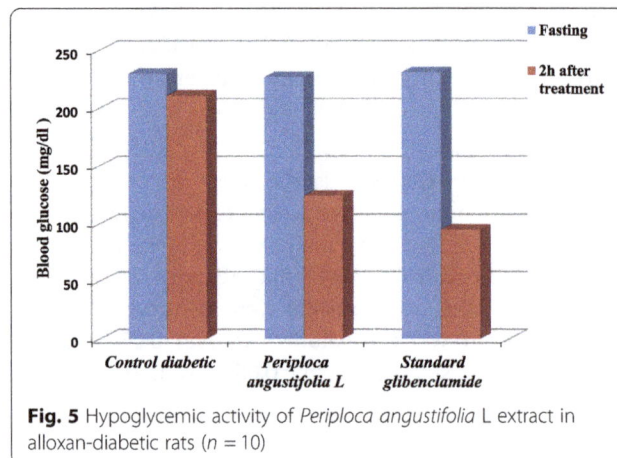

**Fig. 5** Hypoglycemic activity of *Periploca angustifolia* L extract in alloxan-diabetic rats (*n* = 10)

*angustifolia* at the same dose significantly reduced blood glucose level in normoglycemic rats (Table 5 and Fig. 6).

## Discussion

*P. angustifolia* extract had a high safety margin in mice as the $LD_{50}$ was > 5 g/kg. Similarly, Sunil et al. [23] found that alcoholic extract of another plant in the Asclepiadaceae family *Holostemma ada kodien* was non toxic at a dose of 5 g/kg b.wt.

Phenolic compounds increase a plant biological value because they exhibit a range of pharmacological properties, such as anti-diabetic, anti-allergenic, anti-atherogenic, anti-inflammatory, antioxidant, anti-thrombotic, and vasodilator effects [24, 25]. Oxidative stress activates inflammatory pathways in stem cells and progenitor cells, leading to exhaustion of these cells due to increased levels of reactive oxygen species (ROS) [26]. Cellular exhaustion in turn leads to the development of several diseases, such as gastrointestinal ulcers, hyperglycemia, and hepatic dysfunction [27]. Thus, natural antioxidants provide cellular protection and lead to favorable effects in diabetes mellitus [28] and the majority of inflammatory and cardiovascular diseases [29]. Examples of naturally occurring antioxidants are flavonoids, phenolic acids, coumarin, isorhamnetin and quercetin that were separated and identified from *P. angustifolia* extract with promising anti-inflammatory agents. This activity may be due to their inhibitory action on neutrophils infiltration, cyclooxygenase-2 activity and inflammatory cytokines release [30–32]. The anti-ulcerogenic

activity of *P. angustifolia* L. may also be due to the presence of quercetin, as it prevents gastric mucosal damage by increasing mucus production with a comparable regression of gastric lesions [33]. Hyperglycemia is a metabolic disorder that occurs due to the excess production of ROS, which destroy pancreatic β-cells and is associated with vascular complications including neuropathy, retinopathy, and nephropathy [34]. Herbal medicines have long been used for the treatment of diabetes mellitus and have fewer side-effects of toxicity than other hypoglycemic drugs. In the present study, administration of the ethanolic extract of *P. angustifolia* significantly reduced blood glucose levels in normoglycemic and diabetic rats. This promising effect may be attributed to the inhibition of aldose reductase which converts glucose to sorbitol and α-amylase and α-glucosidase (key enzymes linked to type-2 diabetes) by the phenols and flavonoids [35, 36].

Because of its basic chemical structure, quercetin is a antioxidant activity and it is now used as a nutritional supplement for a variety of diseases such as diabetes/obesity and circulatory dysfunction, including inflammation as well as mood disorders [37].

## Conclusion

The crude ethanolic extract of *P. angustifolia* exhibited promising anti-inflammatory, anti-ulcerogenic, and hypoglycemic activities, which are in accordance with

**Table 4** Hypoglycemic activity of *P. angustifolia* L. extract in alloxan-diabetic rats (*n* = 10)

| Group | Blood glucose in alloxan-diabetes rats (mg/dl) | |
| --- | --- | --- |
| | Fasting | 2 h after treatment |
| Control (Diabetic) | 230.66 ± 2.53 | 211.16 ± 3.88 |
| *P. angustifolia* L. extract (500 mg/kg) | 227.50 ± 2.46 | 124.33 ± 4.85** |
| Standard glibenclamide (0.5 mg/kg) | 231.66 ± 2.30 | 95.5 ± 3.74** |

**P < 0.01 as compared to control diabetic

**Table 5** Hypoglycemic activity of *P. angustifolia* L. extract in non-diabetic rats (*n* = 10)

| Group | Blood glucose-in normal rats (mg/dl) | |
| --- | --- | --- |
| | Fasting | 2 h after treatment |
| Control (non-diabetic) | 77.25 ± 0.60 | 73.50 ± 0.85 |
| *P. angustifolia* L. extract (500 mg/kg) | 78.95 ± 0.40 | 67.22 ± 1.20* |
| Standard glibenclamide (0.5 mg/kg) | 76.76 ± 0.30 | 62.85 ± 0.75** |

*P < 0.05 **P < 0.01 as compared to control non-diabetic

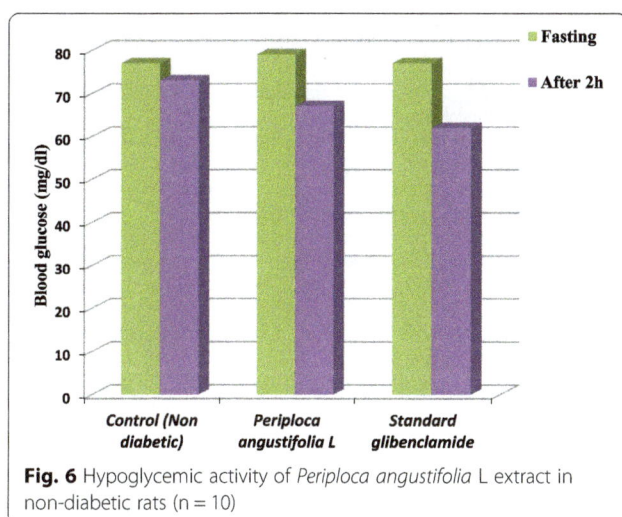

**Fig. 6** Hypoglycemic activity of *Periploca angustifolia* L extract in non-diabetic rats (n = 10)

its use folk medicine. As the extract showed a high, safety profile this study may serve as a guideline for the standardization and validation of natural drugs containing selected medicinal plants ingredients. Moreover, further investigation for the selective activities is required to determine the exact mechanism of action.

### Abbreviations

ABTS: 2, 2'-azino-bis (3-ethylbenzothiazoline-6-sulphonic acid; DPPH: 2,2-diphenyl-1-picrylhydrazyl radical; GAE: Gallic acid equivalent; HPLC: High Performance Liquid Chromatography; LD50: Lethal dose 50; *P. angustifolia*: *Periploca angustifolia*; ROS: Reactive oxygen species

### Acknowledgements

Not applicable.

### About the authors

The corresponding author.
Prof. Khaled Abo-EL-Sooud.
Professor of Pharmacology, Faculty of Veterinary Medicine, Cairo University from 2005 till now. Ph.D. Canadian-Egyptian Scholarship, Cairo University, 1995 at centre for food and animal research, Agriculture Canada, Ottawa, Canada. Teaching Undergraduate and graduate Courses in University of Science and Technology, Irbid, Jordan (2000–2002) and in Qassim University, Buraidah, Saudi Arabia (2005–2007). Supervising and discussing several Master and Ph.D. theses in Egypt and Arabian Countries. Expertise in Radioisotopes and different types of Chromatography (GC-HPLC-TLC etc.) for detection of drug residues in tissues and food. Publishing about 70 papers in different international journals enclosed list of publications. Member of the promotion committee of Supreme Council committee 100 B for Veterinary Pharmacology, Toxicology and Forensic Medicine from 2013 to 2019. Nowadays the research is shifted to ethnopharmacology. Attained a lot of international conferences and obtained several awards and prizes. Member of veterinary drug administration's committee, ministry of Health, Egypt. ASSOCIATE EDITOR.
International Journal of Veterinary Science and Medicine.
GUEST EDITORS IN.
Oxidative Medicine and Cellular Longevity.
https://mts.hindawi.com/guest.editor/journals/omcl/adct/
Evidence-based Complementary and Alternative Medicine.
https://mts.hindawi.com/guest.editor
http://scholar.cu.edu.eg/kasooud
http://scholar.google.com/citations?user=Ww4Vqd8AAAAJ
https://www.scopus.com/authid/detail.uri?authorId=6603356090
http://orcid.org/0000-0001-7636-7018

### Funding

Desert Research Center, Medicinal and Aromatic Plants Department, Cairo, Egypt Supporting Ph.D. Study of Dr. Hanan M. ELTantawy.

### Authors' contributions

KA-E Sooud performed the pharmacological evaluation on animal studies and data collection. Other authors performed the phytochemical analysis. All authors read and approved the final manuscript.

### Competing interests

The authors declare that they have no competing interests.

### Author details

[1]Pharmacology Department, Faculty of Veterinary Medicine, Cairo University, Giza 12211, Egypt. [2]Medicinal and Aromatic Plants Department, Desert Research Center, Cairo, Egypt. [3]Chemistry of Tannins Department, National Research Center, Dokki, Giza, Egypt.

### References

1. Rabei S, Khalik KA. Conventional keys for Convolvulaceae in the flora of Egypt. Flora Mediterr. 2012;22:45–62.
2. Hammiche V, Maiza K. Traditional medicine in Central Sahara: pharmacopoeia of Tassili N'ajjer. J Ethnopharmacol. 2006;105:358–67.
3. Bouhouche N. Conservation and multiplication of an endangered medicinal plant – Caralluma arabica – using tissue culture. Planta Med [Internet]. 2011; 77:PB49. Available from: https://www.thieme-connect.com/products/ejournals/abstract/10.1055/s-0031-1282303
4. Laupattarakasem P, Wangsrimongkol T, Surarit R, Hahnvajanawong C. In vitro and in vivo anti-inflammatory potential of Cryptolepis buchanani. J Ethnopharmacol. 2006;108:349–54.
5. Pandya D, Anand I. A complete review on Oxystelma esculentum R. Br. Pharmacogn J. 2011;3:87–90.
6. Athmouni K, Belhaj D, Mkadmini Hammi K, El Feki A, Ayadi H. Phenolic compounds analysis, antioxidant, and hepatoprotective effects of Periploca angustifolia extract on cadmium-induced oxidative damage in HepG2 cell line and rats. Arch Physiol Biochem. 2017:1–14.
7. Ibrahim A, E O, A. J N, IA U. Combined effect on antioxidant properties of Gymnema Sylvestre and Combretum Micranthum leaf extracts and the relationship to hypoglycemia. Eur Sci J. 2017;13:266–81.
8. Al-Rejaie SS, Abuohashish HM, Ahmed MM, Aleisa AM, Alkhamees O. Possible biochemical effects following inhibition of ethanol-induced gastric mucosa damage by Gymnema sylvestre in male Wistar albino rats. Pharm Biol. 2012;50:1542–50.
9. Bouaziz M, Dhouib A, Loukil S. Polyphenols content, antioxidant and antimicrobial activities of extracts of some wild plants collected from the south of Tunisia. African J. Biotechnol. [Internet]. 2009;8:7017–7027. Available from: http://www.ajol.info/index.php/ajb/article/view/68789
10. Anoop A, Jegadeesan M. Biochemical studies on the anti-ulcerogenic potential of Hemidesmus indicus r.Br. Var. indicus. J Ethnopharmacol. 2003; 84:149–56.
11. Galhena P, Thabrew I, Tammitiyagodage M, Hanna RV. Anti-hepatocarcinogenic Ayurvedic herbal remedy reduces the extent of diethylnitrosamine-induced oxidative stress in rats. Pharmacogn Mag. 2009; 5:19–27.
12. Fairouz D, Sami Z, Mekki B, Mohamed N. Chemical composition of root bark of Periploca angustifolia growing wild in Saharian Tunisia. J Essent Oil-Bearing Plants. 2013;16:338–45.
13. Djeridane A, Yousfi M, Nadjemi B, Boutassouna D, Stocker P, Vidal N. Antioxidant activity of some algerian medicinal plants extracts containing phenolic compounds. Food Chem. 2006;97:654–60.
14. Li C, Feng J, Huang WY, An XT. Composition of polyphenols and antioxidant activity of rabbiteye blueberry (Vaccinium ashei) in Nanjing. J Agric Food Chem. 2013;61:523–31.

15. Ma Y, Kosinska-Cagnazzo A, Kerr WL, Amarowicz R, Swanson RB, Pegg RB. Separation and characterization of phenolic compounds from dry-blanched peanut skins by liquid chromatography-electrospray ionization mass spectrometry. J Chromatogr A. 2014;1356:64–81.

16. Lorke D. A new approach to practical acute toxicity testing. Arch Toxicol. 1983;54:275–87.

17. Dhanarasu S, Selvam M, Al-Shammari NKA. Evaluating the pharmacological dose (Oral ld50) and antibacterial activity of leaf extracts of Mentha piperita Linn. Grown in Kingdom of Saudi Arabia: a pilot study for nephrotoxicity. Int J Pharmacol. 2016;12:195–200.

18. Nalini GK, Patil VM, Ramabhimaiah S, Patil P, Vijayanath V. Anti-inflammatory activity of wheatgrass juice in albino rats. Biomed Pharmacol J. 2011;4:301–4.

19. Hironaka A, Susumu O, Yoshihiko I, Masahiro O, Kazuei I, Seiyu H. Polyamine inhibition of gastric ulceration and secretion in rats. Biochem Pharmacol. 1983;32:1733–6.

20. Nordin N, Salama SM, Golbabapour S, Hajrezaie M, Hassandarvish P, Kamalidehghan B, et al. Anti-ulcerogenic effect of methanolic extracts from Enicosanthellum pulchrum (king) HEUSDEN against ethanol-induced acute gastric lesion in animal models. PLoS One. 2014;9:e111925.

21. Chen S-H, Liang Y-C, Chao JCJ, Tsai L-H, Chang C-C, Wang C-C, et al. Protective effects of Ginkgo biloba extract on the ethanol-induced gastric ulcer in rats. World J Gastroenterol [Internet]. 2005;11:3746–3750. Available from: http://www.ncbi.nlm.nih.gov/pubmed/15968732

22. Tang LQ, Wei W, Chen LM, Liu S. Effects of berberine on diabetes induced by alloxan and a high-fat/high-cholesterol diet in rats. J Ethnopharmacol. 2006;108:109–15.

23. Sunil J, Krishna J, Bramhachari P. Hepatoprotective activity of Holostemma ada Kodien shcult, extract against paracetamol induced hepatic damage in rats. European J Med Plants [Internet]. 2015;6:45–54. Available from: http://www.sciencedomain.org/abstract.php?iid=793&id=13&aid=7471.

24. Abushouk AI, Ismail A, AMA S, Afifi AM, Abdel-Daim MM. Cardioprotective mechanisms of phytochemicals against doxorubicin-induced cardiotoxicity. Biomed Pharmacother. 2017;90:935–46.

25. Ganguly S, Kumar TG, Mantha S, Panda K. Simultaneous determination of black tea-derived catechins and theaflavins in tissues of tea consuming animals using ultra-performance liquid-chromatography tandem mass spectrometry. PLoS One. 2016;11:e0163498.

26. Oh J, Lee YD, Wagers AJ. Stem cell aging: mechanisms, regulators and therapeutic opportunities. Nat Med. 2014;20:870–80.

27. Morris G, Maes M. Oxidative and Nitrosative stress and immune-inflammatory pathways in patients with Myalgic encephalomyelitis (ME)/chronic fatigue syndrome (CFS). Curr Neuropharmacol [Internet]. 2014;12:168–85 Available from: http://www.eurekaselect.com/openurl/content.php?genre=article&issn=1570-159X&volume=12&issue=2&spage=168.

28. Youn J-Y, Siu KL, Lob H, Itani H, Harrison DG, Cai H. Role of vascular oxidative stress in obesity and metabolic syndrome. Diabetes [Internet]. 2014;63:2344–2355. Available from: http://www.ncbi.nlm.nih.gov/pubmed/24550188

29. Bu J, Dou Y, Tian X, Wang Z, Chen G. The role of Omega-3 polyunsaturated fatty acids in stroke. Oxidative Med Cell Logevity. 2016;2016:1–8.

30. Nguyen PH, Zhao BT, Kim O, Lee JH, Choi JS, Min BS, et al. Anti-inflammatory terpenylated coumarins from the leaves of Zanthoxylum schinifolium with α-glucosidase inhibitory activity. J Nat Med. 2016;70:276–81.

31. Antunes-Ricardo M, Gutiérrez-Uribe JA, López-Pacheco F, Alvarez MM, Serna-Saldívar SO. In vivo anti-inflammatory effects of isorhamnetin glycosides isolated from Opuntia ficus-indica (L.) mill cladodes. Ind Crop Prod. 2015;76:803–8.

32. Wang L, Wang B, Li H, Lu H, Qiu F, Xiong L, et al. Quercetin, a flavonoid with anti-inflammatory activity, suppresses the development of abdominal aortic aneurysms in mice. Eur J Pharmacol. 2012;690:133–41.

33. De La Lastra CA, Martín MJ, Motilva V. Antiulcer and gastroprotective effects of quercetin: a gross and histologic study. Pharmacology. 1994;48:56–62.

34. Su S-L, Liao P-Y, Tu S-T, Lin K-C, Tsai D-H, Sia H-K, et al. Correlation analysis of HbAlc and preprandial plasma glucose in diabetes complications. Diabetes [Internet]. 2009:58 Available from: http://www.embase.com/search/results?subaction=viewrecord&from=export&id=L70135710%5Cnhttp://professional.diabetes.org/Abstracts-Display.aspx?TYP=1&CID=73906%5Cnhttp://sfx.library.uu.nl/utrecht?sid=EMBASE&issn=00121797&id=doi:&atitle=Correlation+analysis+.

35. Lee YS, Lee S, Lee HS, Kim BK, Ohuchi K, Shin KH. Inhibitory effects of isorhamnetin-3-O-beta-D-glucoside from Salicornia herbacea on rat lens aldose reductase and sorbitol accumulation in streptozotocin-induced diabetic rat tissues. Biol Pharm Bull. 2005;28:916–8.

36. Adedayo BC, Ademiluyi AO, Oboh G, Akindahunsi AA. Interaction of aqueous extracts of two varieties of yam tubers (Dioscorea spp) on some key enzymes linked to type 2 diabetes in vitro. Int J Food Sci Technol. 2012;47:703–9.

37. D'Andrea G. Quercetin: a flavonol with multifaceted therapeutic applications? Fitoterapia. 2015;106:256–71.

# 23

# Neuropharmacological and antibacterial effects of the ethyl acetate extract of *Diospyros malabarica* (Ebenaceae) seeds

Tusnova Sharmin[1], Razia Sultana[2], Farzana Hossain[3], Shahriar Kabir Shakil[2], Foysal Hossen[4] and Md. Mamun Or Rashid[1]* (iD)

## Abstract

**Background:** *Diospyros malabarica* is a well known flowering plant indigenous to Indian subcontinent which is used in folklore medicine for several purposes. Our study is designed to assess the neuropharmacological and antibacterial efficacy of the ethyl acetate extract of *D. malabarica* seeds.

**Methods:** The behavioral anxiolytic activities of the extract were assessed by using open field (OFT), hole cross (HCT), elevated plus maze (EPZ), hole board (HBT), light dark test (LDT); and antidepressant activities through forced swimming (FST) and tail suspension test (TST). Antimicrobial potential was assessed through disc diffusion method.

**Results:** In OFT and HCT, the extract treated groups significantly (*$p < 0.05$) decrease the movement of animals when compared to vehicle-treated group. Higher dose (400 mg/kg b.w.) of extract greatly increased the spending time in open arm of EPZ, which endorses anxiolytic-like behavior of extract. The observed effect may be due to binding of any phytoconstituent with $GABA_A$ receptor. HBT and LDT results support the exploratory behavior of mice. The extract significantly decreased the immobility time in FST (20.71% for 200 mg/kg, and 31.59% for 400 mg/kg extract) and TST, which indicates the occupancy of antidepressant-active constituents. Gram negative bacteria were susceptible to extract than Gram positive strains; however the antimicrobial effect is not significant, hence trivial to declare.

**Conclusion:** Our study demonstrates the possession of significant anxiolytic and antidepressant effects of *D. malabarica* extract which could be helpful for drug development program. Before potential therapeutic use, finding of the exact phytoconstituents with their mechanisms, and clinical trial are recommended.

**Keywords:** Anxiolytic, Antidepressant, Antibacterial, *D. malabarica*

## Background

Although there is a great advancement of medical science, plants are still considered as important contributors of health care [1]. According to the assessment report of World Health Organization, approximately 80% of the people in the world (especially people of countryside areas) are still dependent on plant based medicine [2]. Last couples of decades, many phytopharmacological compounds have been isolated from the plants; from which a significant number are used as potent therapeutic agents [3].

*Diospyros malabarica* is a medium size, long lived flowering tree belonging to the family of Ebenaceae, which is indigenous to indian subcontinent [4]. Various phytoconstituents are found from the individual parts of this plant- leaves contain triterpenes, betulin, β-sitosterol, oleanolic acid, myricyl alcohol; barks contain tannins, myricyl alcohol, triterpenes, betulinic acid, and saponin; fruits store alkanes, triterpenes, β-sitosterol, tannins, glucoside, betulin, betulinic acid, gallic acid, hexacosane, hexacosanol; and finally seeds possess 32% fatty oil, β-amyrin and betulinic acid etc. [5, 6]. The plant parts are used in folklore medicine

* Correspondence: mamun_nstu@yahoo.com; mamun.orrashid@nstu.edu.bd
[1]Department of Pharmacy, Noakhali Science and Technology University, Sonapur, Noakhali 3814, Bangladesh
Full list of author information is available at the end of the article

as astringent, anti-inflammatory, anti-fertility, hepato-protective, antioxidant, and hypoglycemic agents [7, 8]. In addition, it is used for the treatment of dysentery, fever, and menstrual problems [9].

Although having several uses of *D. malabarica*, it was found through the literature review that there is no claim of research on neuropharmacological effects of the seed of this plant. Similar claim is also true for anti-microbial effectiveness test. The aim of our present study was to assess the neuropharmacological and anti-bacterial activities of the ethyl acetate extract of *D. malabarica* seeds.

## Methods
### Drugs and reagents
Diazepam, ciprofloxacin, imipramine were obtained from Sigma-Aldrich Corporation (USA). Ethyl acetate (Merck, Germany), and other chemicals necessary for experiment were analytical graded which were taken from the labora-tory of Dept. of Pharmacy, NSTU, Bangladesh.

### Plant parts
Fruits of *D. malabarica* were collected from Bahaddar hat, Chittagong, Bangladesh on november, 2016. After col-lection, fruits were washed thoroughly, and later authenti-cated by Naimur Rahman (Taxonomist, Bangladesh National Harberium, Dhaka, Bangladesh); and the speci-men was kept there for future correspondence.

### Preparation of *D. malabarica* extract
The seeds of *D. malabarica* after peeling the fruits were collected. Seeds were allowed to air-dry for 15 days period with shaded condition, which was followed by grinding into course powder. Crude powder materials were macerated into 2000 ml ethyl acetate (> 99% pure) for 18 days at room temperature in a sterilized beaker which was wrapped by aluminum foil to avoid direct ex-posure of sunlight (cold extraction). After the incubation period, solution was filtered through filter cloth and later by Whatman filter paper. Filtrate was allowed to evapor-ate by the rotary vacuum evaporator under the reduced pressure to get concentrated semi-solid filtrate. After few days of drying in room temperature, we found the brownie granular sticky substance which was designated as crude ethyl acetate extract of *D. malabarica* [10].

### Experimental animals
Swiss albino mice (25 ± 5 g) were procured from the ani-mal house of Jahangirnagar University, Bangladesh. These were kept in metal cages (condition: 20 ± 5 °C and light/dark cycle for 12 h), and provided to feed on ro-dent foods and water ad-libitum from seven days before the commencement to finish the experiment.

### Test microorganisms
We have used *Staphylococcus aureus* ATCC 25923, *Sal-monella typhi* ATCC 14028, *Escherichia coli* ATCC 25922 and *Pseudomonas aeruginosa* ATCC 27853 for studying antibacterial activities; these strains were col-lected from the laboratory of the Department of Micro-biology, Noakhali Science and Technology University (NSTU), Bangladesh.

### Behavioral studies of anxiolytic activities
#### Open field test (OFT)
The OFT apparatus was built using white plywood (72 cm × 72 cm × 36 cm). Mice can be seen from the outside wall (made by glass) of the apparatus. 16 squares were drawn on the floor for observing the movement of mice [11]. Mice were divided into four groups (each group consists of 5 mice): control (distilled water: 0.1 ml/mice, oral), standard (diazepam: 1 mg/kg b.w. of mice, i.p.), *D. malabarica* (200 mg/kg b.w. of mice, oral), and *D. malabarica* (400 mg/kg b.w. of mice, oral). After administration of the respective doses, every mouse was observed for 3 min periods at the time of (0, 30, 60, 90, and 120 min) to count the number of squares crossed. After finishing a trail, the OFT apparatus was wiped by (10%) ethanol for cleaning.

#### Hole cross test (HCT)
We have followed the process described by Hossain et al. for HCT [12]. A wood partition was set in center of the cage (30 cm × 20 cm × 14 cm). There was a hole (D-3 cm) at 7.5 cm above from the ground in center of every partition. Animals were divided into four groups (each group consists of 5 mice): control (distilled water: 0.1 ml/mice, oral), standard (diazepam: 1 mg/kg b.w. of mice, i.p.), *D. malabarica* (200 mg/kg b.w. of mice, oral), and *D. malabarica* (400 mg/kg b.w. of mice, oral). Num-ber of transit of mice among the chambers through the hole was recorded for 3 min spell at 0, 30, 60, 90 and 120 min after administering the samples and drug.

#### Elevated plus-maze (EPM) test
EPM test is a widely accepting and authentic research study for finding the new drug with potential anxiolytic effects. The details methodology of this study was de-scribed in our previous paper, Rashid et al. [13]. The ap-paratus consists of two open arms (35 cm × 5 cm × 35 cm) crossed by two closed arms of similar size which are interconnected by a central square of (5 cm × 5 cm). The experimental room was dimly illuminated, and EPM apparatus was kept on approx. 40 cm higher from the ground level. Experimental mice were grouped (each group consists of 5 mice) as control (distilled water: 0.1 ml/mice, oral), standard (diazepam: 1 mg/kg b.w. of mice, i.p.), *D. malabarica* (200 mg/kg b.w. of mice, oral),

and *D. malabarica* (400 mg/kg b.w. of mice, oral). 1 h after treatment, animal was taken individually on the apparatus, and the number of entries in every arm was registered for 5 min spells. After finishing each session, EPM apparatus was cleaned by ethanol (70%) and allow drying for few minutes.

### Hole board test (HBT)
In HBT, head-dipping is generally considered as a measure of exploitation which is somehow distinct from the motor activity. An increase count of head dips compared to control is considered as anxiolytic-like effect. HBT was performed in a box ($40 \times 40 \times 25$ cm) made by wood with 16 equidistant holes (D- 3 cm) was used in this experiment. Apparatus was kept at 35 cm above from the ground [14]. Mice were selected and grouped into 4 groups randomly (each group consists of 5 mice) and administered different samples accordingly. Mouse was kept on board, and its movement and head dipping in the hole was counted for 5 min duration. A single head-dip was counted when a mouse put into the hole at least up to the eye level; repeated dips into same hole were not consider as countable head dips if they can't be separated by locomotion.

### Light--dark transition (LDT) test
LDT test is used for assessing anxiety-like behavior of animal. Natural aversion to bright illumination and exploration in mild stressors of the mice are the basis of this test. We have followed the process described by Hascoet and Bourin for this study [15]. LDT test apparatus consists of a box ($42$ cm $\times 21$ cm $\times 25$ cm), in where there are separated dark chamber and brightly illuminated chamber. Mice were taken in light compartment and allowed to move freely through a ($3$ cm $\times 4$ cm) opening. Animal were select randomly and provide the respective dosages accordingly. Then, the residual time in each chamber for every mouse were recorded.

### Antidepressant activity test

**Forced swimming test (FST)** FCT is another common rodent behavioral model for the exploration of new antidepressant compounds. We have followed the FST method described by Con et al. with minor modification [11, 16]. Cylindrical tanks ($30$ cm $\times 20$ cm) made of glass were used in where water level was kept almost 15 cm from the bottom of tank. We had recorded the immobile time of each mouse (time to keep the head above the water) for 360 s (6 min). The last 240 s data from this recorded period were considered for analysis. Data was taken for each mouse of every group after treating with respective dosages. We used a stopwatch (can measure milliseconds) for counting time.

**Tail suspension test (TST)** TST (a well-known behavioral test of mice) method was adopted from Steru et al. [17]. TST box is made of plastic (Dimension: 55 cm × 60 cm × 11.5 cm). Mouse was suspended from middle of the compartment, so that it can't attach with any wall. Mice were selected and grouped into 4 groups randomly (each group consists of 5 mice) and administered different samples accordingly. Mouse was hung by its tail which was attached on a string (75 cm above the surface) by the help of adhesive tape. Immobile time was counted when mouse hung motionlessly. Observation was done for 6 min period; and the immobile time during this period was recorded.

### Antimicrobial activity test
Antibacterial efficacy of the ethyl acetate extract of *D. malabarica* seeds were assessed through (Kirby-Bauer's disc diffusion method) by following Rashid et al. [18]. Samples were prepared by dissolving them in relevant solvents. Sterilized paper discs (D- 6 mm) of the samples were impregnated into the swab plates (Muller-Hinton agar media) containing microorganisms [$2 \times 10^6$ colony forming units (CFU/mL)]. Aliquot of 50 μL crude extract (concentration: 500 mg/mL) was added in each disc. These plates were stand at 4 °C for 2 h which was followed by incubation at 37 °C for 24 h. Zone of inhibition (in millimeter) on the plates were measured for assessing the antibacterial efficacy of crude extract. Ciprofloxacin (5 μg/disc) and blank (solvents) discs served as positive and negative control respectively.

### Statistical analysis
Data found in the experiment was analyzed statistically using one-way ANOVA followed by Dunnet's t-test. $^*p \leq 0.05$ was considered significant, whereas $^{**}p \leq 0.001$ was highly significant value. Origin Pro (ver. 8.5, Origin Lab. Corp., USA) was used for preparing graphical pre sentations.

## Results
### Open field test
In the OFT, *D. malabarica* extract in both doses significantly ($^*p < 0.05$) reduce the movement of mice when compared with control. Diazepam (1 mg/kg i.p.) also decreased the movement significantly. We found that suppression increases as time goes (Fig. 1). Maximum suppression was found at 120 min after the administration of dosages.

### Hole cross test
The depressant activities of the ethyl acetate extract of *D. malabarica* seeds according to HCT method were shown in Fig. 2. It was found that movements of the mice treated by plant extract (200 mg and 400 mg/kg

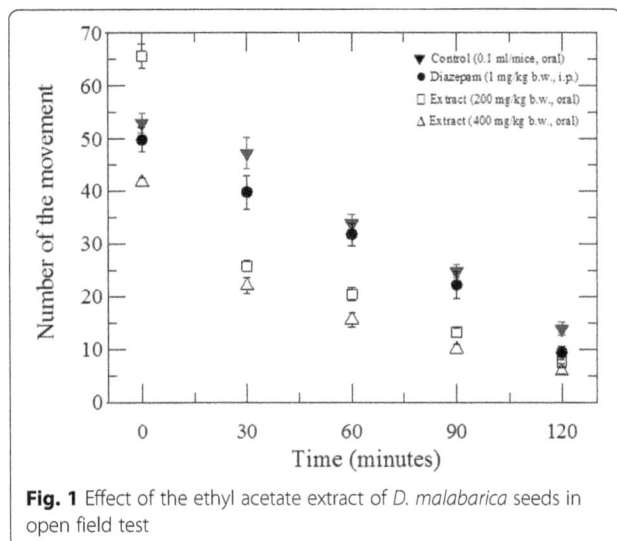

**Fig. 1** Effect of the ethyl acetate extract of *D. malabarica* seeds in open field test

**Table 1** Effect of the ethyl acetate extract of *D. malabarica* seeds on EPM test

| Group | Dose | Time spent by mice in open arms (sec) | Entries of mice in open arms |
|---|---|---|---|
| Distilled water (control) | 0.1 ml/mice (oral) | 93.87 ± 3.73 | 7.34 ± 1.15 |
| Diazepam (standard) | 1 mg/kg b.w. of mice (i.p.) | 120.15 ± 2.42** | 10.55 ± 0.44* |
| *D. malabarica* extract | 200 mg/kg b.w. of mice (oral) | 78.65 ± 2.13 | 6.14 ± 0.93* |
| *D. malabarica* extract | 400 mg/kg b.w. of mice (oral) | 111.24 ± 3.54** | 9.89 ± 1.62** |

Mean ± SEM ($n = 5$); One way ANOVA followed by Dunnet's t-test were performed. *$p < 0.05$, **$p < 0.01$ as compared with control

1.73) for 200 mg/kg b.w., and (4.48 ± 1.02) for 400 mg/kg b.w of mice orally (significant) respectively; whereas this value was (5.53 ± 0.68) for standard (diazepam) (Fig. 3).

### Light –dark transition test

*D. malabarica* extract (at both doses), and diazepam (standard) induced a significant (*$p < 0.05$) increment of spending time and number of transits in illumination side of LDT. Details results were shown in Table 2.

### Tail suspension test

Administration of different dosages of ethyl acetate extract of *D. malabarica* seeds significantly (*$p < 0.05$) and dose dependently decrease the immobility time, which were comparable with imipramine (standard) (Fig. 4). The reductions of immobility time were 20.71%, and 31.59% for 200 and 400 mg/kg dosages (plant extract) respectively which are comparable with the reduction of standard (40%).

### Forced swimming test

Table 3 shows the effect of *D. malabarica* on the immobility time of mice in FST. We found the dose dependent responses of our tested crude extract which were significant

b.w. of mice, oral) decreased significantly from 2nd observation (30 min) to 5th observation (120 min) which is comparable with the reference drug diazepam (1 mg/kg b.w., i.p.) (Fig. 2).

### Elevated plus maze

The outcomes of the EPM test were shown in Table 1. It was found that diazepam (1 mg/kg b.w of mice, i.p.) significantly increased the spending times and entries in open arms when compared to control. Our tested crude extract at higher dosage (400 mg/kg b.w. of mice, oral) significantly (*$p < 0.05$) increased the spending time and entries of mice in open arms of EPM apparatus.

### Hole board test

Ethyl acetate extract of *D. malabarica* seeds decreased the number of head dipping when compared with control. The number of head dipping is (12.17 ±

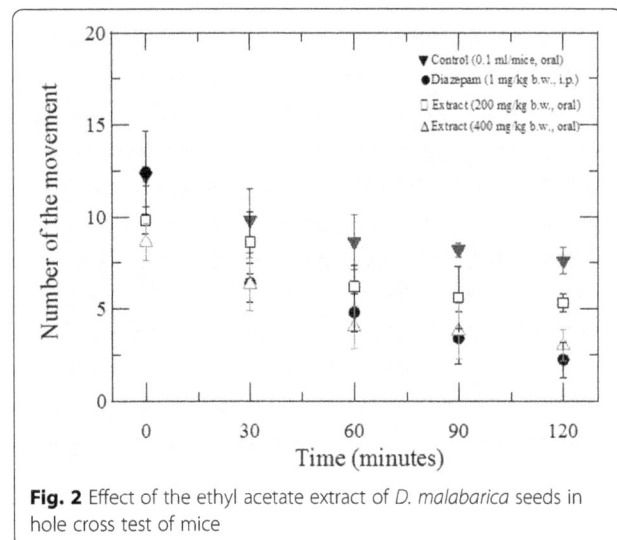

**Fig. 2** Effect of the ethyl acetate extract of *D. malabarica* seeds in hole cross test of mice

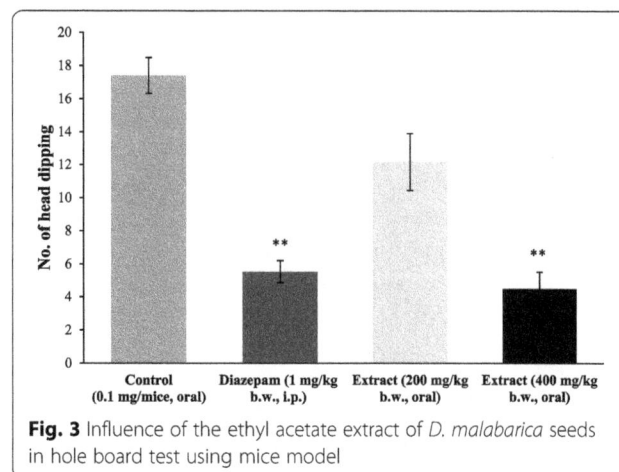

**Fig. 3** Influence of the ethyl acetate extract of *D. malabarica* seeds in hole board test using mice model

**Table 2** Effect of *D. malabarica* extract in LDT test

| Group | Dose | Time (sec) spent by mice in light box | No. of transitions of mice |
|---|---|---|---|
| Distilled water (control) | 0.1 ml/mice (oral) | 74.40 ± 3.36 | 10.24 ± 1.73 |
| Diazepam (standard) | 1 mg/kg b.w. of mice (i.p.) | 178.80 ± 6.56* | 9.73 ± 2.45* |
| *D. malabarica* extract | 200 mg/kg b.w. of mice (oral) | 119.56 ± 5.57 | 14.44 ± 2.36 |
| *D. malabarica* extract | 400 mg/kg b.w. of mice (oral) | 149.75 ± 4.14** | 17.31 ± 2.94* |

Mean ± SEM (*n* = 5); One way ANOVA followed by Dunnet's t-test were performed. *p < 0.05, **p < 0.01 as compared with control

**Table 3** Effect of the ethyl acetate extract of *D. malabarica* seeds on FST in mice

| Group | Dose | Immobility time(sec) |
|---|---|---|
| Distilled water (control) | 0.1 ml/mice (oral) | 168.60 ± 6.06 |
| Diazepam (standard) | 1 mg/kg b.w. of mice (i.p.) | 30.44 ± 2.54* |
| *D. malabarica* extract | 200 mg/kg b.w. of mice (oral) | 57.55 ± 2.73** |
| *D. malabarica* extract | 400 mg/kg b.w. of mice (oral) | 47.12 ± 2.42* |

Mean ± SEM (*n* = 5); One way ANOVA followed by Dunnet's t-test were performed. *p < 0.05, **p < 0.01 as compared with control

when compared with control. Almost (30.44 ± 1.58), and (57.55 ± 2.73) sec immobility time were found for the crude extract of *D. malabarica* (200 mg/kg, oral), and (400 mg/kg, oral) b.w. of the mice respectively; whereas immobile time was (30.44 ± 1.58) for the standard drug (diazepam).

## Antimicrobial activity of crude extract

In-vitro antibacterial efficacy test were performed for the ethyl acetate extract of *D. malabarica* seeds. Overall results (zone of inhibition produced) were summarized in (Table 4), (Fig. 5). We have followed disc diffusion method (conc. 0.1 ml/disc) for studying the antibacterial activities of our tested extract using both Gram positive and Gram negative bacterial strains. Maximum zone of inhibition (12.2 ± 0.8 mm) and (8.9 ± 0.3 mm) were found for the extract when treated against the strains of *E. coli* and *K. pneumonia* respectively. Despite that, zone of inhibition was not noticeable for *P. aeruginosa*. Moreover, we didn't find the antibacterial efficacy for Gram positive bacterial species (*S. aureus*). The zones of inhibitions of the samples were compared with that of ciprofloxacin (Additional file 1).

## Discussion

Our study represents the first step to understand the effects of *D. malabarica* seed extract on CNS using mice model. We found that *D. malabarica* extract possesses significant anxiolytic, antidepressant, and explorative behavioral activities. In OFT and HCT, the extract treated groups significantly (*p < 0.05) decrease the movement of animals when compared with vehicle treated group. Highest decrease was seen after 120 min of administrating the dosages; and this reduction was gradual and somehow follow dose dependent manner. According to the Mechan et al., OFT is a reliable method to assess the anxiety-like behavior characterized through the detestation of mice to bright lit open area. Anxiolytic agents can reduce such fearful attitude of mice in OFT [19, 20]. Similarly reduction of the hole cross number was seen in HCT, where *D. malabarica* extract (both doses) decreased the spontaneous motor activities. As a result, it can be said that our tested extract possess significant anxiolytic-like effect. On the other hand, in EPZ experiment, the natural antipathy of mice to the open arm of EPZ apparatus indicates the anxiolytic-like effect of the compounds. We found that higher dose (400 mg/kg b.w, oral.) of *D. malabarica* extract significantly increased the spending time in open arm of EPZ, which support the anxiolytic-like effect of the extract. Phytochemical

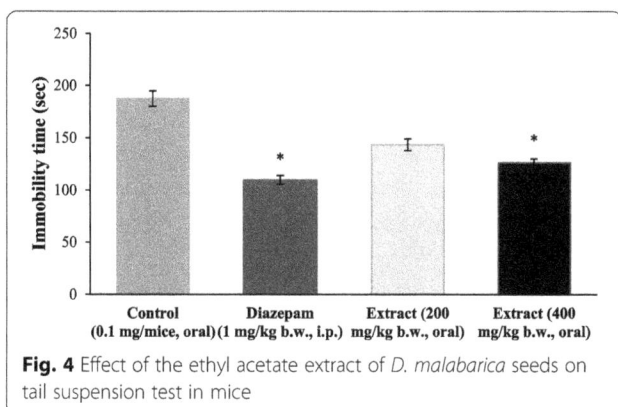

**Fig. 4** Effect of the ethyl acetate extract of *D. malabarica* seeds on tail suspension test in mice

**Table 4** Zone of inhibition of the ethyl acetate extract of *D. malabarica* seeds

| Zone of inhibition (mm) | | |
|---|---|---|
| Test organisms | *D. malabarica* seed extract (500 mg/mL) | Ciprofloxacin (standard) (5 μg/disc) |
| Gram positive bacteria | | |
|   *S. aureus* | 0 | 23.2 ± 1.8 |
| Gram negative bacteria | | |
|   *E. coli* | 12.2 ± 0.8 | 25.6 ± 0.5 |
|   *K. pneumonia* | 8.9 ± 0.3 | 25.6 ± 1.3 |
|   *P. aeruginosa* | 0 | 25.2 ± 0.4 |

Mean ± SEM (*n* = 5); One way ANOVA followed by Dunnet's t-test were performed. *p < 0.05, **p < 0.01 as compared with control

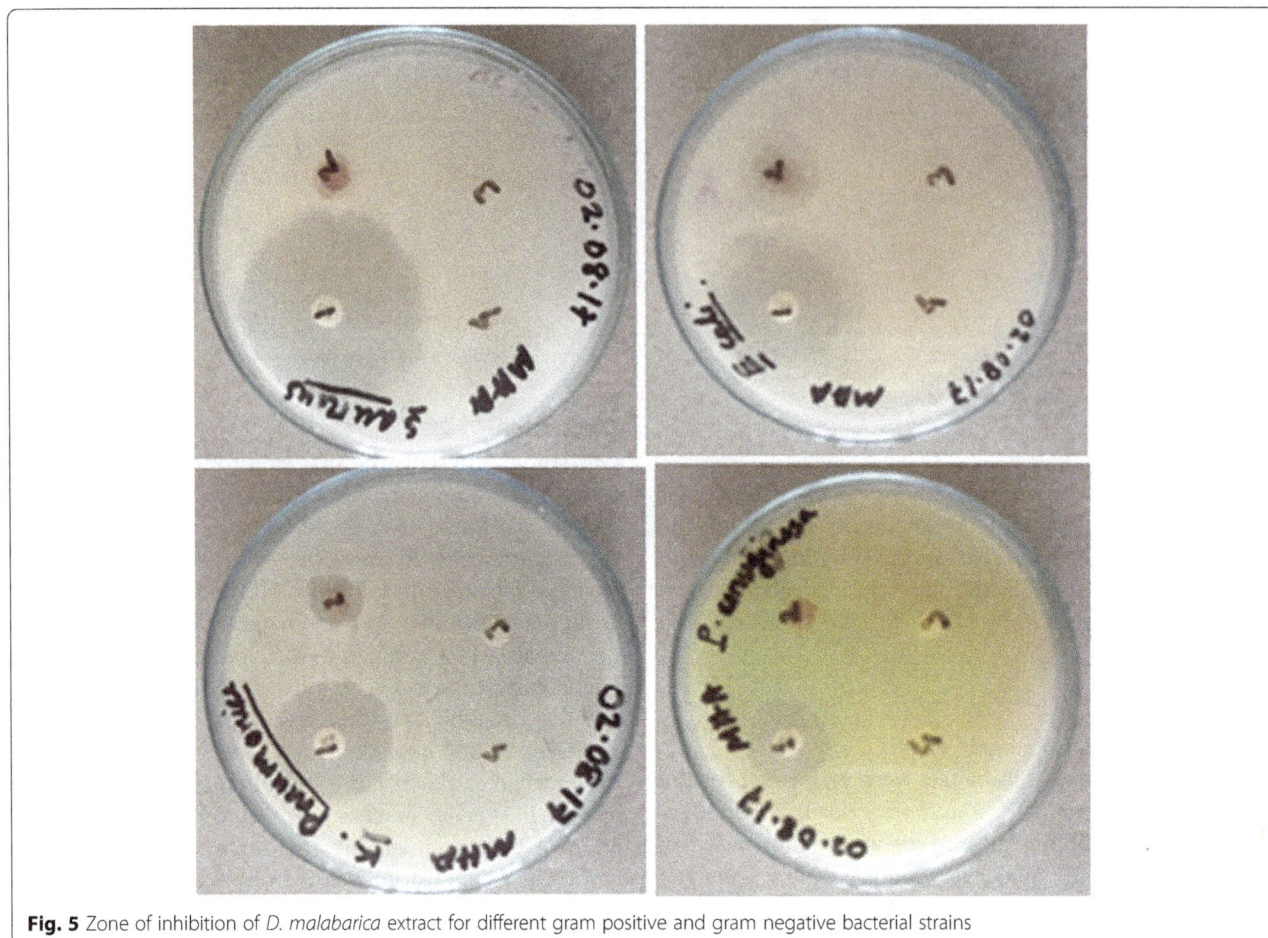

**Fig. 5** Zone of inhibition of *D. malabarica* extract for different gram positive and gram negative bacterial strains

investigation claimed that *D. malabarica* extract possesses flavonoids, alkaloids, phenolic acids, essential oil, saponins, tannins etc. Presence of these phytoconstituent may responsible for CNS effects [21]. The effect may be due to hyperpolarization of CNS through interacting with gamma-amino-butyric acid (GABA$_A$) receptor or benzodiazepine (BZD) receptor. GABA is the major inhibitory neurotransmitter of CNS, and most of the neurological drugs exert their anxiolytic effect by acting on GABA$_A$ receptor [22]. Therefore our hypothesis stand that anxiolytic activity of *D. malabarica* extract may be due to binding of any phytoconstituent with GABA$_A$ [21, 22].

The anxiolytic-like effect of *D. malabarica* extract was also assessed using LDT box. We found that the mice treated with this extract spent more time in lightened side rather than darker one, which clearly indicates the possibility of having anxiolytic efficacy (transition parameter being highly dependent on locomotor activity) of the plants extract [23]. The effect may be due to agonistic effect of extract on GABA/BZD receptor complex, or antagonize 5-HT1B receptor, or agonize 5-HT1A

receptor [20, 24]. In HBT, we found similar decreasing in exploratory behavior pattern of mice.

According to the Riaz et al., shortening of immobility period indicates antidepressant, and prolongation of this period symbolizes the CNS depression-like effect in FST and TST [25]. In both experiments, *D. malabarica* extract significantly decreased the immobility time which indicates the possession of antidepressant active constituents in extract. Approx. 20.71%, and 31.59% of the reductions of immobility time were found for 200 mg/kg and 400 mg/kg doses (crude extract), which were comparable to the reduction of imipramine (40%).

In-vitro antibacterial assay of *D. malabarica* extract has been studied. We found that ethyl acetate extract of this plant seeds possess slight antibacterial efficacy against Gram negative strains; however the effect is not significant. We didn't find any effect of extract on Gram positive strain. The differences of bacterial cell wall compositions may responsible for the variation of antibacterial effect. Perhaps, the antimicrobial effect was found due to the attachment of phytoconstituents (present in the extract) with cell proteins of bacteria, which was followed by the disruption of microbial protein synthesis [18, 22]. Our results partially support the finding of Taranath et al., although the observed antibacterial effect is not significant to declare according to our experimental result [26].

## Conclusion

In conclusion, based on our experimental data it can be said that mice treated with ethyl acetate extract of *D. malabarica* seeds offered significant antidepressant and anxiolytic activities. However, the antimicrobial effect of this extract is trivial to declare. For confirming the neurological effects and using as potential source of drug, further researches especially clinical trial is suggested of this plant part.

## Abbreviations

BZD: Benzodiazepine; *D. malabarica*: *Diospyros malabarica*; EPZ: Elevated plus maze; FST: Forced swimming test; GABA: Gamma amino butyric acid; HBT: Hole board test; HCT: Hole cross test; LDT: Light dark test; OFT: Open field test; TST: Tail suspension test

## Acknowledgements

Authors are grateful to the staffs (technical/non-technical) of the Dept. of Microbiology, and Dept. of Pharmacy, NSTU, Bangladesh for giving valuable support and lab facilities during research works. In addition, heartiest thanks to the authority of JU, Bangladesh for providing mice during this research.

## Funding

TS got fund from the institutional research budget (Noakhali Science and Technology University, Bangladesh) for conducting this research work as part of her graduation degree.

## Author's contributions

Study design and writing of the manuscript were done by MMOR. TS, and FH participated in all the experiments under the supervision of MMOR, except antibacterial efficacy test. RS, and SKS activity participated into the antibacterial test where FH guided them. RS, and SKS helped to improve the writing, and revised the manuscript in current version. All authors read and approved the final version of the manuscript.

## Competing interests

The authors declare that they have no competing interests.

## Author details

[1]Department of Pharmacy, Noakhali Science and Technology University, Sonapur, Noakhali 3814, Bangladesh. [2]Department of Biotechnology and Genetic Engineering, Noakhali Science and Technology University, Sonapur, Noakhali 3814, Bangladesh. [3]Department of Microbiology, University of Dhaka, Dhaka 1000, Bangladesh. [4]Department of Microbiology, Noakhali Science and Technology University, Sonapur, Noakhali 3814, Bangladesh.

## References

1. Calixto JB, Beirith A, Ferreira J, Santos AR, Cechinel FV, Yunes RA. Naturally occurring antinociceptive substances from plants. Phytother Res. 2000;14:401–18.
2. World Health Organization. WHO Guideline for the Assessment of herbal Medicines, WHO expert committee on specification for pharmaceutical preparation. In: Technical Report series No 863- Thirty fourth Report, Geneva. 1996.
3. Calixto JB. Efficacy, safety, quality control, marketing and regulatory guidelines for herbal medicines (phytotherapeutic agents). Braz J Med Biol Res. 2000;33:179–89.
4. Mondal SK, Chakraborty G, Gupata M, Mszumder UK. *In-vitro* antioxidant activity of *Diospyros malabarica* Kostel bark. Indian J Exp Biol. 2006;44:39–44.
5. Kaushik V, Saini V, Pandurangan A, Khosa RL, Parcha V. A review of phytochemical and biological studies of *Diospyros malabarica*. Int J Pharm Sci Let. 2013;2(6):167–9.
6. Ghani A. Medicinal plants of Bangladesh with chemical constituents and uses. In: 2nd edition, Asiatic society of Bangladesh, 5 old secretariat road, Nimtali, Dhaka, Bangladesh; 2003.
7. Rode MS, Kalaskar MG, Gond NY, Surana SJ. Evaluation of anti-diarrheal activity of *Diospyros malabarica* bark extract. Bangladesh J Pharmacol. 2013;8:49–53.
8. Choudhary DN, Singh JN, Verma SK, Singh BP. Antifertility effects of leaf extracts of some plants in male rats. Indian J Exp Biol. 1990;28(8):714–6.
9. Chopra RN, Chopra IC, Handa KL, Kapur LD. Chopra's indigenous drugs of India. 2nd ed. Calcutta, India: Academic publishers; 1994. p. 505.
10. Haque SS, Rashid MMO, Prodhan MA, Noor S, Das A. *In vitro* evaluation of antimicrobial, cytotoxic and antioxidant activities of crude methanolic extract and other fractions of *Sterculia villosa* barks. J Appl Pharm Sci. 2014;4(03):35–40.
11. Amin KMR, Uddin MG, Rashid MMO, Sharmin T. New insight in neuropharmacological activities of *Dioscorea alata*. Discovery Phytomedicine. 2018;5(1):1–6.
12. Hossain MF, Talukder B, Rana MN, Tasnim R, Nipun TS, Uddin SMN, Hossen SMM. *In vivo* sedative activity of methanolic extract of *Stericulia villosa* Roxb leaves. BMC Complement Altern Med. 2016;16:398.
13. Rashid MM, Hussain MS, Rashid MMO, Halim MA, Sen N, Millat MS, Sarker MA. *In vivo* analgesic potential in swiss albino mice and *in vitro* thrombolytic and membrane stabilizing activities of methanolic extract from *Suaeda maritima* whole plant. Bagcilar Med Bull. 2017;2(1):13–8.
14. Salahdeen HM, Yemitan OK. Neuropharmacological effects of aqueous leaf extract of *Bryophyllum pinnatum* in mice. Afr J Biomed Res. 2006;9:101–7.
15. Bourin M, Hascoët M. The mouse light/dark box test. Eur J Pharmacol. 2003;463(1–3):55–65.
16. Can A, Dao DT, Arad M, Terrillion CE, Piantadosi SC, Gould TD. The mouse forced swim test. J Vis Exp. 2012;59:3638.
17. Steru L, Chermat R, Thierry B, Simon P. The tail suspension test: a new method for screening antidepressants in mice. Psychopharmacology (Berl). 1985;85:367–70.
18. Rashid MMO, Akhter KN, Chowdhury JA, Hossen F, Hussain MS, Hossain MT. Characterization of phytoconstituents and evaluation of antimicrobial activity of silver extract nanoparticles synthesized from *Momordica charantia* fruit extract. BMC Complement Altern Med. 2017;17:336.
19. Mechan AO, Moran PM, Elliott M, Young AJ, Joseph MH, Green R. A comparison between dark Agouti and Sprague-Dawley rats in their behaviour on the elevated plus-maze, open-field apparatus and activity meters, and their response to diazepam. Psychopharmacology. 2002;159(2):188–95.
20. Thippeswamy BS, Mishra B, Veerapur VP, Gupta G. Anxiolytic activity of *Nymphaea alba* Linn in mice as experimental models of anxiety. Indian J Pharmacol. 2011;43(1):50–5.
21. Dolai N, Karmakar I, Kumar RBS, Haldar PK. CNS depressant activity of *Castanopsis indica* leaves. Orient Pharm Exp Med. 2012;12:135–40.
22. Maridass M, Ghanthikumar S, Raju G. Preliminary phytochemical analysis of *Diospyros* species. Ethnobot Leaflets. 2008;12:868–72.
23. Zaretsky DV, Zaretskaia MV, DiMicco JA. Characterization of the relationship between spontaneous locomotor activity and cardiovascular parameters in conscious freely moving rats. Physiol Behav. 2016;154:60–7.

24. Nishikava H, Hata T, Funakami Y. A role for corticotropin-releasing factor in repeated cold stress-induced anxiety-like behavior during forced swimming and elevated plus-maze test in mice. Biol Pharm Bull. 2004;27:352–6.

25. Riaz M, Zia-Ul-Huq M, Ur-Rahman N, Ahmad M. Neuropharmacological effects of methanolic extracts of *Rubus fruticosus* L. Turk J Med Sci. 2014;44:454–60.

26. Taranath TC, Hedaginal BR, Rajani P, Sindhu M. Phytosynthesis of silver nanoparticles using the leaf extract of *Diospyros malabarica* (desr.) Kostel and its antibacterial activity against human pathogenic gram negative *Escherichia coli* and *Pseudomonas aeruginosa*. Int J Pharm Sci Rev Res. 2015;30(2):109–14.

# 24

# Diuretic effect of chlorogenic acid from traditional medicinal plant *Merremia emarginata* (Burm. F.) and its by product hippuric acid

Rameshkumar Angappan[1], Arul Ananth Devanesan[1,2] and Sivasudha Thilagar[1]*

## Abstract

**Background:** Medicinal and aromatic plants exhibit important pharmacological activities to human. The present study evaluates the diuretic activity of aqueous extract of *Merremia emarginata* (MEAE).

**Methods:** Female Wistar albino rats were used for diuretic activity in vivo studies. Urinary hippuric acid of treated animal group was successfully quantified by RP-HPLC. UPLC-MS/MS is used for the identification of important bioactive compound in MEAE.

**Results:** Diuretic activity was confirmed through analyzing the disparity in total volume and diuretic markers (total sodium and potassium concentration of urine) which was compared to normal group rats. MEAE plays a crucial role for inducing diuretics without side effects such as glycosuria or proteinuria. This activity was significantly high ($p < 0.05$) compared to control group rats and diuretic responsible polyphenolic compound chlorogenic acid was identified in MEAE through RP-HPLC and UPLC-MS/MS.

**Conclusion:** Hippuric acid is a byproduct of chlorogenic acid and reported to be responsible for inducing diuretics. Secondary metabolites such as chlorogenic acid and their byproducts might be responsible for diuretic activity. Hippuric acid can act as a diuretic agent as well as it could be used as a biomarker to detect the polyphenolics induced diuretic activity. *M. emarginata* can act as an excellent diuretic agent, without causing any harmful side effects.

**Keywords:** *M. emarginata*, RP-HPLC, UPLC-MS/MS, Diuretic activity, Chlorogenic acid, Hippuric acid

## Background

*Merremia emarginata* (Burm. f.) belongs to family Convolvulaceae is prevalent throughout India and tropical region of Asia. This plant is uncultivated food crop used by people in India as green leaf vegetable and creeping perennial herb rooting at the nodes. *M. emarginata* traditionally used as diuretic, deobstruent, rheumatism, neuralgia, cough and headache [1]. Previous reports suggested that *M. emarginata* leaves have strong antioxidant property and antibacterial activity against both gram positive and gram negative bacterial [2, 3].

A diuretic drug is any substance that elevates the urine excretion, they are widely used for treatment of edema, congestive heart failure, hypertension, liver and kidney diseases [4]. Now a day's many commercial diuretic drugs available in the market are class of thiazide (chlorothiazide, hydrochlorothiazide etc), loop (furosemide, bumetanide etc), K+ sparing (amiloride, eplerenone etc) and CA inhibitors (acetazolamide, dichlorphenamideetc). These commercial diuretics drugs have variety of side effects such as hypokalemia, metabolic alkalosis, dehydration (hypovolemia), leading to hypotension, fever, cough, unusual bleeding, excessive weight loss, nausea, vomiting [5]. Diuretic drugs of medicinal plants origin are a better alternative to commercial diuretic drugs. Wright et al. [6] reported that about hundreds of medicinal plants

* Correspondence: sudha@bdu.ac.in; sudacoli@yahoo.com
[1]Department of Environmental Biotechnology, Bharathidasan University, Tiruchirappalli, Tamil Nadu 620024, India
Full list of author information is available at the end of the article

and its extracts were successfully investigated for their diuretic property. The most successful and most potential diuretic medicinal plant genus includes *Spergularia purpurea*, *Petroselinum sativum*, *Foeniculum vulgare* and *Hibiscus sabdariffa* [7–10]. These medicinal plants contain secondary metabolites (alkaloids, phenolics and flavonoids etc.) which might be responsible for diuretic activity [11, 12]. But there is no previous report about specific phenolic compound and its byproduct for diuretic activity. The mechanism of medicinal plant induces diuretic activity is still unclear. Further, Kaur, [13] reported that, cow urine containing hippuric acid responsible for induced diuretic activity. Based on this, the present study was carried out to study the diuretic activity of MEAE. Chlorogenic acid which is one of the phenolic compounds found in MEAE and hippuric acid is a byproduct of chlorogenic acid was detected in our plant extract treated rat urine sample through RP-HPLC which indirectly reveals about the role of polyphenolics present in the plant extract in inducing diuretics.

## Methods

### Plant collection

Fresh leaves of *M. emarginata* were collected from Dharmapuri, Tamil Nadu in India. The identity of the plant was authenticated by the Department of Plant Science, Bharathidasan University, Tiruchirappalli. The leaves were picked and washed with distilled water to remove all the unwanted debris and shade dried under room temperature of 30 °C for 10 days, ground into powder using electronic grinder and stored in an airtight container until further use.

### Preparation aqueous extract

Ten gram of powdered plant material was extracted with distilled water (250 ml; 27–30 °C) on shaker (*Orbitec-scigenics Biotech*, India) for 48 h. The extract was filtered and quickly frozen at – 80 °C and dried for 48 h using a vacuum freeze dryer (Christ alpha *1-2 / LD plus*, Germany) to give a yield of 8.87% of dry extract. The resulting extract was reconstituted with distilled water to give desired concentrations and used for further analysis.

### In vivo studies

Adult female Wistar albino rats weighing 150–200 g were housed in standard cages with good feed and water access. Experimental procedures and protocols were approved by the committee (BDU/IAEC/2012/33/28/03/2012) for the purpose of CPCSEA, Chennai, Tamil Nadu, India.

### Experimental method

Diuretic activity was carried out by Biswas et al. [14] method. Animals were divided into five groups each with five rats. Before starting the experiment, the rats were starved for 18 h. Among the five groups, group one served as a control which was fed normal drinking water only (10 ml/kg b.w.). Second group served as a commercial diuretic drug treated (furosemide 20 mg/kg b.w.). The third, fourth and fifth groups received MEAE orally at the doses of 200, 400 and 600 mg/kg b.w. respectively. After administration of drugs (orally), animals were caged immediately under sterile condition. Urine samples were collected up to 5 h, during the experiment, food and water was not given to the animals in cages. After collection, urine samples were preserved with sodium azide to avoid microbial contamination. Further, urine $Na^+$ and $K^+$ ions were analyzed by flame photometer (*Elico. CL 378*, India) [15]. Total protein was estimated by Bradford standard protocol [16] and glucose was analyzed through Ortho tolludine method [17].

### Identification and quantification of hippuric acid through RP-HPLC

Rat urine was centrifuged at 13000 rpm for 4 min at 4 °C. The resulting supernatant was used for further analysis. The RP-HPLC on a $C_{18}$ column (4.6 × 250 mm, 5 μm particle size) was used for hippuric acid identification. Analytical HPLC system employed consists of Waters high performance liquid chromatography coupled with a photodiode array detector (PDA-2998), USA. Mobile phase consist of water with 0.1% formic acid (Solvent A) and 100% methanol (Solvent B), the gradient program followed; Solvent A and B was 0–10% (5 min), 10–15% (5 min), 15–20% (5 min), 20–30% (5 min), 30–40% (10 min); Flow rate was 1 ml/min. Detection was carried out in the multi wavelength detection range of 210 to 400 [18]. Hippuric acid presence in urine sample was confirmed by comparing its retention time and λ max of an authentic standard.

### Chlorogenic acid identification by UPLC-MS/MS

UPLC was carried out using Waters UPLC system with PDA detector by Waters Corporation, USA. $C_{18}$ UPLC column (150 mm X 2.1 mm dia X 1.7 μm particle size) used for chlorogenic acid identification. The mobile phase was similar as followed in RP-HPLC analysis. Gradient program was optimized according to UPLC condition. Mass Spectrometric analysis of phenolic compounds carried out by SYNAPT Mass Spectrometer from Waters, USA with ESI mode. Compounds were analyzed both positive and negative modes.

### Statistical analysis

All the statistical data were analyzed through SPSS 16.0 and Origin 6.0. The significance of difference between the groups was determined using one way ANOVA. All data were expressed as mean ± standard deviation (SD). The significance level was expresses as $p < 0.05$.

**Table 1** Effect of MEAE on diuretic excretion parameters of albino Wistar rat urine

| Treatment Groups | Total volume of Urine (ml/5 h) | Total Sodium (mEq/l) | Total Potassium (mEq/l) | Total Protein (μmol/dl) | Total Glucose (mg/dl) |
|---|---|---|---|---|---|
| Control | 1.55 ± 0.03[d] | 120.3 ± 1.2[e] | 210.6 ± 1.1[e] | 1.162 ± 0.1[c] | 2.3 ± 0.5[d] |
| Furosemide (20 mg/kg b.w.) | 3.58 ± 0.08[a] | 225.7 ± 1.9[d] | 365.1 ± 1.8[a] | 1.249 ± 0.02[a] | 6.3 ± 0.07[a] |
| MEAE (200 mg/kg b.w.) | 1.46 ± 0.02[e] | 309.1 ± 2.2[c] | 243.1 ± 1.5[d] | 0.667 ± 0.01[e] | 3.4 ± 0.12[c,b] |
| MEAE (400 mg/kg b.w.) | 1.83 ± 0.04[c] | 325.3 ± 1.8[b] | 289.4 ± 2.1[c] | 0.817 ± 0.01[d] | 3.5 ± 0.07[c,a] |
| MEAE (600 mg/kg b.w.) | 2.61 ± 0.05[b] | 345.1 ± 1.3[a] | 349.4 ± 1.7[b] | 1.218 ± 0.01[b] | 4.1 ± 0.04[b] |

Mean ± SD obtained from analysis of three independent samples, in duplicate
[abcde]; In each column, the superscript letters significantly differences in the mean at ($P < 0.05$) level

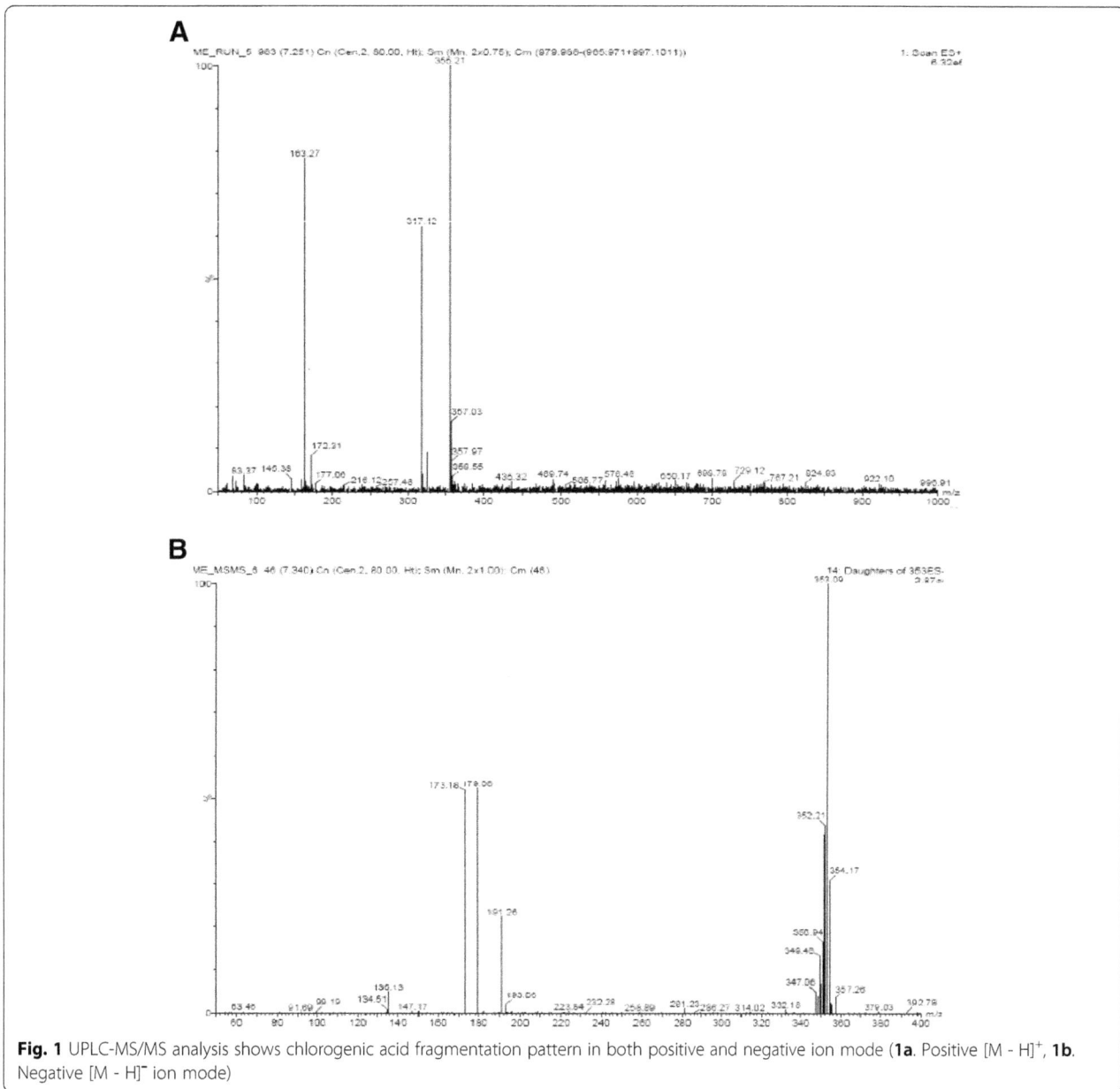

**Fig. 1** UPLC-MS/MS analysis shows chlorogenic acid fragmentation pattern in both positive and negative ion mode (**1a**. Positive [M - H]$^+$, **1b**. Negative [M - H]$^-$ ion mode)

## Results and discussion
### Diuretic and excretion parameters analysis
The volume of urine measured up to 5 h. Table 1 shows total volume of urine excretion, total sodium, total potassium, total protein and total glucose concentration in the rat urine samples. Total volume of urine excretion data shows (MEAE) and furosemide (Lasix) treated rat group excreted high volume of urine compared to untreated control group. MEAE treated rat groups urine excretion had increased in a dose dependant manner. Furosemide (20 mg/kg b.w) treated animal group urine volume ($3.55 \pm 0.03$ ml/5 h) is very high when compared

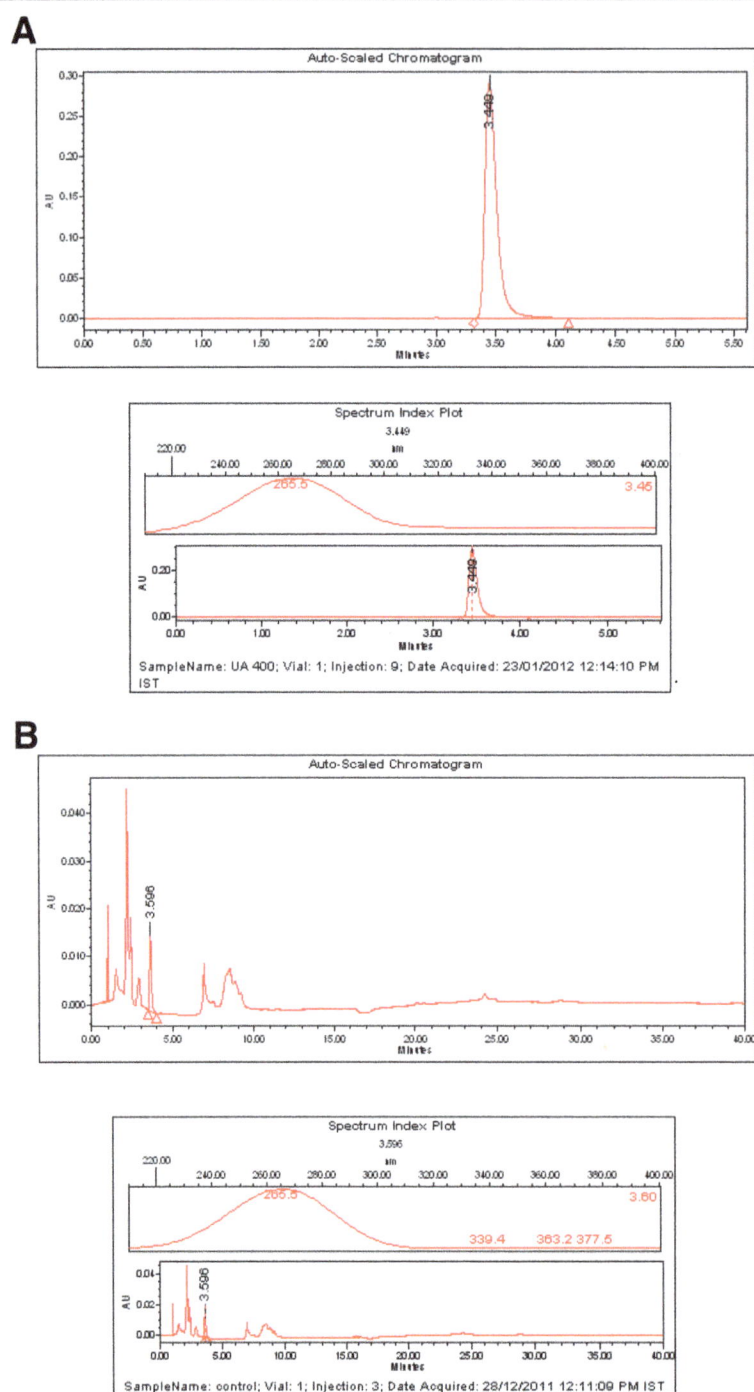

**Fig. 2 a** RP-HPLC chromatograms (photo-diode array detector set at 200–400 nm). Hippuric acid (HA) standard maximum absorption (λ max) is at 265.5 nm and Retention time is 3.4 min. **b** RP-HPLC chromatograms (PDA detector set at 200–500 nm). Hippuric acid (HA) analysis from MEAE treated albino Wistar rat urine sample. Maximum absorption (λ max) is at 265.5 nm and Retention time is at 3.5 min

to 600 mg/kg b.w MEAE treated group, (2.61 ± 0.05 ml/5 h), volume of urine at when the total sodium and potassium levels were significantly increased ($p < 0.05$) in the treated animal group when compared to control group. Total protein and glucose levels in urine samples of MEAE treated animal groups were similar to control group. These results clearly indicate that the plant doesn't produce side effects such as either proteinuria or glycosuria.

### Identification of chlorogenic acid through RP-HPLC and UPLC-MS/MS

Occurrence of chlorogenic acid in the MEAE was confirmed by comparing with chlorogenic acid standard (HPLC grade, Sigma) retention time, absorbance spectrum and mass analysis through MS/MS fragmentation (Fig. 1a and b). The presence of chlorogenic acid in MEAE was detected through UPLC-MS/MS and confirmed by MS/MS fragmentation pattern in both positive $[M-H]^+$ and negative $[M - H]^-$ mode ionization. The chlorogenic acid exact molar mass is 354.09. Fig. 1a shows chlorogenic acid in $[M-H]^+$ mode, the mass of base peak gave $[M-H]^+$ ion at $m/z$ is 355.21, and $MS^2$ fragmentation $[M-H]^+$ ion shows at 163.07. In negative $[M - H]^-$ ion mode (Fig. 1b), chlorogenic acid shows a base peak at 353.09, and $MS^2$ fragmentation $[M-H]^-$ ion shows at 191.26, 173.18 and 135.13 respectively. It was same fragmentation pattern previously reported [19, 20].

### Detection and quantification of hippuric acid through RP-HPLC analysis

Gonthier et al. [21] studied about chlorogenic acid degradation through gut microbial pathway. Their result shows the chlorogenic acid degradation or digestion through gut microorganisms, from this microbial degradation, chlorogenic acid produced byproducts namely hippuric acid and 3- hydroxyhippuric acid. This hippuric acid can act as diuretic agent [13], but the mechanism of hippuric acid acting as diuretics is still unclear.

The filtered urine sample was injected into RP-HPLC to determine the hippuric acid content. The presence of hippuric acid in the urine was confirmed by comparing the peak with retention time and absorbance spectrum of commercial hippuric acid standard. The absorbance maximum at 265.5 nm and retention time of 3.449 ± 0.1 min was observed in both commercial hippuric acid standard and urine sample (Fig. 2a and b). Hippuric acid content of the urine samples (control and drug treated) were determined based on the hippuric acid standard curve ($y = 5342.x - 35,193$, $R^2 = 0.999$). Hippuric acid content of control and furosemide treated was 97.25 and 566.3 ng/ml respectively. MEAE treated (200, 400 and 600 mg/kg b.w) groups showed hippuric acid content 240.8, 494.9 and

620.7 ng/ml respectively (Table 2). Control and furosemide treated excretion of hippuric acid perhaps due to benzoic acid conjugated hippuric acid excretion [22], because generally hippuric acid is the glycine conjugate of benzoic acid. Because, hippuric acid synthesized in the liver and its production is greatly increased from benzoic acid based food substance or substances which generate benzoic acid during intermediate metabolism (e.g. polyphenols such as chlorogenic acid, quinic acid and caffeic acid) [20, 21]. Perhaps, based on the polyphenolic concentration, the hippuric acid elution was increased in the MEAE treated group urine sample, the hippuric acid excretion in the urine got increased with increase in MEAE dose in a dose depended manner. The commercial drug furosemide chemical name is (4-Chloro-N-furfuryl-5-sulfamoylanthranilic acid 5-(Aminosulfonyl)-4-chloro-2-([2 furanylmethyl] amino) benzoic acid) and the furosemide functional group benzoic acid conjugated with glycine may induce diuretics through hippuric acid formation, but that mechanism is still unclear.

On the other hand, secondary metabolites profile of MEAE by UPLC-MS/MS shows the presence of chlorogenic acid. Chlorogenic acid is well known plant secondary metabolite, which is responsible for inducing diuretic activity [23]. Similarly, plant secondary metabolites altered the diuretic markers like sodium, potassium and chloride levels in human urine [24, 25]. From these results, the total volume of urine, sodium and potassium levels clearly indicate that the plant M. emarginata play crucial role for inducing diuretic activity. The presence of chlorogenic acid has been confirmed through RP-HPLC and UPLC-MS/MS and it might be responsible for inducing diuretics in animal model.

### Conclusion

Based on the results we conclude that the M. emarginata can act as a good diuretic agent, without causing any side effects such as proteinuria or glycosuria. M. emarginata secondary metabolites may act as diuretic agents, especially chlorogenic acid and their byproducts. Chlorogenic acid byproduct, hippuric acid can act as a

**Table 2** Effect of MEAE on hippuric acid concentration in urine samples collected from MEAE treated rats

| Treatment Groups | Hippuric Acid (ng/ml) |
|---|---|
| Control | 97.25 ± 1.0[e] |
| Furosemide (20 mg/kg b.w.) | 566.3 ± 5.87[b] |
| MEAE (200 mg/kg b.w.) | 240.8 ± 4.04[d] |
| MEAE (400 mg/kg b.w.) | 494.9 ± 3.51[c] |
| MEAE (600 mg/kg b.w.) | 620.7 ± 8.38[a] |

Mean ± SD obtained from analysis of three independent samples, in duplicate [abcde]; in column, the superscript letters significantly differences in the mean at ($P < 0.05$) level

diuretic agent as well as it could be used as a biomarker to detect the polyphenolics induced diuretic activity. However, the mechanism of chlorogenic acid inducing diuretics is unclear. Furthermore, additional studies need to be carried out to purify the bioactive compounds to evaluate diuretic activity and hippuric acid excretion analysis using animal as model system.

## Abbreviations
CA inhibitors: Carbonic anhydrase inhibitors; CPCSEA: Control and supervision of experiments on animals; ESI: Electron Spray Ionization; MEAE: *M. emarginata* aqueous extract; PDA: Photo Diode Array; RP-HPLC: Reverse Phase High Performance Liquid Chromatography; UPLC-MS: Ultra Performance Liquid Chromatography; USA: United States of America; λ max: Maximum Absorbance

## Acknowledgements
A.R thanks University Grants Commission (UGC), India for UGC Research Fellowship in Science for Meritorious students under Non-SAP programme and Bharathidasan University for providing University research scholar fellowship. Authors sincerely thank Department of Science and Technology (DST-FIST) and UGC-SAP, India for providing instrumental facilities to our department.

## Authors' contributions
RA & AAD have conducted all the experiments. ST has edited the manuscript. All authors read and approved the final manuscript.

## Competing interests
The authors declare that they have no competing interests.

## Author details
[1]Department of Environmental Biotechnology, Bharathidasan University, Tiruchirappalli, Tamil Nadu 620024, India. [2]Department of Food Quality and Safety, Gilat Research Center, Agricultural Research Organization, M.P. Negev - 85280, Tifrah, Israel.

## References
1. Singh AK, Raghubanshi AS, Singh JS. Medical ethnobotany of the tribals of Sonaghati of Sonbhadra district, Uttar Pradesh, India. J Ethnopharmacol. 2002;81:31–41.
2. Babu AV, Rao RSC, Kumar KG, Babu BH, Satyanarayanan PW. Biological activity of Merremia emarginata crude extracts in different solvents. Res J Med Plant. 2009;3:134–40.
3. Elumalai EK, Ramachandran M, Thirumalai T, Vinothkumar P. Antibacterial activity of various leaf extracts of Merremia emarginata. Asian Pac J Trop Biomed. 2011;1:406–8.
4. Flavio DF. Diuretics: drugs of choice for the initial management of patients with hypertension. Expert Rev Cardiovasc Ther. 2003;1:35–41.
5. Maland LJ, Lutz LJ, Castle CH. Effects of withdrawing diuretic therapy on blood pressure in mild hypertension. Hypertension. 1983;5:539–44.
6. Wright CI, Van-Buren L, Kroner CI, Koning MMG. Herbal medicines as diuretics: a review of the scientific evidence. J Ethnopharmacol. 2007; 114:1–31.
7. Jouad H, Lacaille-Dubois MA, Eddouks M. Chronic diuretic effect of the water extract of Spergularia purpurea in normal rats. J Ethnopharmacol. 2001;75:219–23.
8. Kreydiyyeh SI, Usta J. Diuretic effect and mechanism of action of parsley. J Ethnopharmacol. 2002;79:353–7.
9. El Bardai S, Lyoussi B, Wibo M, Morel N. Pharmacological evidence of hypotensive activity of Marrubium vulgare and Foeniculum vulgare in spontaneously hypertensive rat. Clin Exp Hypertens. 2001;23:329–43.
10. Odigie IP, Ettarh RR, Adigun SA. Chronic administration of aqueous extract of Hibiscus sabdariffa attenuates hypertension and reverses cardiac hypertrophy in 2K-1C hypertensive rats. J Ethnopharmacol. 2003;86:181–5.
11. Consolini AE, Baldini OA, Amat AG. Pharmacological basis for the empirical use of Eugenia uniflora L. (Myrtaceae) as antihypertensive. J Ethnopharmacol. 1999;66:33–9.
12. Navarro E, Alonso J, Rodriguez R, Trujillo J, Boada J. Diuretic action of an aqueous extract of Lepidium latifolium L. J Ethnopharmacol. 1994;41:65–9.
13. Kaur RG. Cow urine distillate as bioenhancer. J Ayurveda Integr Med. 2010;1:240–1.
14. Biswas S, Murugesan T, Maiti K, Ghosh L, Pal M, Saha BP. Study on the diuretic activity of Strychnos potatorum Linn. Seed extract in albino rats. Phytomedicine. 2001;8:469–71.
15. Souleymane M, Bahi C, Yéo D, Datte JY, Djaman JA, Nguessan DJ. Laxative activities of Mareya micrantha (Benth.) Mull. Arg. (Euphorbiaceae) leaf aqueous extract in rats. BMC Compliment Altern Med. 2010;10:2–6.
16. Bradford MM. A rapid and sensitive method for the quantitation of microgram quantities of protein utilizing the principle of protein-dye binding. Anal Biochem. 1976;7:248–54.
17. Dubowski KM. An o-toluidine method for body-fluid glucose determination. Clin Chem. 1962;8:215–35.
18. Rameshkumar A, Sivasudha T, Jeyadevi R, Ananth DA, Pradeepha G. Effect of environmental factors [air and UV-C irradiation] on some fresh fruit juices. Eur Food Res Technol. 2012;234:1063–70.
19. Clifford MN, Knight S, Kuhnert N. Discriminating between the six isomers of dicaffeoylquinic acid by LC-MS(n). J Agric Food Chem. 2005;18:3821–32.
20. Pältinean R, Mocan A, Vlase L, Gheldiu A, Crisan G, Ielciu I, et al. Evaluation of polyphenolic content, antioxidant and diuretic activities of six Fumaria species. Molecules. 2017;22:639.
21. Gonthier MP, Verny MA, Besson C, Remesy C, Scalbert A. Chlorogenic acid bioavailability largely depends on its metabolism by the gut microflora in rats. J Nutr. 2003;133:1853–9.
22. Rahim YA, Raizul ZM. Spectrophotometry semiquantitation method hippuric acid in urine for demonstration of toluene abuse. Indian J Forensic Med Toxicol. 2010;4:68–70.
23. Daly JW. Caffeine analogs: biomedical impact. Review Cell Mol Life Sci. 2007; 64:2153–69.
24. Lawrence EA, Pumerantz AC, Roti MW, Judelson DA, Watson G, Dias JC, et al. Fluid, electrolyte, and renal indices of hydration during 11 days of controlled caffeine consumption. Int J Sport Nutr Exerc Metab. 2005;15:252–65.
25. Hailu H, Engidawork E. Evaluation of the diuretic activity of the aqueous and 80% methanol extracts of Ajuga remota Benth (Lamiaceae) leaves in mice. BMC Compliment Altern Med. 2014;14:135.

# 25

# Pharmacological influences of natural products as bioenhancers of silymarin against carbon tetrachloride-induced hepatotoxicity in rats

Shamama Javed[1], Waquar Ahsan[2] and Kanchan Kohli[1*]

## Abstract

**Background:** Popularity of herbal remedies is increasing day by day despite the presence of synthetic drugs to treat the Liver Diseases owing to the adverse effects and high cost of synthetic drugs. Silymarin has tremendous potential for the treatment of various liver disorders because of its high antioxidant potential as liver diseases are associated with increased oxidative stress. The low oral bioavailability of Silymarin continues to be a major challenge in the development of its formulations having clinical efficacy. Our idea was to constitute a pharmaceutical composition of Silymarin with natural products as bioenhancers that might work positively and synergistically in the control of hepatotoxicity.

**Methods:** In this work, various combinations of Silymarin with natural bioenhancers such as Lysergol (L), Piperine (P) and Fulvic acid (FA) were prepared and their hepatoprotective activities were evaluated against carbon tetrachloride (CCl4) induced hepatotoxicity in animal model.

**Results:** Although, all the combinations decreased the liver enzymes and changed protein level significantly, group G (silymarin:FA (1:1) + P (10%) was found to be most significant as compared to the toxic control. It also displayed better protection when compared to the marketed tablet containing silymarin alone. None of the combinations showed any signs of cytotoxicity when screened on MCF-7 cells by MTT assay.

**Conclusions:** Group G (silymarin:FA (1:1) + P (10%) appeared to be the most effective combination in treating the liver diseases envisaging an industrially viable product of Silymarin as a contemporary therapeutic agent with enhanced bioavailability and medicinal value. Further this combination can be examined for safety and efficacy in clinical studies.

**Keywords:** Silymarin, Bioenhancers, Piperine, Fulvic acid, Lysergol, Bioavailability, Hepatoprotection, MTT assay

## Background

Liver, a vital organ (organ of metabolism and excretion) in the human body, plays an astounding array of functions vital for the maintenance as well as performance of the body. Unfortunately, liver is exposed to a variety of xenobiotics, chemotherapeutic agents, drug-drug interactions and environmental pollutants which weaken and damage the liver leading to hazardous liver diseases such as Hepatitis, Cirrhosis and Cancer etc. [1]. LDs and their complications are often linked with imbalance between the production of free radicals (ROS) and body's antioxidant defense mechanism that result into increased oxidative stress. These ROS have an important role in the etiology of LDs andthe antioxidant therapy is expected to impart beneficial effects in treating these. Liver disease (LD), a multi-factorial disease remains one of the most serious health problems and millions of people world-wide are suffering from one form or the other. High cost of treatment and adverse effects are the disadvantages associated with synthetic drugs when used for prolonged periods [2]. Therefore, it is logical to think of herbal remedies for the treatment of LD. Silymarin, a known

* Correspondence: kanchankohli2010@gmail.com
[1]Department of Pharmaceutics, School of Pharmaceutical Education and Research, Jamia Hamdard, New Delhi 110062, India
Full list of author information is available at the end of the article

hepatoprotective drug has well defined hepatoprotective, free radical scavenging and antioxidant properties, that improves the antioxidant defense by preventing the glutathione depletion as well as antifibrotic activity. It has been investigated through in-vitro and in-vivo experimental studies by Radko and Cybulski 2007 [3]. Although, clinical trials suggested the safety of silymarin at higher doses (up to 1500 mg/day) in humans, but the pharmacokinetic studies have revealed poor absorption, rapid metabolism and excretion in bile and urine and all these ultimately results in poor oral bioavailability of silymarin [4].

Generally, all pharmacokinetic parameters of silymarin are referred to, and standardized as, silybin. According to Wu et al. 2007, silymarin (silybin), when administered orally, is rapidly absorbed with a $T_{max}$ (2–4 h) and $t_{1/2}$ (6 h). Due to extensive enterohepatic circulation, only 20–50% of oral silymarin is absorbed from the gastrointestinal tract and 0.73% oral bioavailability of silymarin (silybin) in rat plasma was reported [5, 6].

*Silybum marianum* (milk thistle, family: Asteraceae), is one of the oldest and thoroughly researched plants of ancient times used in the treatment of liver and gall bladder disorders, including jaundice, cirrhosis and hepatitis and Silymarin is the active constituent of this plant which is a 70–80% standardized extract consisting of silymarin flavonolignans (silybin A & B, isosilybin A & B, silydianin, and silychristin) and flavonoids (taxifolin and quercetin), and the remaining 20–30% consists of chemically undefined fraction comprising polymeric and oxidized polyphenolic compounds [7]. There are as many as 75 brands of silymarin available in market in different dosage forms such as tablets, capsules, syrups, etc. Some of the important brands are Legalon capsules, Carsil Tablets and Alrin-B syrup etc. An array of methods are available in the literature that can improve the bioavailability of silymarin like formation of microparticles, nanoparticles, self- emulsifying drug delivery systems, phytosomes, liposomes and micelles as summarized by Javed et al. 2012 [7]. But they suffer from disadvantages of using a large amount of surfactants, co-surfactants, exogenous compounds as these cause irritation to patients suffering from gastric disorders and ulcers and thus leading to abdominal discomfort [8]. The concept of using the bioenhancers to increase the drug bioavailability is one of the newest approaches. The discovery of first bioenhancer piperine in 1979 by scientists in RRL, Jammu, India introduced a new concept in science [9]. Non-toxicity, effectiveness at low concentrations, easy to formulate with the drug, enhanced uptake and absorption of drug and lastly, synergizing the activity of the drug are the advantages associated with the bioenhancers. Bioenhancers increase in the bioavailability of nutraceuticals by acting through several mechanisms, which include acting on gastrointestinal tract to enhance absorption, or by altering the drug metabolism process [10].

In our study, three natural products as bioenhancers were selected based on their mechanism of action: first, Fulvic acid (FA) – a water soluble carrier for increasing the solubility of silymarin by complex formation [11], second piperine (P) – a known inhibitor of hepatic and intestinal glucoronidation inhibitor [12] and third, lysergol (L) – a permeability enhancer of drugs across intestinal epithelial cells for better absorption and efficacy [13]. All the formulations no. 1–5 were subjected to accelerated stability studies as per ICH guidelines Q1A. The carbon tetrachloride induced hepatotoxicity study in rats was performed to evaluate the effect of silymarin alone and with bioenhancers in all the tablet formulations. Previously, researchers from all over the world have demonstrated the hepatoprotective activity of silymarin against various toxic models and partial hepatectomy models in experimental animals by using chemical toxins such as carbon tetrachloride ($CCl_4$), acetaminophen, D-galactosamine, ethanol, and *Amanita phalloides* toxin [14]. In cellular events that modulate hepatotoxicity, $CCl_4$ is metabolized by CYP450 enzymes in liver endoplasmic reticulum in reactive trichloromethyl free radicals which in turn react with oxygen and form trichloromethylperoxy radicals. These radicals attack lipids on endoplasmic reticulum of liver cells and leads to elevation of liver enzymes and ultimately cell death. $CCl_4$ interferes with the transport function of the liver cells, leading to leakage of SGOT and SGPT from the cell cytoplasm into the serum, thereby increasing their levels in serum and reduces the capacity of liver to synthesize albumin, leading to decreased serum levels [15].

Recent studies conducted in the past decade have shown the hepatoprotective potential of silymarin against $CCl_4$ induced liver injury. Silymarin and garlic oil were reported as highly promising compounds in protecting the hepatic tissue against oxidative damage and preventing hepatic dysfunction due to $CCl_4$ induced hepatotoxicity in rats [16]. In another study, the restoration of the $CCl_4$–induced hepatic fibrosis was reported due to high doses of silymarin in rats [17]. The biochemical parameters returned to normal values in $CCl_4$ intoxicated rats after treating with silymarin and/or ginger for one month [18]. A significant reduction in enzyme levels in silymarin lipid microspheres treated group was reported by Abrol et al. 2005 when compared to toxic control, normal control (plain lipid microspheres) as well as groups treated with silymarin solution [19]. In another study conducted by El-Samaligy et al. 2006, silymarin hybrid liposomes produced a significant decrease in both the transaminase levels (SGOT and SGPT) when challenged with intraperitonial $CCl_4$ () in comparison to the orally administered silymarin suspension [20]. Synergistic effects of silymarin and standardized extract of

*Phyllanthus amarus* against CCl$_4$ induced hepatotoxicity in rat model was also reported previously [21].

## Results

### MTT cytotoxicity studies of Silymarin, fulvic acid, Piperine and lysergol on MCF-7 cells

MTT cell viability assay is a versatile, quantitative, significantly advanced measurement of cell viability, proliferation and cell population's response to external factors. This test was based on the formation of water-insoluble purple formazan product from the yellow water- soluble tetrazolium dye by live cells. The amount of formazan generated is directly proportional to the number of viable cells [22]. This test was performed to evaluate the cytoxicity profile of silymarin and all the three bioenhancers on human breast adrenocarcinoma MCF-7 cell lines. Figure 1 shows the photomicrographs of control/untreated cells (a) and cells treated with silymarin, P, L and FA (b, c, d, e) respectively. No cell death, rupture, necrosis was visible in them and morphology and integrity remained intact. Figure 2 shows the Percentage cell death vs. Concentration (µg/mL) bar graph and it was found that neither the drug silymarin nor any of the bioenhancers appeared to be cytotoxic on MCF-7 cells over the concentration range of 25–500 µg/mL. Upto 12% and 18% cell death with P and L was observed at the concentration 500 µg/mL respectively. From this study, it was concluded that no cell death, rupture, necrosis was visible, morphology and integrity remained intact on MCF-7 cells. A higher cell viability throughout the experiment ensured non-cytotoxic behavior of drug and bioenhancers. The bioenhancers were considered non-cytotoxic and were carried forward for further studies.

### Carbon tetrachloride (CCl$_4$) induced hepatotoxicity in rats

CCl$_4$ induces hepatotoxicity by interfering with the transport functions of the liver cells which leads to leakage of SGOT and SGPT from the cell cytoplasm into the serum. Also, enzymatic activation of CCl$_4$ by CYP P450 generates free radicals (ROS) which combine with proteins and cellular lipids in presence of oxygen resulting in liver necrosis [23, 24]. The results in this experiment showed marked increase in plasma SGOT and SGPT levels in toxic control group after CCl$_4$ treatment as compared to the normal control group signifying that the experiment was successful to induce liver injury in rats. Bilirubin is a metabolite of heme and is an important means to excrete the unwanted and toxic heme from body. It is found to be increased in a variety of liver disorders such as cirrhosis and jaundice.

### Statistical analysis

The pharmacodynamic data analysis was carried out using the GraphPad Prism version 6.02 (Registered trademark of GraphPad software, Inc). All the numeric variables were expressed as Mean ± Standard Error of Mean (SEM) and results were statistically analyzed using One Way-Analysis of Variance (ANOVA) followed by Dunnett's Multiple Comparison Test. For all tests a probability ($p < 0.0001$) was considered significant.

### Biochemical estimation

Levels of SGOT, SGPT, ALKP and Serum Bilirubin were found to be significantly reduced in all treatment groups with most significant results obtained for Silymarin–FA–P formulation treated group when compared to toxic

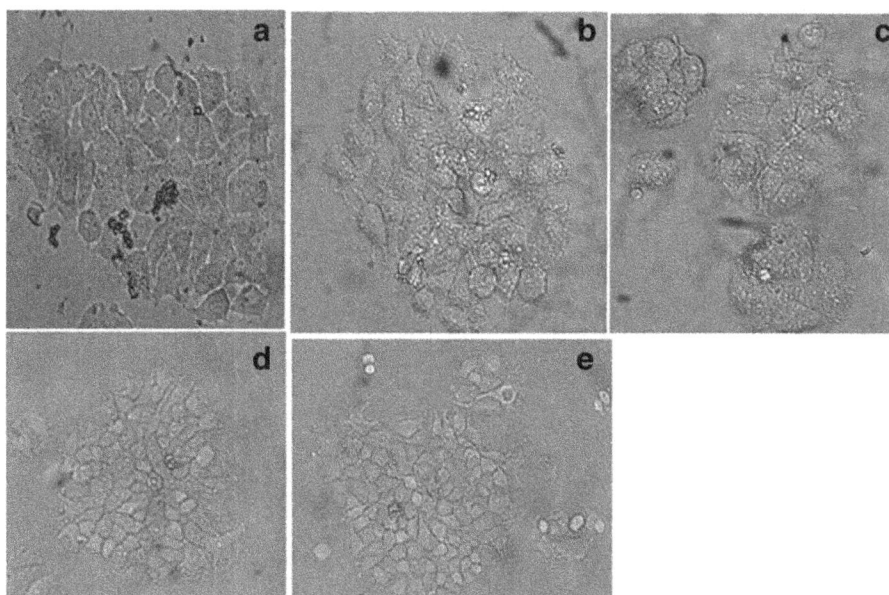

**Fig. 1** Photomicrographs of control cells (**a**), silymarin (**b**), piperine (**c**), lysergol (**d**), and fulvic acid (**e**) treated MCF-7 cells respectively

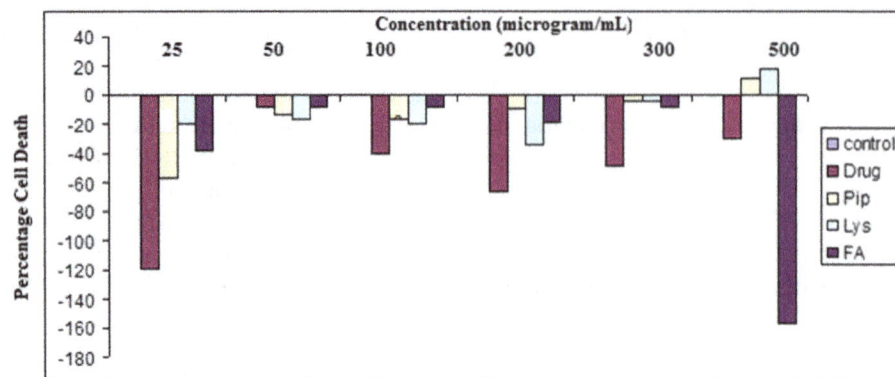

**Fig. 2** Bar-graph between Percentage cell death vs. Concentration (μg/mL) shows that neither the drug silymarin nor any of the bioenhancers appeared to be cytotoxic on MCF-7 cells over the concentration range of 25–500 μg/mL

control. Table 1 indicates different degrees of hepatoprotection showed by these groups. The levels of total plasma protein were observed to be decreased in toxic control group which seconded the findings reported by Tanaka et al., 1998 in LDs [25]. This decrease in plasma proteins reflects decreased hepatic synthesis, which is often attributed to the hepatic impairment of albumin synthesis. The decrease may also be due to leakage in kidney function leading to the release of albumin in urine [18]. Hepatotoxin also decreases serum albumin levels by reducing the capacity of liver to synthesize albumin. Administration of Silymarin- FA- P (group G) formulation significantly counteracts CCl4 induced changes suggesting that it provided better hepatoprotection by improving both synthetic and metabolic activities of the liver as compared to silymarin alone (group C).

The results of percent recovery of serum parameters showed that the combinations of silymarin and bioenhancers had a higher recovery of serum parameters in comparison to plain silymarin tablet (Table 2). Silymarin-L (10%) tablet formulation showed improved (50–70%) percent recovery of serum parameters when compared to plain silymarin formulation. Lysergol is an important constituent of

Ipomoea sp. and two species of Ipomoea namely Ipomoea hederacea and Ipomoea asarifolia (Desr.) have been reported to have antioxidant and hepatoprotective potential against CCl4 induced hepatotoxicity [26, 27]. It has been reported that lysergol modifies the drug transport across the cell membranes and has its own antioxidant and hepatoprotective activity.

Similarly, silymarin–P (10%) tablet formulation showed improved percent recovery of serum parameters (70–75%) in comparison to treatment by plain Silymarin tablet. Piperine is a known inhibitor of CYP 450 enzymes and thus inhibits the hepatic and intestinal glucoronidation thereby increasing the drug concentration. Furthermore, the antioxidant and hepatoprotective activity of Piper longum and Piper nigrum against the CCl4 induced liver injury has been reported previously [28, 29]. Our findings are concordant with these findings and suggest that silymarin and P together in the formulation might have exhibited synergistic hepatoprotective and antioxidant activity.

Thirdly, silymarin – FA tablet formulation also showed improved percent recovery of serum parameters (upto 80%) in comparison to the treatment by our plain silymarin tablet. As, FA is a known enhancer of water

**Table 1** Summary of biochemical parameters for all treatment groups

| Parameters | Group A | Group B | Group C | Group D | Group E | Group F | Group G | Group H |
|---|---|---|---|---|---|---|---|---|
| | Normal control | Toxic control | Plain Sily tab | Sily + Lys (10%) tab | Sily + Pip (10%) tab | Sily + FA (1:1) tab | Sily + FA (1:1) + Pip (10%) tab | Marketed Tab |
| SGOT (IU/L) | 67.25 ± 4.29 | 303.3 ± 1.85[a] | 225.3 ± 6.02[b] | 175.2 ± 4.55[b] | 125.4 ± 5.58[b] | 106.2 ± 3.89[b] | 83.03 ± 2.08[b] | 199.2 ± 8.62[b] |
| SGPT (IU/L) | 55.34 ± 4.27 | 195.6 ± 2.87[a] | 123.5 ± 6.92[b] | 99.14 ± 6.58[b] | 82.89 ± 1.88[b] | 78.90 ± 4.26 [b] | 66.82 ± 3.14[b] | 107.2 ± 6.56 [b] |
| ALKP (IU/L) | 85.08 ± 5.17 | 353.3 ± 8.91[a] | 183.5 ± 5.14[b] | 163.8 ± 3.59[b] | 145.0 ± 4.04[b] | 133.3 ± 3.69[b] | 109.8 ± 4.76[b] | 172.2 ± 2.53[b] |
| Total Bilirubin (mg/100 mL) | 0.38 ± 0.02 | 1.18 ± 0.04[a] | 0.65 ± 0.03[b] | 0.60 ± 0.01[b] | 0.57 ± 0.02[b] | 0.53 ± 0.03[b] | 0.43 ± 0.04[b] | 0.65 ± 0.03[b] |
| Total protein (g/dL) | 7.37 ± 0.16 | 5.06 ± 0.33[a] | 8.74 ± 0.05[b] | 8.06 ± 0.11[b] | 7.93 ± 0.13[b] | 7.70 ± 0.13[b] | 7.45 ± 0.33[b] | 8.66 ± 0.08[b] |

Dunnett's Multiple Comparison Tests showed that all values of group A, C, D, E, F, G, H exhibited significant changes when compared to toxic control with 99.9% CI of difference. For each group n = 5, the values are expressed as mean ± SEM. 'a' exhibits significant (p < 0.05) changes from normal control, whereas, 'b' exhibits significant (p < 0.05) change when compared to toxic control

**Table 2** Percent recovery of serum parameters

| Parameters | Plain Sily tablet (No. 1) | Sily + L (10%) tablet (No. 2) | Sily + P (10%) tablet (No. 3) | Sily + FA (1:1) tablet (No. 4) | Sily + FA (1:1) + P (10%) tablet (No. 5) | Marketed tab |
|---|---|---|---|---|---|---|
| SGOT (IU/L) | 33.17 | 54.26 | 75.36 | 83.49 | 93.31 | 44.10 |
| SGPT (IU/L) | 51.40 | 68.77 | 80.35 | 83.20 | 91.81 | 63.02 |
| ALKP (IU/L) | 63.30 | 70.65 | 77.60 | 82.02 | 90.78 | 67.51 |
| Total Bilirubin (mg/100 mL) | 66.25 | 72.51 | 76.25 | 81.25 | 93.75 | 66.21 |
| Total Protein (g/dL) | 45.84 | 72.72 | 77.86 | 86.95 | 96.83 | 49.01 |

% Recovery = (Toxin group – Treated group)/ (Toxin group – Control group) × 100

solubility by complexation, the increase in activity of silymarin can be attributed to this fact [30]. Recently, the antioxidant potential of FA was unearthed and researched by Rodriguez et al. 2011 who attributed the health benefits of FA to its antioxidant nature and categorized it as a good candidate in pharmaceutical and food industry [31].

Lastly, the administration of Silymarin-FA- P tablet formulation attenuated the increased levels of the serum SGOT, SGPT, ALKP and Total Bilirubin caused by $CCl_4$ and produced most subsequent recovery towards normalization (upto 90%).

Our findings suggest that FA and P exert bioenhancing effects on silymarin by dual mechanism. Firstly, FA might have improved the solubility of silymarin by its solubilizing nature [11] and P a known hepatic and intestinal glucoronidation inhibitor might have inhibited the metabolism of silymarin [12]. Secondly, as all the three components have antioxidant properties, the highest recovery conferred by this tablet formulation can be attributed to the antioxidant potential of their combination. Thus, it can be concluded that combination of silymarin with FA and P exhibited significant hepatoprotection as indicated by significant changes in various liver biochemical parameters.

*Histopathology of liver*

Histopathological examination of rat livers observed no alterations in normal control group, while necrosis and diffused kupffer cells proliferation among the hepatocytes of toxic group was seen (Fig. 3a and b). The liver sections of $CCl_4$ exposed rats showed major necrosis and degeneration of hepatocytes, and infiltration of inflammatory cells, when compared to the normal control which had normal lobular architecture with central vein and radiating hepatic cords. Fig. 3a shows normal hepatocytes where no alteration in the hepatocyte architecture was observed, while, in Fig. 3b enormous damage of the liver cells could be seen due to $CCl_4$ intoxication in between the hepatocytes because of focal necrosis and diffused kupffer cells proliferation. The results were concordant with those in the literature [32].

However, the $CCl_4$-induced destruction of liver architecture was not significantly improved in case of marketed tablet formulation and our plain silymarin tablet. A non-significant protection of hepatocytes against the hepatotoxin was seen as depicted in photomicrograph (Fig. 3c and d). Dilatation in the hepatic sinusoids associated with inflammatory cells infiltration and diffused kupffer cells proliferation in between the damaged hepatocytes was seen. This might be due to the incomplete or lesser bioavailability of plain silymarin to the liver cells from both these formulations.

Some improvements in results for silymarin in terms of partial protection against hepatotoxin were obtained in case of silymarin – L (Fig. 3e) and silymarin – P (Fig. 3f) formulation groups where lesser amount of necrosis was observed. The degree of vacuolation also decreased in these groups as compared to $CCl_4$ treated group showing better protection and improvement.

It is worthy to state that as the antioxidant potential of silymarin increased the most when used in combination with both FA and P and even better hepatoprotective results were observed with least liver damage. It suggested the superior hepatoprotective activity of this formulation over rest of the drug-bioenhancer combinations. The antioxidant property might have helped the hepatocytes counteract the oxidative stress and this might have contributed to blocking the progression of LD (Fig. 3g and h).

**Discussion**

In recent times, several studies have been carried out to demonstrate the efficacy of herbal drugs and nutraceuticals in LDs and most of these studies showed significant hepatoprotectivity with lesser side effects and good efficacy [33].

By now, it is well understood that silymarin has significant antioxidant and hepatoprotective potential if it is bioavailable [34]. The only limitation in its use is its poor bioavailability that leads to higher daily doses in order to observe some of its pharmacological activity. If by some approach, the bioavailability increases, it would lead to lesser amount and frequency of dosing and better pharmacological activity of silymarin. The aim of our work was to use natural products as bioenhancers along

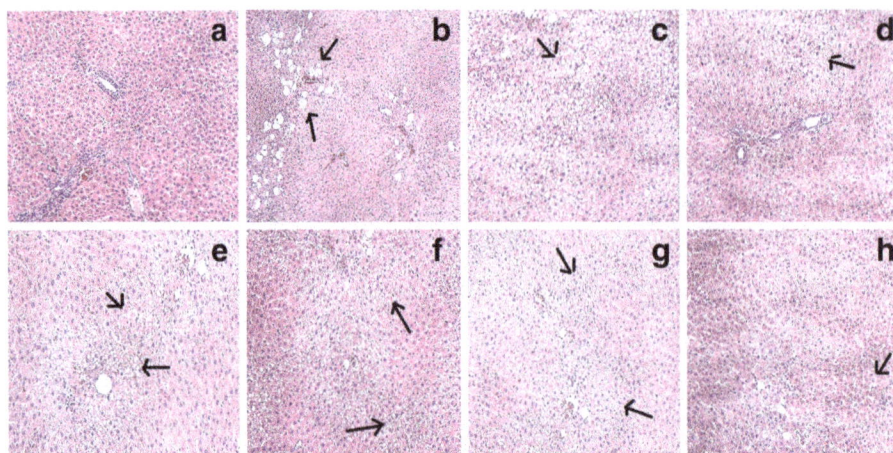

**Fig. 3** Liver histological structure of rats in normal control (**a**), toxic control (**b**), plain silymarin tablet (**c**), marketed formulation (**d**), Silymarin – Lysergol (**e**), Silymarin – Piperine (**f**), Silymarin – Fulvic acid (**g**) and Silymarin – Fulvic acid- Piperine (**h**) (H + E × 100). The small arrows are used to show the extent of necrosis and presence of vacuoles

with silymarin in order to increase its bioavailability either by increasing its water solubility, increasing its permeability or by inhibiting its metabolism. Silymarin can also modify the plasma membrane phospholipid content therefore, protects against the $CCl_4$ induced alterations of the liver plasma membrane through its antioxidant properties [35].

Our systematic study brought up the results that if the bioavailability of silymarin is increased with the help of bioenhancers like FA and P, together these three compounds may act as strong antioxidants and provide synergistic and additive hepatoprotective effects. So we suggest, a formulation with good anti–inflammatory and antioxidant potential and is anticipated to show good hepatoprotective activity if used properly. We hypothesized that silymarin along with FA and P in a definite concentration in a pharmaceutical dosage form would provide much better hepatoprotection because of two reasons: Firstly, with their bioenhancing effects on silymarin and secondly, together with silymarin they proved to be a good antioxidant combination which is important for the protection against the injury caused by $CCl_4$.

The results obtained from the present study indicated that SGOT, SGPT, ALKP and Total Bilirubin levels were markedly increased in toxic group after $CCl_4$ treatment as compared to the normal group signifying the induction of liver injury in rats ($p < 0.05$). Silymarin along with bioenhancers ameliorated the hepatotoxic effect of $CCl_4$ and exhibited significant hepatoprotective activity against $CCl_4$-induced liver injury in the following order: silymarin- FA- P formulation, > silymarin – FA > silymarin – P > silymarin – Lformulation by normalizing the elevated levels of hepatic enzymes when compared to plain silymarin formulation. A novel treatment of LDs by the use of a strong antioxidant silymarin in combination with FA

and P in a tablet dosage form is anticipated. To further prove this point and idea, the safety as well as the efficacy must be evaluated in pre-clinical and clinical studies.

## Conclusions

In addressing the current status of the treatment of LDs, there is a need for development of new hepatoprotective formulation with higher efficacy and safety. We intended to focus on a novel approach for the treatment of LD by increasing the bioavailability of silymarin with the help of natural products as bioenhancers. Bioenhancers when combined together proved to be a potential antioxidant combination and are proposed to have synergistic and additive effects with silymarin. A number of LDs are commonly associated with oxidative stress which plays a vital role in the pathogenesis of ailments such as alcoholic liver disease, chronic hepatitis C, non-alcoholic steatohepatitis (NASH), haemochromatosis, and Wilson's disease. Thus, antioxidant therapy has been believed to have beneficial effects in managing these diseases. Both FA and P work by different mechanisms in order to increase the bioavailability of silymarin and a pilot scale study is required to determine the optimal dose of the combination that shows highest safety and efficacy, and if worthwhile effects are revealed in preclinical studies clinical studies can also be designed.

## Methods
### Tablet manufacturing techniques
Silymarin tablets were made by the three techniques viz. Direct Compression Technique, Foam Granulation Technique and Solid Dispersion Technique as shown in Fig. 4. Direct compression plain silymarin tablet formulation (no.1) was used as control. Foam granulation technique was used to make silymarin – L (no. 2) and

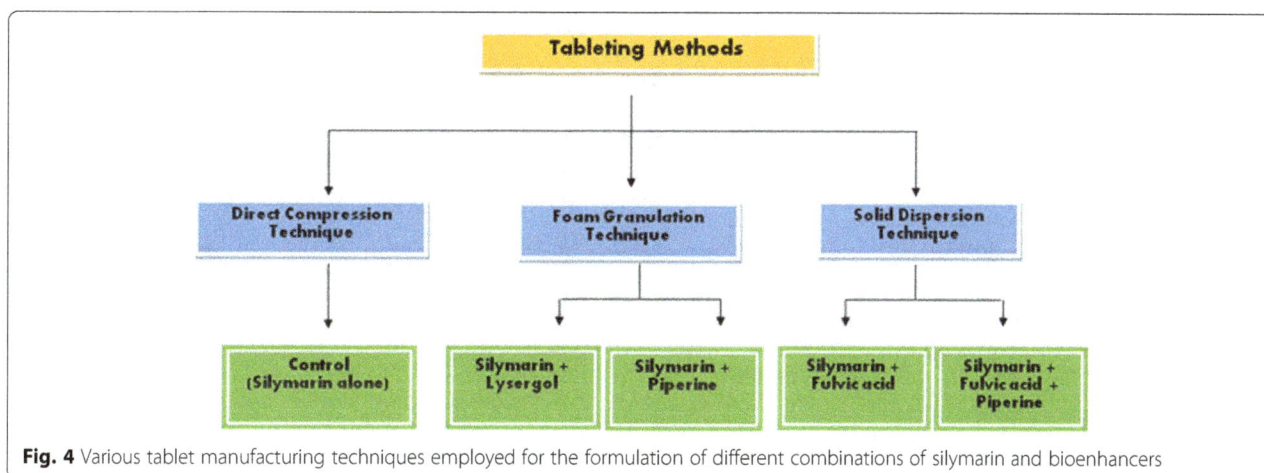

**Fig. 4** Various tablet manufacturing techniques employed for the formulation of different combinations of silymarin and bioenhancers

silymarin-P (no. 3) tablets. Methocel E6 PLV was used as foam binder that aided in improved dissolution profile of silymarin because of its surfactant properties [36]. Solid dispersion technique was used to make silymarin – FA (no. 4) and silymarin-FA-P (no. 5) tablets. FA used as carrier moiety for silymarin, aided in improved solubility and enhanced dissolution profile because of its water soluble nature [30].

## MTT cytotoxicity studies of Silymarin, fulvic acid, Piperine and lysergol on MCF-7 cells

MTT assay was employed to evaluate the cytotoxic effect of the free drug silymarin and the bioenhancers P, FA and L on MCF-7 cells. For MTT assay, MCF-7 cells were grown using DMEM media mixed with 10% Fetal Bovine Serum (FBS), seeded on 96 well plate and allowed to adhere. Concentrations of free drug and the bioenhancers amounting to 25–500 μg/mL respectively were added to the 96 well tissue culture plate (Falcon Plate) in duplicates. MTT assay was performed after 24 h of treatment to assess cell viability. The respective media was removed from all the wells and 10 μL of MTT reagent (Chemicon International, from Millipore) was added in each well from a working stock (5 mg/mL) solution and the plates were kept in incubator for 2–3 h. The reagent was then removed and the remaining crystals were solubilized in DMSO. Formazan gets dissolved to give homogeneous purple solution and its absorbance was measured at a test wavelength of 570 nm and reference wavelength 630 nm using ELISA plate reader. The absorbance value is a direct measure of the number of live cells. The corresponding values for O.D. for different drug and bioenhancer concentrations were recorded [24].

## Carbon tetrachloride induced hepatotoxicity in rats
### Animal protocol

For the experimental purpose, male wistar rats, weighing approximately $250 \pm 10$ g, fasted over night with free

access to water were used. The protocol of the study was approved by Jamia Hamdard Institutional Animal Ethics Committee (Registration No – 173/CPCSEA). The guidelines provided by the institutional ethics committee for the usage of animals in scientific research were strictly followed [37]. All the painful procedures were performed under anesthesia and the animals which cannot be relieved or repaired at the end of the study were sacrificed ethically under anesthesia. Throughout the study, animals were hygienically kept in a controlled environment in large polypropylene cages at air conditioned temperature ($25 \pm 2$ °C) with a 12 h light/dark cycle in Central Animal House, Jamia Hamdard, New Delhi (India). Principle of 4 Rs (replacement, reduction, refinement, and rehabilitation) given by the Committee for the Purpose of Control and Supervision of Experiments on Animals (CPCSEA) in India was followed in this study.

### In-vivo hepatoprotective study protocol

The $CCl_4$ induced hepatotoxicity model as described by Yadav et al. 2008, was employed with some modifications in order to assess the hepatoprotective potential of our various formulation groups [23]. For this purpose, the rats were divided into eight groups (A, B, C, D, E, F, G, H) with five animals each ($n = 5$). The rats were assigned treatment as follows:

I.   Group A assigned as normal control group and was fed with light liquid paraffin (1 mL/kg b. w.) orally for six days.
II.  Group B marked as toxic control group and toxicity was induced using $CCl_4$ (1 mL/kg b. w.), in light liquid paraffin orally on day 3rd and 4th and with plain vehicle on rest of the days.
III. Group C received plain silymarin formulation (equivalent to 100 mg/kg/mL) for all six days and $CCl_4$ (1 mL/kg b.w.) orally on day 3rd and 4th.

IV. Group D received silymarin + L formulation (equivalent to 100 mg/kg/mL) for all six days and CCl$_4$ (1 mL/kg b.w.) orally on day 3rd and 4th.

V. Group E received silymarin + P formulation (equivalent to 100 mg/kg/mL) for all six days and CCl$_4$ (1 mL/kg b.w.) orally on day 3rd and 4th.

VI. Group F received silymarin + FA formulation (equivalent to 100 mg/kg/mL) for all six days and CCl$_4$ (1 mL/kg b.w.) orally on day 3rd and 4th.

VII. Group G received silymarin + FA + P formulation (equivalent to 100 mg/kg/mL) for all six days and CCl$_4$ (1 mL/kg b.w.) orally on day 3rd and 4th.

VIII. Group H received silymarin marketed formulation (equivalent to 100 mg/kg/mL) for all six days and CCl$_4$ (1 mL/kg b.w.) orally on day 3rd and 4th.

On 7th day, blood was collected in separator tubes from retro orbital plexus of each animal, allowed to clot and centrifuged at 3000 rpm for 15–20 min. Serum was separated and stored at – 20 °C till further analysis. All the samples were analyzed for various biochemical parameters namely SGOT, SGPT, ALKP, Total Bilirubin and Total Proteins by using diagnostic kits and manufacturers' protocol present therein.

### Biochemical analysis

In vitro determination of SGOT and SGPT in rat plasma/serum was carried out by 2, 4- DNPH Reitman and Frankel Method – an end point colorimetric method for the estimation of enzyme activity. Alkaline phosphatase determination in rat serum was carried out by King and King's method. Bilirubin analysis in rat serum was carried out by Malloy and Evelyn method and Total Protein Analysis in rat serum/plasma was carried out by Modified Biuret End point Assay by using diagnostic kits and manufacturers' protocol.

### Histopathological assessment

The liver tissue specimens taken from rats of all groups were placed in 10% formalin solution for 24 h, blocked in paraffin and sectioned at 5 μm thickness with a microtome followed by staining with hematoxylin-eosin dye stains. Microscopic images were taken through the light microscope.

### Abbreviations

ALKP: Alkaline Phosphatase; ANOVA: Analysis of Variance; BW: Body Weight; CCl$_4$: Carbon tetrachloride; CYP450: Cytochrome P450; DMEM: Dulbecco's Modified Eagle Medium; DMSO: Dimethylsulfoxide; DNPH: Dinitrophenylhydrazine; ELISA: Enzyme-linked Immune Sorbent Assay; FBS: Fetal Bovine Serum; ICH: International Council for Harmonization; LD: Liver Disease; MCF-7: Michigan Cancer Foundation-7; MTT: [3-(4,5-dimethylthiazol-2-yl)-2,5-diphenyltetrazolium bromide]; OD: Optical Density; RRL: Regional Research Laboratories; SEM: Standard Error of Mean; SGOT: Serum Glutamic Oxaloacetic Transaminase; SGPT: Serum Glutamic Pyruvic Transaminase; T$_{1/2}$: Terminal Half Life; T$_{max}$: Time to reach Peak Concentration

### Acknowledgements

Authors wish to acknowledge Maneesh Pharmaceuticals Pvt. Ltd. India for providing the Silymarin 70% extract.

### Funding

Research work was funded by Indian Council of Medical Research (ICMR), New Delhi, India in the form of Senior Research Fellowship to one of the author (S. Javed).

### Authors' contributions

SJ: Carried out the experimental work. Also involved in writing the manuscript. WA: Worked as consultant to the work, helped SJ in writing the manuscript. KK: Designed the work, guided the whole project. All authors read and approved the final manuscript.

### Competing interests

The authors declare that they have no competing interests.

### Author details

[1]Department of Pharmaceutics, School of Pharmaceutical Education and Research, Jamia Hamdard, New Delhi 110062, India. [2]Department of Pharmaceutical Chemistry, College of Pharmacy, Jazan University, P. Box No. 114, Jazan, Saudi Arabia.

### References

1. Williams R. Global challenges in liver disease. Hepatol. 2006;44:521–6.
2. Muriel P, Rivera-Espinoza Y. Beneficial drugs for liver diseases. J App Toxicol. 2008;28:93–103.
3. Radko L, Cybulski W. Application of silymarin in human and animal medicine. J Pre-Clin Clin Res. 2007;1:22–6.
4. Kren V, Walterova D. Silybin and silymarin – new effects and applications. Biomed Papers. 2005;149:29–41.
5. Wu JY, Lin LC, Hung SC, Chi CW, Tsai TH. Analysis of silibinin in rat plasma and bile for hepatobiliary excretion and oral bioavailability application. J Pharm Biomed Anal. 2007;45:635–41.
6. Wu JW, Lin LC, Hung SC, Lin CH, Chi CW, Tsai TH. Hepatobiliary excretion of silibinin in normal and liver cirrhotic rats. Drug Met Disp. 2008;36:589–96.
7. Javed S, Kohli K, Ali M. Reassessing bioavailability of silymarin. Altern Med Rev. 2012;16:239–49.
8. Porter CJ, Pouton CW, Cuine JF, Charman WN. Enhancing intestinal drug solubilization using lipid-based delivery systems. Adv Drug Deliv Rev. 2008; 60:673–91.
9. Navin A, Bedi KL. Bioenhancers: revolutionary concept to market. J Ayurv Integ Med. 2010;1:96–9.
10. Javed S, Ahsan W, Kohli K. The concept of bioenhancers in bioavailability enhancement of drugs – a patent review. J Sci Lett. 2016;1:143–65.
11. Ghosal S. Delivery system for pharmaceutical, nutritional and cosmetic ingredients. United States Patent 6. 2003;558:712.
12. Majeed M, Badmaev V, Rajendran R. Use of piperine as a bioavailability enhancer. In: United States Patent Number- 5744161; 1998.
13. Khanuja SPS, Arya JS, Srivastava SK, et al. Antibiotic pharmaceutical composition with lysergol as bioenhancer and method of treatment. In: United States patent number-20070060604A1; 2007.
14. Pradhan SC, Girish C. Hepatoprotective herbal drug, silymarin from experimental pharmacology to clinical medicine. Indian J Med Res. 2006; 124:491–504.
15. Mehendale HM, Roth RA, Gandolfi RA, Klaunig JE, Lemasters JJ, Curtis LR. Novel mechanisms in chemically induced hepatotoxicity. FASEB J. 1994;8: 1285–95.
16. Wafay H, El-Saeed G, El-Toukhy S, Youness E, Ellaithy N, Agaibi M, Eldaly S. Potential effect of garlic oil and silymarin on carbon tetrachloride –induced liver injury. Aust J Basic Appl Sci. 2012;6:409–14.

Pharmacological influences of natural products as bioenhancers of silymarin against carbon...

203

17. Tsai JH, Liu JY, Wu TT, Ho PC, Huang CY, Shyu JC, Hsieh YS, Tsai CC, Liu YC. Effects of silymarin on the resolution of liver fibrosis induced by carbon tetrachloride in rats. J Vir Hep. 2008;15:508–14.

18. El-Gendy H. Evaluation of silymarin and/or ginger effect on induced hepatotoxicity by carbon tetrachloride in male albino rats. Egypt. J Hosp Med. 2003;12:101–12.

19. Abrol S, Trehan A, Katare OP. Comparative study of different silymarin formulations: formulation, characterization and in vitro/in vivo evaluation. Curr Drug Deliv. 2005;2:45–51.

20. El-Samaligy MS, Afifi NN, Mahmoud EA. Evaluation of hybrid liposomes-encapsulated silymarin regarding physical stability and in vivo performance. Int J Pharm. 2006;319:121–9.

21. Yadav NP, Pal A, Shaker K, Bawankule DU, Gupta AK, Darokar MP, Khanuja SPS. Synergistic effect of silymarin and standardized extract of *Phyllanthus amarus* against CCl$_4$-induced hepatotoxicity in *Rattus norvegicus*. Phytomed. 2008;15:1053–61.

22. Mosmann T. Rapid colorimetric assay for cellular growth and survival: application to proliferation and cytotoxicity assays. J Immunol Met. 1983;65: 55–63.

23. Aterman K. Toxic effect of carbon tetrachloride on the liver cell. Br J Pharmacol. 1962;19:219–25.

24. Clawson GA. Mechanism of carbon tetrachloride hepatotoxicity. Path Immunopath Res. 1989;8:104–12.

25. Tanaka K, Sakal H, Hashizume M, Hirohata T. A long term follow up study on risk factors for hepatocellular carcinoma among Japanese patients with liver cirrhosis. Jap J Canc Res. 1998;89:1241–50.

26. Devi RS, Chitra M, Jayamathi P. Hepatoprotectivity and an antioxidant study of *Ipomoea hederacea* on experimentally induced hepatotoxic rats. Rec Res Sci Tech. 2010;2:17–9.

27. Farida T, Salawu OA, Tijani AY, Ejiofor JI. Pharmacological evaluation of *Ipomoea Asarifolia* (Desr.) against carbon tetrachloride–induced hepatotoxicity in rats. J Ethnopharmacol. 2012;142:642–6.

28. Patel JA, Shah US. Hepatoprotective activity of *Piper longum* traditional milk extract on carbon tetrachloride induced liver toxicity in Wistar rats. Bol Latinoam Caribe Plant Med Aromat. 2009;8:121–8.

29. Bai X, Zhang W, Chen W, Zong W, Guo Z, Liu X. Antihepatotoxic and antioxidant effects of extracts from *Piper nigrum* L. root Afr J Biotechnol. 2011;10:267–72.

30. Javed S, Kohli K, Ahsan W. Solubility and dissolution enhancement of Silymarin with fulvic acid carrier. Int J Drug Dev Res. 2016;8:9–14.

31. Rodriguez NC, Urrutia EC, Gertrudis BH, Chaverri JP, Mejia GB. Antioxidant activity of fulvic acid: a living matter-derived bioactive compound. J Food Agric Environ. 2011;9:123–7.

32. Shaker E, Mahmoud H, Manaa S. Silymarin, the antioxidant component and *Silybum marianum* extracts prevent liver damage. Food Chem Toxicol. 2010; 48:803–6.

33. Muriel P, Mourelle M. Prevention by silymarin of membrane alterations in acute CCl$_4$ liver damage. J Appl Toxicol. 1990;10:275–9.

34. Castro JA, Ferrya GC, Castro CR, Sasama H, Fenos OM, Gillette JR. Prevention of carbon tetrachloride induced necrosis by inhibitors of drug metabolism. Further studies on the metabolism of their action. Biochem Pharmacol. 1974;23:295–302.

35. Ozturk M, Akdogan M, Keskin I, Kisioglu AN, Oztas S, Yildiz K. Effect of *Silybum marianum* on acute hepatic damage caused by carbon tetrachloride in rats. Biomed Res. 2012;23:268–74.

36. Javed S, Kohli K, Ahsan W. Incorporation of Methocel E6 PLV by a novel foam granulation technique for dissolution augmentation of poor soluble silymarin. J Pharm Res. 2016;10:79–89.

37. Sahni SK. Guidelines for care and use of animals in scientific research. 1st ed. New Delhi: Bengal Offset Works; 2000. p. 1–31.

# Permissions

# List of Contributors

**Maksim Sabadash**
Institute of Urology of NAMS of Ukraine, 04053Str. V. Vinnichenko, 9-a, Kiev, Ukraine

**Alexander Shulyak**
Institute of Urology Cystitis in Women, 04053Str. V. Vinnichenko, 9-a, Kiev, Ukraine

**Tania Sultana, Md. Abdul Mannan and Tajnin Ahmed**
Department of Pharmacy, Stamford University Bangladesh, 51, Siddeswari Road, Dhaka -1217, Bangladesh

**Mitchel Otieno Okumu, James Mucunu Mbaria and Laetitia Wakonyu Kanja**
Department of Public Health, Pharmacology and Toxicology, Faculty of Veterinary Medicine, University of Nairobi, Nairobi, Kenya

**Francis Okumu Ochola**
Department of Pharmacology and Toxicology, Faculty of Medicine, MoiUniversity, Eldoret, Kenya

**Daniel Waweru Gakuya and Alice Wairimu Kinyua**
Department of Clinical Studies, Faculty of Veterinary Medicine, University of Nairobi, Nairobi, Kenya

**Paul Onyango Okumu**
Department of Veterinary Pathology, Microbiology and Parasitology, Faculty of Veterinary Medicine, University of Nairobi, Nairobi, Kenya

**Stephen Gitahi Kiama**
Department of Veterinary Anatomy and Physiology, Faculty of Veterinary Medicine, University of Nairobi, Nairobi, Kenya

**Sk Moquammel Haque, Avijit Chakraborty and Biswajit Ghosh**
Plant Biotechnology Laboratory, Post Graduate Department of Botany, Ramakrishna Mission Vivekananda Centenary College, Rahara, Kolkata 700118, India

**Diganta Dey**
Department of Microbiology, Ashok Laboratory Clinical Testing Centre Private Limited, Kolkata 700068, India

**Swapna Mukherjee**
Department of Microbiology, Dinabandhu Andrews College, Garia, Kolkata 700084, India

**Sanghamitra Nayak**
Centre of Biotechnology, Siksha O Anusandhan University, Bhubaneswar 751030, India

**Kingsley Omage**
Department of Biochemistry, College of Basic Medical Sciences, Igbinedion University, Okada, Edo State, Nigeria

**Marshall A. Azeke**
Department of Biochemistry, Faculty of Natural Sciences, Ambrose Alli University, Ekpoma, Edo State, Nigeria

**Sylvia O. Omage**
Department of Biochemistry, Faculty of Life Sciences, University of Benin, Benin, Edo State, Nigeria

**Imtiaz Mahmud, Md. Nazmul Hasan Zilani, Nripendra Nath Biswas and Bishwajit Bokshi**
Pharmacy Discipline, Life Science School, Khulna University, Khulna 9208, Bangladesh

**Ankita Joshi, Harsha Lad, Harsha Sharma and Deepak Bhatnagar**
School of Biochemistry, Devi Ahilya University, Khandwa Road, Indore, MP 452017, India

**Michael Katotomichelakis**
Department of Otorhinolaryngology, Medical School, Democritus University of Thrace, Alexandroupolis, Greece

**K. Van Crombruggen, G. Holtappels, C. Bachert and N. Zhang**
Upper Airways Research Laboratory (URL), Ghent University Hospital, Ghent, Belgium

**F. A. Kuhn, C. E. Fichandler, C. A. Kuhn-Glendye and C. T. Melroy**
Georgia Nasal and Sinus Institute, Savannah, GA, USA

**J. B. Anon**
ENT Specialists of Northwest Pennsylvania, Erie, PA, USA

**B. Karanfilov**
Ohio Sinus Institute, Dublin, OH, USA

**T. W. Haegen**
Arizona Sinus Center, Phoenix, AZ, USA

**I. Kastanioudakis**
Department of Otorhinolaryngology, Medical School, University of Ioannina, Ioannina, Greece

T. Dons and S. Soosairaj
Department of Botany, St. Joseph's College, Trichy, India

Kingsley Omage
Department of Biochemistry, College of Basic Medical Sciences, Igbinedion University, Okada, Edo State, Nigeria

Marshall A. Azeke
Department of Biochemistry, Faculty of Natural Sciences, Ambrose Alli University, Ekpoma, Edo State, Nigeria

Jerry N. E. Orhue and Sylvia O. Iseghohi
Department of Biochemistry, Faculty of Life Sciences, University of Benin, Benin City, Edo State, Nigeria

Vasyl I. Popovich
Department of Otorhinolaryngology, Ivano-Frankivsk University, Ivano-Frankivsk, Ukraine

Ivanna V. Koshel
Ivano-Frankivsk University, Galitskaya str. 2, 76000, Ivano-Frankivsk, Ukraine

Md. Zahidul Islam, Md. Tanvir Hossain, Nahid Sultana and Shujit Chandra Paul
Department of Applied Chemistry and Chemical Engineering, Noakhali Science and Technology University, Noakhali, Bangladesh

Foysal Hossen and Sanjoy Kumar Mukharjee
Department of Microbiology, Noakhali Science and Technology University, Noakhali, Bangladesh

Theanmalar Masilamani and Thavamanithevi Subramaniam
SIRIM Bhd, Industrial Biotechnology Research Centre (IBRC), No 1, Persiaran Dato Menteri Seksyen 2, 40700 Shah Alam, Selangor, Malaysia

Norshariza Nordin
Genetics and Regenerative Medicine Research Centre, Faculty of Medicine and Health Sciences, Universiti Putra Malaysia, 43400 Serdang, Selangor, Malaysia

Rozita Rosli
MAKNA-Cancer Research Laboratory, Institute Bioscience (IBS), Universiti Putra Malaysia, 43400 Serdang, Selangor, Malaysia

Ashfique Rizwan and Md. Sohel Rana
Department of Pharmacy, Jahangirnagar University, Savar, Dhaka 1342, Bangladesh

Artyom Zinchenko
Max Planck Institute for Human Cognitive and Brain Sciences, Stephanstraße 1A, 04103 Leipzig, Germany

Ceyona Özdem
Department of Psychology, Vrije Universiteit Brussel, Pleinlaan 2, B - 1050 Brussel, Belgium

Md. Mamun Al-Amin
Department of Pharmaceutical Sciences, North South University, Plot-15, Block-B, Bashundhara, Dhaka 1229, Bangladesh

Niloy Sen, Latifa Bulbul, Md. Saddam Hussain and Sujan Banik
Department of Pharmacy, Noakhali Science and Technology University, Noakhali-3814, Bangladesh

Md. Shahbuddin Kabir Choudhuri
Department of Pharmacy, Jahangirnagar University, Dhaka-1342, Bangladesh

Afifa Qidwai, Manisha Pandey and Rajesh Kumar
Department of Botany, University of Allahabad, Allahabad 211002, Uttar Pradesh, India

Anupam Dikshit
Department of Botany, University of Allahabad, Allahabad 211002, Uttar Pradesh, India
Biological Product Laboratory, Department of Botany, University of Allahabad, Allahabad 211002, Uttar Pradesh, India

Md Ashraful Alam, Abu Taher Sagor, Nabila Tabassum, Anayt Ulla, Manik Chandra Shill, Ghazi Muhammad Sayedur Rahman and Hasan Mahmud Reza
Department of Pharmaceutical Sciences, North South University, Dhaka, Bangladesh

Hemayet Hossain
BCSIR Laboratories, Bangladesh Council of Scientific and Industrial Research (BCSIR), Dhaka, Bangladesh

Hammad Ahmed
Department of Pharmacology, Faculty of Pharmacy, Ziauddin University, Karachi 75600, Pakistan

Muhammad Aslam
Department of Pharmacology, Faculty of Pharmacy, Ziauddin University, Karachi 75600, Pakistan
Department of Pharmacology, Faculty of Pharmacy, University of Sindh, Jamshoro 76080, Pakistan

Arkajyoti Paul
Drug Discovery, GUSTO A Research Group, Chittagong 4000, Bangladesh
Department of Microbiology, Jagannath University, Dhaka 1100, Bangladesh

Md. Adnan
Department of Pharmacy, International Islamic University Chittagong, Chittagong 4318, Bangladesh

**Mohuya Majumder and Nishat Rahman**
Drug Discovery, GUSTO A Research Group, Chittagong 4000, Bangladesh
Department of Pharmacy, BGC Trust University Bangladesh, Chittagong 4000, Bangladesh

**Niloy Kar and Muntasir Meem**
Department of Pharmacy, East West University, Dhaka 1212, Bangladesh

**Mohammed Shahariar Rahman**
Department of Pharmacy, University of Science and Technology Chittagong, Chittagong 4202, Bangladesh

**Akash Kumar Rauniyar**
Department of information technology, MDP Bioinformatics, University of Turku, 20500 Turku, Finland

**Md. Nazim Uddin Chy and Mohammad Shah Hafez Kabir**
Drug Discovery, GUSTO A Research Group, Chittagong 4000, Bangladesh
Department of Pharmacy, International Islamic University Chittagong, Chittagong 4318, Bangladesh

**Shovon Bhattacharjee, Azhar Waqar, Kishan Barua and Shukanta Bhowmik**
Department of Applied Chemistry and Chemical Engineering, Noakhali Science and Technology University, Noakhali 3814, Bangladesh

**Abhijit Das**
Department of Pharmacy, Noakhali Science and Technology University, Noakhali 3814, Bangladesh

**Sumitra Rani Debi**
Department of Environmental Science and Disaster Management, Noakhali Science and Technology University, Noakhali 3814, Bangladesh

**Kelly Oriakhi**
Department of Medical Biochemistry, School of Basic Medical Sciences, University of Benin, Benin City, Nigeria

**Patrick O. Uadia**
Department of Biochemistry, Faculty of Life Sciences, University of Benin, Benin City, Nigeria

**Ikechi G. Eze**
Department of Anatomy, School of Basic Medical Sciences, University of Benin, Benin City, Nigeria

**Mahadi Hasan, Rabeya Akter and Laizuman Nahar**
Department of Pharmacy, School of Science and Engineering, Southeast University, Banani, Dhaka 1213, Bangladesh

**Mohammad Tuhin Ali and Parag Palit**
Department of Biochemistry and Molecular Biology, Faculty of Biological Sciences, University of Dhaka, Dhaka 1000, Bangladesh

**Aminul Islam and Rifat Khan**
Department of Pharmacy, Faculty of Sciences and Engineering, East West University, Dhaka 1212, Bangladesh

**Veronique Seidel**
Natural Products Drug Discovery Research Group, Strathclyde Institute of Pharmacy and Biomedical Sciences, University of Strathclyde, Glasgow, UK

**Khaled Abo-EL-Sooud**
Pharmacology Department, Faculty of Veterinary Medicine, Cairo University, Giza 12211, Egypt

**Fatma A. Ahmed, Hanona S. Yaecob and Hanan M. ELTantawy**
Medicinal and Aromatic Plants Department, Desert Research Center, Cairo, Egypt

**Sayed A. El-Toumy**
Chemistry of Tannins Department, National Research Center, Dokki, Giza, Egypt

**Tusnova Sharmin and Md. Mamun Or Rashid**
Department of Pharmacy, Noakhali Science and Technology University, Sonapur, Noakhali 3814, Bangladesh

**Razia Sultana and Shahriar Kabir Shakil**
Department of Biotechnology and Genetic Engineering, Noakhali Science and Technology University, Sonapur, Noakhali 3814, Bangladesh

**Farzana Hossain**
Department of Microbiology, University of Dhaka, Dhaka 1000, Bangladesh

**Foysal Hossen**
Department of Microbiology, Noakhali Science and Technology University, Sonapur, Noakhali 3814, Bangladesh

**Rameshkumar Angappan and Sivasudha Thilagar**
Department of Environmental Biotechnology, Bharathidasan University, Tiruchirappalli, Tamil Nadu 620024, India

**Arul Ananth Devanesan**
Department of Environmental Biotechnology, Bharathidasan University, Tiruchirappalli, Tamil Nadu 620024, India
Department of Food Quality and Safety, Gilat Research Center, Agricultural Research Organization, M.P. Negev - 85280, Tifrah, Israel

**Shamama Javed and Kanchan Kohli**
Department of Pharmaceutics, School of Pharmaceutical
Education and Research, Jamia Hamdard, New Delhi
110062, India

**Waquar Ahsan**
Department of Pharmaceutical Chemistry, College of
Pharmacy, Jazan University, Jazan, Saudi Arabia

# Index